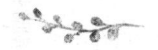

ALSO BY DR MARY CLAIRE HAVER

The Galveston Diet
The New Menopause

the new perimenopause

An Evidence-Based Guide to Surviving the Zone of Chaos and Feeling Like Yourself Again

the new perimenopause

Dr Mary Claire Haver

Vermilion
LONDON

VERMILION

UK | USA | Canada | Ireland | Australia
India | New Zealand | South Africa

Vermilion is part of the Penguin Random House group of companies whose
addresses can be found at global.penguinrandomhouse.com

Penguin Random House UK
One Embassy Gardens, 8 Viaduct Gardens, London SW11 7BW

penguin.co.uk

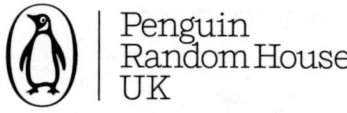

First published in the United States of America by Rodale Books in 2026
First published in Great Britain by Vermilion in 2026

1

Copyright © Mary Claire Haver 2026

The moral right of the author has been asserted.

Penguin Random House values and supports copyright. Copyright fuels creativity, encourages diverse voices, promotes freedom of expression and supports a vibrant culture. Thank you for purchasing an authorised edition of this book and for respecting intellectual property laws by not reproducing, scanning or distributing any part of it by any means without permission. You are supporting authors and enabling Penguin Random House to continue to publish books for everyone. No part of this book may be used or reproduced in any manner for the purpose of training artificial intelligence technologies or systems. In accordance with Article 4(3) of the DSM Directive 2019/790, Penguin Random House expressly reserves this work from the text and data mining exception.

Printed and bound in Great Britain by Clays Ltd, Elcograf S.p.A.

The authorised representative in the EEA is Penguin Random House Ireland,
Morrison Chambers, 32 Nassau Street, Dublin D02 YH68

A CIP catalogue record for this book is available from the British Library

Hardback ISBN 9781785046308
Trade Paperback ISBN 9781785046315

Penguin Random House is committed to a sustainable future
for our business, our readers and our planet. This book is made
from Forest Stewardship Council® certified paper.

FOR EVERY WOMAN WHO WAS TOLD IT WAS ALL IN HER HEAD.

For those who were dismissed, misdiagnosed, or handed a vague label
and a bottle of antidepressants instead of real answers.

For the clinicians who are listening, truly listening and learning
alongside their patients, even when the textbooks
come up short.

For the researchers who dared to challenge the early conclusions of
the Women's Health Initiative. You faced resistance, skepticism,
and institutional inertia, but you pressed on in pursuit of
the truth. Because of your courage, an entire generation of
women may finally be seen, heard, and cared for
with the rigor they deserve.

And for my daughters and yours.
May they enter this transition armed with knowledge,
supported by science, and empowered by a healthcare system
that no longer treats midlife as invisible.

Contents

LETTER TO THE READER   xi

INTRODUCTION: Let's Begin   xv

Part One: You Are Here

1: The Status Quo Experience of Perimenopause   3

2: The Zone of Chaos   24

3: The Troubling Pattern of Misdiagnosis (and Gaslighting)   39

Part Two: A Window of Vulnerability

4: This Is Your Brain on Perimenopause   55

5: The Mental Health Changes You May Notice   64

6: Strange Cognition: The Rise of Brain Fog and ADHD-Like Symptoms   76

7: Perimenopause and Metabolic Syndrome   92

8: Osteoporosis: The Debilitating Bone Disease That Starts Sooner Than You Think   122

9: Sarcopenia: The Muscle Loss No One Warned You About   142

10: Dreaming of Sleep in Perimenopause   155

Part Three: Sex, Pregnancy, and Periods in Perimenopause

11: When Desire Shifts: Perimenopause and Sexual Function — 173

12: Fertility Changes and Challenges: The Clock Is Real, but So Is Your Power — 198

13: When the Bleeding Becomes a Mystery: Uterine Changes in Perimenopause — 209

Part Four: A Window of Opportunity (for Prevention)

14: Treating Hormonal Fluctuation with Hormones: A Deep Dive into MHT to Treat Perimenopause — 223

15: The Foundation for Resilience: The Lifestyle Factors That Matter Most — 249

16: Talking Points and Lab Tests: Everything You Need for Your Next Appointment — 270

CONCLUSION: What I Wish I'd Known at Thirty-Five — 279

ACKNOWLEDGMENTS — 283

APPENDIX A: Selected Resources — 285

APPENDIX B: The New Perimenopause Five-Day Meal Plan — 289

REFERENCES — 307

INDEX — 339

Letter to the Reader

I've written this book with my two daughters, now in their early twenties, in mind. I hope to empower them with knowledge, insight, and confidence. I want them to understand beyond a shadow of a doubt that their experiences are seen and validated. And that by learning how to approach their health with intention and resilience, they can secure the foundation for their well-being and vibrancy far into the future.

I want the very same for you.

Because here's the truth: You all deserve so much more than what was offered to your mothers, grandmothers, and great-grandmothers. You deserve more than vague answers and dismissed symptoms. You need the tools for radical thriving through every stage of life, especially in perimenopause and beyond. You need a guide toward a future in which you are fully informed, supported, and confident in taking charge of your health on your terms. It's all here in *The New Perimenopause*.

In many ways, this book is a representation of the very best I have to offer. It is a joint production from my doctor's brain, a relentless pursuer of life-changing science, and my heart, an organ I can't keep from promising only the best for my daughters. It's also in many ways a love letter to my younger self. This is the guide I wish I'd had, filled as it is with insight and knowledge, before I reached my own perimenopause. The confusion, frustration, and uncertainty often tied to this phase of life would have been so much easier to navigate with the right support and information. Information that even as an OB-GYN physician I wasn't taught. I hope that because I'm sharing this with you, you won't have to face the same struggles.

One of the most valuable lessons I've learned in the years since I dedicated my medical practice to the care of women in middle age is that every woman's experience with perimenopause and menopause is unique. Each journey is valid. What may feel manageable for one person could be overwhelming for another. Our bodies respond differently, and we should honor without judgment the path each woman walks.

For too long, women's health has been underserved, with science treating us as smaller, more emotional versions of men. This approach has left a tremendous gap in knowledge and care, resulting in women's health issues, including perimenopause and menopause, being significantly underfunded and overlooked.

But this book isn't just about identifying what's been missing. It's about filling those gaps with the research, knowledge, and tools you need to navigate midlife and beyond. My goal is to help you lay a foundation for aging as healthily and vibrantly as possible.

I'm fifty-seven years old, and I'm living my best life. I'm healthier and happier, with stronger boundaries and more fulfilling relationships, than ever before. This is what I want for each of you reading this book: to step into each stage of life with confidence, clarity, and vitality.

Together, we can rewrite the narrative around women's health. We can demand better research, more comprehensive care, and a compassionate, informed approach that supports women at every age. It's time for a change, and it starts with each of us asking for what we deserve: informed, personalized care that respects our unique experiences. Let's create a future where every woman feels supported, valued, and fully prepared to thrive, no matter where she is in her journey.

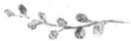

What's to come: *The New Perimenopause* is divided into four parts. The first part will establish some historical and clinical context for the current state of perimenopausal care. The second lays out the vulnerabilities introduced by the hormonal changes that are the hallmark of this transitional stage. In part three, I will detail physiological and reproductive changes you may experience in areas related to sex, pregnancy, and menstruation. And in the final part of the book, you will find everything you want to know about hormone therapy in perimenopause, the habits that matter most to support your health now and in the future, and how to get what you need out of your appointments with healthcare practitioners.

INTRODUCTION

Let's Begin

"I feel fatigued and anxious all the time."
"I'm irritable and less resilient."
"I feel so disconnected from who I once was."
"I don't know what's going on."
"I don't know what to do."
"What's wrong with me?"

As a practicing obstetrician-gynecologist, I've heard these sentiments expressed by many patients between the ages of thirty-five and fifty. For years, I responded based on my medical education, which at the time had taught me only that this constellation of complaints was embedded in the female experience, an aspect of aging that had no explanation or cure and was meant to be endured. I regretfully offered little more than dismissive condolences: "Sorry—it's just part of being a woman" or "Sorry—life is just stressful at this age and stage."

These words provided no comfort or solutions and, I now realize, only reinforced my patients' feelings of helplessness. I could see the disappointment in their faces, but I had no tools to offer. With my administrators demanding that I see an additional thirty patients a day, all while managing my laboring patients in the hospital, taking night calls, and navigating the demands I faced as a wife and mother, I had no time to dive deeper.

Medicine has a long-standing history of training physicians to interpret many symptoms in women through the framework of somatization, a concept that attributes physical symptoms to psychological or emotional distress. In essence, doctors have been conditioned to diagnose women with an implicit bias that whispers, "It's all in her head." I wish I were kidding.

Most of my patients who came into the clinic describing these symptoms were, in many ways, in a sweet spot of their lives. They were experiencing no more than the usual stress they had managed for years, yet they were being besieged by an unnamed existential disruption. For some, this disruption was subtle yet noticeable; for others, it was a tidal wave of change and discomfort. They were united by the need to fend for themselves and find ways to overcome this vague yet very real, however clinically unrecognized or undiagnosed, state of being.

Fortunately, recent research is starting to affirm that these emotional shifts, feelings of disconnection, and challenges to resilience aren't imagined or solely situational; they are real, with a physiological basis rooted in hormonal changes. Some of the newest findings have confirmed that clusters of symptoms that may include fatigue, increased irritability, difficulty with concentration and decisions, the feeling of not being able to calm down on the inside, and increased crying and worry are probably some of the first key indicators that your hormones are shifting into perimenopause.

When I first saw this research published in the journal *Menopause* in May 2024, the title alone hit me like a bolt of lightning: "'Not feeling like myself' in perimenopause." There it was right in front of my eyes. The lived patient experience being given an academic stamp. It felt like a turning point in the history of women's health—could it be that we were finally moving away from assigning a psychological cause to something biological in nature?

Now, before I get ahead of myself, it's important that I back up a little to give you some context for this moment. So much had happened before I read this study. I had gone through my own menopause, which turned my world upside down and put me in the position of the patients who for so long had been telling me of their symptoms.

I finally *got it* in a whole new way.

I also started posting about my experience on social media and was flooded by responses from followers. Their responses and their desperate need for help drove me to expand my own medical knowledge outside the standard OB-GYN curriculum and continuing medical education. I attended seminars on the state of menopausal care; I dug in to do the work on making myself a better practitioner. I was floored by what I learned, especially by the revelation that my own treatment practices had been informed by one of the most erroneous misinterpretations of scientific data in history. This misinterpretation came about from the Women's Health Initiative in 2002, which, like a tsunami, wiped out any progress that had been made up to that point in the treatment of women in their postreproductive era. I felt like I had been misled by my medical education and by the gatekeepers of scientific guidelines.

I was *angry*: A moral failure had occurred, and legions of patients had been abandoned in the wake; they were struggling to stay above water and offered nothing more than a "sorry" to help them stay afloat. This awareness pained me, but it also gave me a renewed purpose—to educate myself and in turn the millions of women who, like my patients and so many of the followers I had connected with on social media, were left in the dark or denied treatment options or even a *discussion* of treatment options for their symptoms. The "it's all in her head" mantra needed to be buried for good. The truth about the multi-organ system involvement of the menopause transition and the use of hormone therapy needed to be revealed—again (I wasn't the first to share it)—this time from a bigger platform.

I poured all my energy, my emotions, my intellectual resources, into researching and writing a book called *The New Menopause*. Nothing could have prepared me for the response to the book. The outpouring of gratitude, the thousands of women I met in person who waited to get a picture with me, give me a hug, or just tell me, "Thank you. I feel seen. I feel validated. I have the tools I need now."

Amid all the excitement, I still managed to keep my mind on the larger mission, which became clearer as my conversations with women across the world continued and my connections to influential and trailblazing doctors increased. *My aim is to revolutionize menopause care and education.* I want to empower women with evidence-based knowledge and ensure they feel informed, validated, and supported as they navigate this transformative stage of life.

It was clear in a lot of ways that the work was just getting started. My research revealed that perimenopause, which I also refer to as the zone of chaos, still needed so much more attention. Even though I had addressed it some in *The New Menopause,* perimenopause wasn't in the spotlight, and it needed to be. Especially because little more than a slow drip of scientific research was coming out on the topic (more on the abysmal number of studies on perimenopause in chapter 1). What I did discover made it clear that, for premenopausal and perimenopausal women, there was no time to waste. So many women in Gen X are playing catch-up as we try to override cultural programming around dieting for thinness; a big percentage of us are over fifty and for the first time in our lives learning to prioritize building muscle and strength, the real keys to health and longevity that are critically important to staving off frailty in older age. We missed out on our peak muscle-building and bone-fortifying years because we were too busy cutting calories and counting points, but you're in a different place, and you have a once-in-a-lifetime opportunity to get ahead of the aging game and win.

It's this opportunity, *your* opportunity, that makes me so excited to be meeting you here in *The New Perimenopause.* Of course, I should be asking: How are *you* feeling? Perhaps you, too, are excited because you're eager to soak up the support, science, and strategies in the pages ahead. Or like many of my patients and the thousands of women surveyed for research and better understanding, you may be saying, *I'm just not feeling like myself.* To which I can finally respond with the words I so desperately wish I had access to several years ago: Based on what you're telling me, I can say there's a good chance you're in perimenopause—and there's much we can do together to proactively support your health and well-being during this transition.

Part One

YOU ARE HERE

CHAPTER 1

The Status Quo Experience of Perimenopause

Amy had lived her life with purpose and determination. At forty-three, she was successfully juggling the roles of wife, mother, and career professional, raising her kids with care, and navigating the everyday challenges of life with a sense of accomplishment. Her health had always been steady with no major issues to speak of. Like many other women, she followed the cultural prescription for staying healthy: years of dieting and regular exercise, mostly walking. It was a struggle, but she managed. Additional cardio from her spin class kept her happy, and though she sometimes wished for an easier path, she was proud of her ability to stay disciplined.

But then, seemingly out of nowhere, something changed. She began to feel off, as if she wasn't herself anymore. At first, it was subtle. Weight started accumulating around her midsection, an area that for her had never been an issue. It was frustrating. Everything she had done in the past to maintain her figure now seemed futile. She doubled down, cutting calories and increasing exercise, but nothing worked. Alongside the weight gain came irritability; she began snapping at her loved ones over minor things. At work, she felt perpetually frustrated. She chalked it up to stress, but deep down, she knew something wasn't right.

Her first visit to her doctor to try to get to the bottom of things didn't yield a satisfying answer. "This is just what women go through," her doctor said. "Work out more and eat less. We can prescribe an antidepressant for your mood." She left feeling dismissed, unseen. Her irritability worsened, and then her sleep began to falter. She would wake up at 3 A.M., staring at the ceiling, unable to drift back into rest. Exhaustion became her constant companion, and the weight gain continued.

Back at the doctor's office, she received a prescription for sleeping pills. The physician noted an additional five-pound weight gain and recommended a 1,200-calorie diet and more exercise. She wanted to scream as she was already eating 1,000 calories a day and now attending high-intensity interval training classes three times a week. Her hair began to thin, and her libido vanished. At her next well-woman exam, she hesitantly mentioned her loss of sexual desire. "Just relax more and have some wine," her doctor advised, looking over her glasses and adding, "If you don't use it, you'll lose it."

Her frustration turned to despair when a nurse called to inform her that her cholesterol levels had risen and she was now prediabetic. The nurse offered her prescriptions for metformin and a statin, with the familiar advice: "Eat low fat and continue with your efforts to lose some weight." Brain fog at work and her constant exhaustion kept her from applying for the promotion she had worked toward for years. Her husband grew frustrated with her lack of interest in intimacy, which only deepened her feelings of inadequacy and isolation.

Next, her periods became heavy and unpredictable, often waking her in the middle of the night to deal with excessive bleeding. Her gynecologist ordered two tests; a painful in-office biopsy and an ultrasound, but each showed no abnormalities. Still, the recommended solution was a hysterectomy, though they advised that because of her age she should remove only her uterus. Her healthy ovaries would continue to produce important hormones, they explained. Anemic and desperate for relief, she agreed to the major surgery.

Afterward, the bleeding stopped, but new problems emerged. A few months later, she began experiencing severe hot flashes and night sweats, and a worsening sense of exhaustion. It occurred to her that this might be menopause, but when she mentioned it to her physician, she dismissed the idea; she still had her ovaries, after all. "You are too young for that," she said, again advising weight loss.

Desperation drove her to social media, where ads for "hot flash cures" and "libido boosters" filled her feeds. She ordered herbal supplements, each promising relief, but none delivered. Intercourse, when she managed it, became unbearable. The pain was sharp, like razors cutting into her, leaving her in tears. She braved another doctor's visit and mentioned the pain, only to be told it might be herpes. Mortified, she waited for test results, which eventually came back negative.

Late one night, scrolling through her phone in yet another bout of sleeplessness, she saw an ad for a telemedicine company specializing in menopause care. Feeling both skeptical and hopeful, she reached out. For the first time, a clinician truly listened. After a thorough evaluation, they diagnosed her with menopause and the genitourinary syndrome of menopause (GSM). They discussed hormone therapy, systemic and local, and together they reviewed the risks and benefits. Finally, she felt seen, heard, and validated. She began treatment, and slowly, her life started to shift.

The unfortunate truth is that it's not hyperbolic to define this story as status quo; in fact, I would bet that if you don't identify with parts of it directly, you've got to stretch out only one or two degrees to connect with someone who does.

I'm here to deliver a critical message: This doesn't have to be your story. Together we can rewrite the status quo experience of women in perimenopause and create a movement that changes the trajectory of women's health. Your task in the push for change is simple: You must no longer be willing to accept the brand of treatment that is defined by dismissive condolences from doctors and other clinicians. Our movement, created for you and with you, is defined instead by active listening and proactive practices that improve quality of life and protect against the effects of inevitable hormone loss.

Perimenopause Symptoms Stats

In 2024, I conducted a community survey to get a clear sense of the most common symptoms reported by women in perimenopause. More than eight hundred women participated. Perhaps you'll see yourself in this feedback.

Top Five Most Common Symptoms

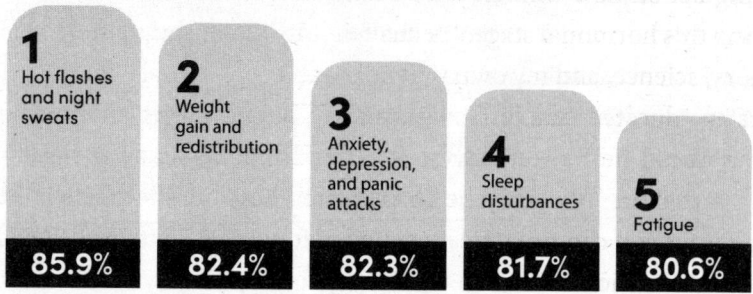

1. Hot flashes and night sweats — 85.9%
2. Weight gain and redistribution — 82.4%
3. Anxiety, depression, and panic attacks — 82.3%
4. Sleep disturbances — 81.7%
5. Fatigue — 80.6%

Additional Symptoms Reported

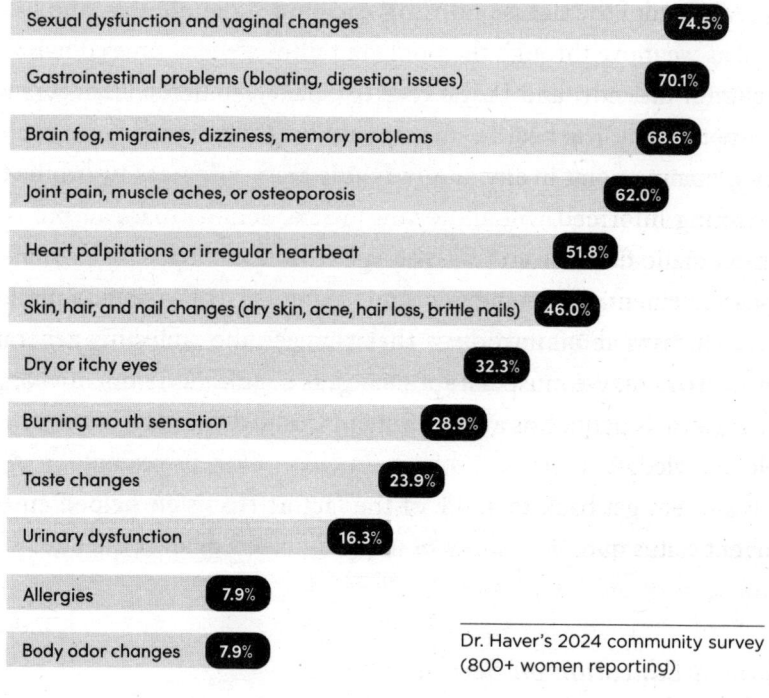

- Sexual dysfunction and vaginal changes — 74.5%
- Gastrointestinal problems (bloating, digestion issues) — 70.1%
- Brain fog, migraines, dizziness, memory problems — 68.6%
- Joint pain, muscle aches, or osteoporosis — 62.0%
- Heart palpitations or irregular heartbeat — 51.8%
- Skin, hair, and nail changes (dry skin, acne, hair loss, brittle nails) — 46.0%
- Dry or itchy eyes — 32.3%
- Burning mouth sensation — 28.9%
- Taste changes — 23.9%
- Urinary dysfunction — 16.3%
- Allergies — 7.9%
- Body odor changes — 7.9%

Dr. Haver's 2024 community survey (800+ women reporting)

How the Status Quo Was Born

A standard experience doesn't come into existence by chance. It's instead the result of several factors that over time converge and coalesce into *this is just how it's done*. In the case of perimenopause, it's challenging to say for certain which factors, because there are so many, have had the greatest impact on how women have been treated (or more like *not* treated) during this hormonal stage. It's challenging but not impossible. Based on history, science, and my own personal and professional experience, I can offer an educated take on how it came to be that a woman in perimenopause would be more likely to win the lottery than hear these words from a doctor: "You may be in perimenopause. Let's together explore some ways you can proactively support your health and well-being during this transition."

It's important first to acknowledge what's at stake when you aren't offered a clinical discussion on perimenopause—that is, why is it so critical that we disrupt the status quo? I have a lot to say about this, and I will expand as we move through the book, but ultimately it comes down to your quality of life, now and in the future. Quality of life concerns emotional well-being, physical health, and sexual health. Perimenopause can represent a turning point in any or all of these areas, and not toward the better. Becoming informed will allow you to take actions that can put out the symptomatic fire *now* and set you up with habits that may prevent heart disease, dementia, osteoporosis, and sarcopenia (age-related muscle loss) *later*. This isn't about introducing fear; it's about establishing generational empowerment. We must disrupt the status quo so that, from now on, perimenopause is defined as a transition invigorated by awareness and actionable knowledge.

Now, let's get back to some of the factors that have helped create the current status quo.

Limited Education on Perimenopause

To become a doctor, you generally complete four years of undergraduate study and then four years of medical school. After that, if you choose to specialize in an area of medicine, you need to successfully undergo additional education in that area. In my case, I chose to specialize in obstetrics and gynecology. Women are used to seeing one doctor, an OB-GYN, for these two specialties, but they address distinct elements of female health.

Obstetrics involves treating women through pregnancy, childbirth, and postpartum, while gynecology includes providing care as it relates to the reproductive system consisting of the vagina, uterus, cervix, ovaries, and breasts.

When you specialize in obstetrics and gynecology, you must complete a four-year residency working under the supervision of practicing physicians. Over this course of time, doctors in training spend thousands of hours treating the female reproductive system, downloading all there is to know about the organs and hormones involved in menstruation and pregnancy, and learning about the environmental, cultural, and genetic factors that can influence disease in women. We become encyclopedias of knowledge on the topics of diseased organs and reproduction. Yet the education seems to dry up when it comes time to discuss women's health as the reproductive years wane and eventually end.

Do you want to know how much of that time in medical school and residency was spent learning about perimenopause? About as long as it takes you to say the word *perimenopause*. It's baffling, but it was barely even a thing.

Of course, I did learn about perimenopause, but I was taught little more than the definition of it as the transitional phase that occurs before menopause. Any meaningful education I got on the subject would come much later when I experienced my own disruptive perimenopausal symptoms and began to research this stage of hormonal change.

The unfortunate reality is that not a lot has changed as it relates to education on perimenopause since I went to medical school almost twenty-eight years ago. Yet outside the hallowed halls of medicine, *so much* has changed and women in perimenopause want more information and guidance than most clinicians have been prepared to provide. A lot of doctors realize this fact, and they want the education, they want to do more for their patients, yet they feel stuck; the traditional channels don't currently offer the education needed to thoroughly treat the perimenopausal patient.

It's this conundrum that's led a lot of doctors who want to treat perimenopause and menopause away from traditional practice. Well, that and the current hospital system, which employs most doctors and which doesn't allow for the time or flexibility needed for the highest standard of treatment. Guess how much time your doctor is allotted for your appointment if they're working with an insurance company? Fifteen minutes. Honestly, this is barely enough time for most doctors to get through handwashing and a pelvic exam. (This problem isn't unique to perimenopause; the rigidity around allotted appointment times for patient treatment creates substandard care across the medical world.) Most of the doctors—including me—who have moved to the independent-practice model don't have multiple levels of administrators dictating how much time they can spend with patients or telling them what they can or can't prescribe.

How This Helped Shape the Status Quo: Doctors offer diagnoses and discuss treatment protocols based on the extensive education they've received. Perimenopause has never been given adequate attention in the curriculum taught early in medical schools, a fact that leaves most clinicians lacking a foundational understanding of this stage of change. Patients and doctors suffer as a result.

I think what's best for patients and for OB-GYNs is for the menopausal transition to be recognized as a multi-organ issue because, as I'll explain more in part 2, that's what it is—hormonal changes that begin in perimenopause affect the vast majority of organs and tissues throughout the body. Because of this systemic impact, perimenopause and menopause should frankly become their own specialty, one that focuses on the holistic health of a woman as she nears or enters her post-reproductive era. Until then, undereducated OB-GYNs will be unfairly scrutinized for their inadequate treatment of patients in perimenopause and beyond. And those patients in turn will struggle, sometimes for years, to receive clinical validation of their symptoms and a protocol that produces relief in the present and protection for the future.

Disruption in Progress: In 2025, I co-authored *A Citizen's Guide to Menopause Advocacy* with Jennifer Weiss-Wolf, the executive director of the Birnbaum Women's Leadership Center at NYU Law. Part of our motivation in creating this resource was to demand legislation requiring better care for women as they approach, enter, and surpass the menopause transition. At the time of this writing, there are twenty-six pro-menopause bills in sixteen states (red and blue) that mandate education and improve healthcare coverage.

> ## Defining Perimenopause, Menopause, and More
>
> Before you read on, I want to make sure you're aware of some important definitions related to perimenopause.
>
> **Perimenopause:** A transitional stage that happens before menopause and is heralded by fluctuations in hormone levels, primarily estrogen and progesterone. This stage may also be referred to as the menopausal transition and can begin in the forties or even in the mid-thirties. The duration of perimenopause varies, with the average being reported to be around four years, but it can last as long as ten.
>
> **Menopause:** One moment in time that happens when you've reached twelve months after your last period. This date will mark the end of your menstrual cycle and natural reproductive capabilities. The average age of menopause is fifty-one, with normal menopause falling between forty-five and fifty-five years of age. Early menopause is defined as menopause that happens before age forty-five, and premature menopause, before age forty.
>
> **Postmenopause:** The rest of your life after menopause. In postmenopause, we see the highest prevalence of vasomotor symptoms, such as hot flashes, heart palpitations, and sweating. Such symptoms may last between 4.5 and 9.5 years after the final menstrual period.
>
> In some cases, the word *menopausal* is used in the scientific literature to refer broadly to any or all of the above stages.

Promotion of Outdated Guidelines by Medical Organizations

I want to be crystal clear about one thing: I am and have been throughout my career board-certified by the American College of Obstetricians and Gynecologists (ACOG), and this is something of which I am very proud.

But ACOG, like all other professional medical organizations, suffers from what's referred to as a knowledge-translation or evidence-to-practice gap. What this means is that when new evidence is produced within the scientific research field, there's a gap between when this evidence comes to light and when it's incorporated into clinical guidelines. This matters because only once it's in the guidelines does it become part of a doctor's required continuing education and have the potential to be implemented into the treatment of patients.

So, how big of a time gap are we talking about? You'll be shocked to discover that it takes an average of *seventeen years* for evidence to change clinical practice. Yes, at a time when within seconds we can jump on a video call with a friend half a world away or order a new pair of our favorite leggings and get them delivered the same day, it takes in some cases more than seventeen years for your doctor to learn about and incorporate new scientific developments.

Let's think about this in terms of a woman in perimenopause. If you're forty years old when there's a groundbreaking scientific development on the use of hormone therapy in perimenopause, you could be fifty-seven before your doctor starts to implement this information into their practice. And at age fifty-seven, you're most likely postmenopausal already and beyond the time frame in which the information would have been relevant, even potentially life changing.

The other part of this that we must consider is how woefully underrepresented menopause and perimenopause are in the research that OB-GYNs are required to review to keep their board certification up to date. Using my own medical career as an example, in the thousands of papers that I have had to review for continuing medical education, less than 3 percent were clinically significant to a woman's menopause or perimenopause; they were instead focused on pregnancy and gynecologic disease. This isn't to say that the guideline updates I was presented with were unimportant, but they were clearly unbalanced and didn't allow me to sufficiently treat patients in perimenopause or beyond.

Thankfully, a small but mighty collection of doctors and researchers have been saying for years, "We refuse to accept this glacial pace of change, and we're going to accelerate progress because it's what our patients deserve." This includes people like the clinicians who in 1989 founded a forward-thinking coalition, the North American Menopause Society (now The Menopause Society), in response to the lack of progress being made by the longer-standing professional organizations. In 2022, the Menopause Society presented updated guidelines with prescribing practices that are based on the most current research. Sadly, these guidelines weren't and haven't yet been recognized or adopted by ACOG; as of this writing, ACOG is still using 2014 guidelines, which focus solely on hot flashes and vaginal dryness and don't mention perimenopause or the prevention of osteoporosis.

How This Helped Shape the Status Quo: Professional medical organizations are perpetuating the scarcity of perimenopausal education by failing to fast-track evidence-based practices into clinical guidelines. After reproduction ends or wanes, no one has taken the reins.

Disruption in Progress: I have been honored to find myself alongside a group of doctors, scientists, and other thought leaders promoting an overhaul of clinical practice based on emerging evidence. Sure, we're spending a lot of time swimming upstream, but we're starting to see the direction of the current change. We can't do this alone, however. We need *you*. We need citizen advocacy in the form of patients and other activists who are engaged in the disruption of the status quo. We need patients to refuse to settle for outdated information being passed off as an acceptable standard of care.

Who Is the Menoposse?

We've been talking about the menopause movement, but let me tell you about the menopause posse, a.k.a. the Menoposse. It's not a trend or a club. It's a global coalition of more than 250 scientists, clinicians, and other thought leaders: OB-GYNs, general practitioners, cardiologists, psychiatrists, oncologists, urologists, endocrinologists, internal medicine physicians, obesity medicine specialists, nurse practitioners, and researchers. We first came together to challenge the flawed, reductive narrative published in *The Lancet*'s menopause series.

We didn't start as a team; we found one another through urgency and purpose: a shared, unshakable belief that women in menopause deserve more: more science, more accurate care, and more respect, especially from the clinicians doing the work, day in and day out. The status quo didn't include us. So, we built something of our own.

And this isn't just about data; it's about what happens when women-centered science, advocacy, and empathy collide. Dr. Kelly Casperson dared to say what too many doctors were trained to avoid: Women deserve pleasure, and shame has no place in the exam room. Dr. Emily Nagoski reframed desire through the lens of neuroscience and compassion. Dr. Lauren Streicher gave us strategies we could use the next day in clinic. Dr. Rachel Rubin set the record straight on anatomy, testosterone, and sexual health with a firebomb appearance on *The Drive*.

We're also standing on the shoulders of brilliant colleagues who have been calling for change for years: Dr. Avrum Bluming and Dr. Carol Tavris, whose fearless book, *Estrogen Matters,* helped dismantle the fear-based narrative around hormone therapy. Dr. Sharon Malone, who has used her platform and clinical expertise to bring menopause to the national stage. Dr. Corinne Menn, whose nuanced, evidence-based voice continues to guide patients and practitioners alike. Dr. Suzanne Gilberg, who blends science with soul in her advocacy for integrative care. Dr. Rocio Salas-Whalen, a leader in obesity medicine, who brings clarity and compassion to treating metabolic health in midlife women.

And there are *so many more*.

We share research, patient cases, complications, triumphs, books, stages, and microphones. We support one another and hold the line because we know that when clinicians and scientists band together, we don't just push back against outdated norms. We build new ones.

Underfunded Women's Health

The National Institutes of Health (NIH) is an agency of the U.S. government that funds biomedical and behavioral research within the United

States and throughout the world. It has an annual budget of around fifty billion dollars (yes, that's *billion* with a *b*), and each year these funds are divided among areas of health. The percentage of this mega-budget that is dedicated exclusively to women's health is typically less than 10 percent. A 2024 report from the National Academies of Sciences, Engineering, and Medicine, a nonprofit think tank based in Washington, D.C., found that just 8.8 percent of NIH grant spending from 2013 to 2023 focused on women's health research. They also noted that despite steady increases in the agency's budget, the percentage dedicated to women's health has lessened over time.

I'm giving you this background because inadequate funding has a direct link to the medical treatment someone will receive across her lifespan. The gaps in our understanding around female-specific conditions, such as uterine fibroids, endometriosis, and polycystic ovary syndrome, exist because of insufficient funding. We know far too little about the distinct ways certain diseases, such as cardiovascular disease, affect women (even though women face worse outcomes than men after heart attack or stroke), because of lack of funding. We don't fully understand yet how complications during pregnancy may be associated with chronic disease later in life, because of lack of funding. I could go on, but you get my point.

When it comes to menopause and perimenopause, the story is much the same, if not even worse. Matters related to reproductive transitions and aging fall lowest on the funding priority list. Menopause is estimated to get less than 1 percent of the women's health research budget (and remember, that's 1 percent of an already-small slice of the pie). The result is limited scope and depth of studies on perimenopause, as well as a limited number of studies period. When I looked at the number of studies with a perimenopause focus, the results were shocking: Until 1977, there were only thirty-five medical research articles that even mentioned perimenopause. Since then, things have improved, and that number is around 7,000.

On the surface, this seems like a significant increase, and it is. However, if we consider this number in comparison with other topics that fall under the umbrella of women's health, it's minuscule, *especially* when we weigh it against mentions of pregnancy, the topic that by far gets the most attention as it relates to women. A search of the PubMed database today reveals nearly 1.2 million mentions of pregnancy, 102,000 mentions of menopause, and around 7,000 mentions of perimenopause. Perimenopause and menopause are also *not* among the 292 topics listed in the NIH Research Portfolio Online Reporting Tools system, making it difficult to track and prioritize research investment in this area.

How This Helped Shape the Status Quo: Perimenopause involves multiple organ systems and symptoms. To understand it fully, we need rigorous and comprehensive scientific studies that offer insight into the biological processes taking place and help us better connect the dots. The problem is that these studies cost money. The bulk of the funding for scientific research comes from the National Institutes of Health, which has historically underfunded matters related to women's health, perimenopause being no exception.

Disruption in Progress: Despite the continued lack of NIH funding in the United States, incredible research is being conducted worldwide and the results are getting broadcast across the world to doctors and other clinicians who care. We're also seeing the funding landscape change as private organizations begin to invest in research in new and exciting ways. Plus, incredible funding work is happening internationally. In just one example, Australia voted in 2025 to put five hundred million dollars toward menopause education initiatives and expanding coverage of menopause treatment.

Again, there is room here for you to get involved and advocate for increased funding. I encourage you to visit thepauselife.com to review *A Citizen's Guide to Menopause Advocacy* for ways to take action. You are not without a voice and influence!

No Standard Criteria for Diagnosis

I've made it clear that it's uncommon to hear about a woman in midlife who's gone to her doctor to report symptoms of deep fatigue, increased anxiety, and not feeling like herself and emerged with the understanding that she may be in perimenopause. She is far more likely to hear "This is just what women go through" or a similarly dismissive phrase.

The lack of education and funding and outdated guidelines are indeed contributing factors in creating this status quo experience. But another complicating factor is that perimenopause requires a *symptom-based* diagnosis rather than a *lab-test-based* one. There are currently *no lab tests that allow for a conclusive and straightforward diagnosis of perimenopause,* so a doctor must rely on their knowledge of symptoms related to this reproductive transition to make that diagnosis. Well, this is a big problem since doctors aren't being educated about symptoms. I was never taught during my residency that perimenopause had any symptoms other than disrupted periods. The majority of clinicians don't have a bank of knowledge to rely on for the diagnosis and treatment of perimenopause, so many sadly default to dismissive condolences.

It's true that changes to your menstrual cycle do occur in response to underlying hormone fluctuations taking place, but emerging research is revealing that this isn't always the first symptom, and it's certainly not the only symptom you may experience.

What scientists are beginning to understand is that the *brain* is often the first organ to recognize that something is changing, even before the menstrual cycle becomes irregular. Although ovulation may still be occurring, hormone levels aren't reaching the same peaks they once did. This lack of adequate hormonal feedback tells the brain that *something is changing* and leads to a cascade of effects. On an endocrinological level, you've entered what I refer to as the zone of chaos. The stage during which your hormones are erratic and so, too, may be your ability to focus, your energy level, and your moods. In fact, research suggests that greater than 70 percent of women in perimenopause report anxiety, depression, and/or mood swings. (See the the "Zone of Chaos Up Close" graphic in chapter 2—and read the entire chapter—if you want to understand in detail the hormonal volatility of perimenopause and why it's no mystery that you may start to feel unlike yourself during this time.)

The issue again is that most clinicians haven't been taught that the focus, energy, and mood symptoms, along with abdominal weight gain, low libido, and fatigue, can be signs of perimenopause. As a result, many patients, in pursuing a diagnosis and relief, seek alternative practitioners who offer a variety of extensive and expensive tests and protocols (see chapter 3 for common misdiagnoses in perimenopause). Effective lifestyle-based protocols, on the other hand, do exist, but they are built around tried-and-true practices such as reducing stress, getting adequate sleep, eating more fiber, ensuring optimal vitamin D levels, and lifting weights. No hard-to-pronounce supplements or gimmicks required; in other words, it's tough to "wellness" your way through your perimenopause.

How This Helped Shape the Status Quo: The clinical diagnostic criteria for perimenopause consists of a very short list: irregular periods and hot flashes. If you don't have either of these, it will be very challenging to get a clinician to discuss the possibility of perimenopause. Especially because there is no specific blood test for perimenopause. This fact alone has led countless women down the status quo path, defined by multiple doctor's visits during which the same symptoms are repeatedly dismissed because they don't match the short "symptoms of perimenopause" checklist.

If you've been down this path, you know how distressing it can be, especially if you are included in the high percentage of women who suffer from disruptive mental health changes during the menopause transition. These changes, including some of the most common symptoms such as increased anxiety, depressive thoughts, and trouble focusing, can be incredibly isolating and often come with the most fear and concern around what may be causing such disruptive changes.

If you report any of these symptoms, you are statistically much more likely to be offered an antidepressant than to be offered a discussion on your fluctuating hormones. In fact, use of selective serotonin reuptake inhibitors (SSRIs), the most common type of antidepressant, doubles for women during the menopausal transition. While, in some cases, clinical depression is present and this is the correct treatment protocol, the bulk of the mental health changes we see happen in perimenopause are related to hormone fluctuations rather than clinical mood disorders. For this reason, patients should be offered a discussion of hormone therapy as first-line treatment alongside a referral to a mental health professional. Not only is hormone therapy more effective in stabilizing the hormones that most affect mood in perimenopause, but it also has fewer side effects than SSRIs or other types of antidepressants.

Disruption in Progress: People are no longer willing to settle for treatment based on stagnant clinical definitions that refuse to align with a woman's lived experience in perimenopause. And this is creating a push to change not only how perimenopause is defined but also who does the defining.

This is a grassroots movement born out of necessity.

Doctors are listening to their patients and realizing what should have been obvious all along. Women in perimenopause are profoundly underserved, and those entrusted with their care have been profoundly undereducated.

By seeking knowledge beyond the limits of traditional medical training, these clinicians are gaining deeper insight into the lived realities of women during the menopause transition. Together, they are building a dynamic and evolving body of real-world evidence, a living and breathing database of symptoms, patterns, and treatments that actually work.

This work takes time. It requires patience, persistence, and often a fair amount of trial and error. But this movement is gaining momentum, earning legitimacy, and challenging outdated frameworks. My hope is that it will ultimately help redefine perimenopause to reflect the complexity, nuance, and urgency of what women are truly experiencing.

We also have telemedicine platforms to thank for expanding our understanding of women's lived experience. Many of these platforms, such as Midi and Alloy Health, have created interactive questionnaires that collect data directly from women. The larger this data set grows, the stronger the conclusions are about the prevalence of certain symptoms and the effectiveness of treatment options. While these companies use the information they obtain to improve the products and services they offer at a cost, they also freely add any insight gained to the public domain and this benefits all of us.

There are promising developments, too, in the area of diagnostic testing for perimenopause. New studies have found that rising levels of anti-Mullerian hormone (AMH) and a type of LDL cholesterol called small dense low-density lipoprotein cholesterol (sdLDL-C) may be indicative of having reached perimenopausal status. (Anyone's cholesterol suddenly begin to rise in perimenopause? Yep, most of us will experience this.) Other research has noted that an increase in NSUN4, a sign of mitochondrial dysfunction, may serve as a potential biomarker for ovarian aging. This research is ongoing, and nothing conclusive has resulted, but I'm hopeful that we will someday soon have one or more markers that help eliminate both the difficulty of diagnosis and the unnecessary prevalence of misdiagnosis.

A Poor Understanding of the Impact of Aging While Female

In the United States, our healthcare system operates off a sick-care model, which means that the standard practice is to fix something only when it breaks. This is the status quo, and we must fall in line if we, the doctors, want to get paid or if you, the patient, want insurance-supported coverage of your medical care.

There are some efforts at prevention incorporated into our current system. For example, if you are a female patient, you typically get an annual physical, a well-woman exam, and at age forty a mammogram covered by insurance. These important screenings aim to catch early evidence of diabetes or cervical or breast cancer at a time when intervention may be most effective. What is missing from these appointments, however, is a screening for signs and symptoms of perimenopause and tests to check for subclinical changes related to bone, heart, and brain health, which occur as your hormones fluctuate regardless of whether you have noticeable symptoms.

It's becoming increasingly clear that the hormonal volatility associated with perimenopause activates changes that affect a woman's health, and that these changes happen at an accelerated rate independent of aging. For example, our greatest acceleration of bone density loss happens in perimenopause. Levels of LDL, the worst kind of cholesterol for your risk of atherosclerosis, jump up more than 18 percent at or around perimenopause. And it's difficult to acknowledge this statistic, but the most likely time for a woman to commit suicide is between the ages of forty-five and fifty-five; there is no clearer sign that entering a state of hormonal upheaval can initiate disruptive mental health changes. (Let me take this moment to make sure you know one thing for certain: You are *not* alone if you feel unmoored during this time of your life. Help is here on these pages, and it's critical to remember that the 988 Lifeline is always available. You can call or text 988 any day of the year, twenty-four hours a day, and you will be connected to someone you can talk to confidentially and at no cost.)

How This Helped Shape the Status Quo: For far too long, scientific research was androcentric—that is, focused on men. As a result, conclusions about male biology were assumed to represent the norm for all humans, and distinctions created by female biology and endocrinology weren't even considered. You might think of this another way: If you were born female with a male twin, most of the understanding about your health would have been based on how *his* body operates and ages, not yours.

What we know now is that women age differently from men (as Dr. Stacy Sims so brilliantly put it, "women are not small men"). In fact, during the menopause transition, we experience an accelerated window of aging that can put us on a path to certain diseases that preferentially affect us. Returning to your hypothetical twin for a moment—even if you were to have lived your lives identically, you would still have a much higher risk for developing dementia, osteoporotic fracture, and depression.

Disruption in Progress: My hope is that we will someday soon have screenings in place for the disease paths that can be initiated throughout the menopause transition. Until then, consider this your notice that you can and should be proactive about your health. If you are thirty-five, you aren't too young to start thinking about the impact hormone changes can have on the rest of your life. You can get a head start on avoiding the diseases that disproportionately affect women as they age, and you can do this not because you are afraid but because you want to be informed about and awake to the possibilities of becoming the boss of your own healthcare.

In part 4, I'll detail the early-prevention measures you should consider and why. The items at the top of the list include . . .

- Tracking your cholesterol to spot any unexplained or sudden increases in LDL levels.

- Getting a bone density scan earlier than what is currently recommended. Many guidelines suggest that unless you have a specific risk factor, bone density scans should begin at age sixty-five (this is also when insurance will start covering the cost without a risk factor). The cost is between one hundred and three hundred dollars and varies based on your location.

- Obtaining your HOMA-IR score to check for insulin resistance. HOMA-IR stands for "homeostatic model assessment for insulin resistance," which is a calculation that looks at your glucose and insulin levels to determine metabolic health and risk for type 2 diabetes.

Again, there's so much more on this to come. For now, the key thing to remember is this: Your health and wellness are in your hands.

Why It's So Important That We Disrupt the Status Quo

Perimenopause is a universal physiological process for females that can bring about a litany of changes that affect mental and physical health—and often not for the better. For a number of reasons, these changes haven't been fully acknowledged by professional medical organizations or discussed and treated by clinicians.

The tragedy in this lies in the trajectory. If we fail to intervene, what we see in the future is millions of women who continue to be disproportionately affected by illness and disability; we see women who live longer but sicker lives compared with men. It's true that women have a longevity edge: We live an average of 80.2 years compared with 74.8 years for men.

Recent research reveals, however, that this advantage is lost when it comes to health span, which is the portion of your life that you spend in good health, free from serious disease or disability. Women in this case are behind the curve.

In *Closing the Women's Health Gap,* the World Economic Forum in collaboration with the McKinsey Health Institute reported that as women we spend on average 25 percent more of our lives in poor health compared with men. "A woman will spend an average of nine years in poor health," the report revealed. This time that is consumed by disability, chronic pain, reduced mobility, and cognitive decline is part of what's referred to as the gender health gap.

The gender health gap doesn't exist simply because we live longer. The years of poor health can occur throughout a woman's life, with nearly half the burden reported to occur between the ages of twenty and sixty-four. Poor health at this time of your life can be wholly disruptive, pulling you away from family, shutting you out of opportunities at work, such as pay raises and promotions, and downgrading quality of life significantly.

Raising awareness of the gender health gap is critical because it allows us to quantify the consequences of the status quo. The lack of education on women's health; the perpetually underfunded scientific study of conditions that disproportionately or only affect women, such as autoimmune diseases, depression, and endometriosis; and gender biases that lead to the dismissal or misdiagnosis of symptoms and often delay treatment. These are not theoretical concepts but real factors that convert to irreplaceable lost time, years eaten up by complex or chronic health issues.

I see patients in my clinical practice every day who have been burdened by such issues, and I see the gap as being largely to blame for their reliance on multiple medications for blood pressure, osteoporosis, and insulin resistance and for their need to take antidepressants, sleeping pills, or pain medications. My patient demographic includes women ranging in age from thirty to eighty, and those who are now in their late sixties and older come into my office and say, "I wish I had known." They wish they had known that many of the health challenges they are now facing could have been mitigated or delayed if preventative habits had been implemented in their forties or sooner.

Before you get too concerned, I have some good news: You have the power to change the trajectory, and I'm here to help you do it. Perimenopause presents a once-in-a-lifetime opportunity to get ahead of the health changes on the horizon. There are habits that, if adopted, can keep you strong and support the pursuit of a long and healthy life. We will get to all of it. But first, if you are like most of my patients, your priority is getting through today without collapsing from exhaustion or crying, without feeling intense angst or anxiety, or without wishing you could disappear. Your priority is to feel more like yourself again, whatever that looks like. Let me share what's going on within your body that may be causing you to feel unlike yourself, and then we will get to what you can do to start feeling better.

CHAPTER 2

The Zone of Chaos

I entered my forties feeling amazing, fit, healthy, full of energy, and most importantly happy. Fast-forward three years, and just before my forty-third birthday, my life feels drastically different.

Over the past year, symptoms started to appear. I experienced itchy and irritated skin and eyes and started feeling warmer at nighttime, almost like my blood was simmering. I noticed painful sex and a decline in sex drive. I am also irrationally irritated; my ability to handle stress is terrible. I feel so much apathy for life, low moods, and increased anxiety. My husband has noticed and asked, "Do you not like us anymore?" This question made me feel so sad because my inner turmoil was affecting those around me—but mostly because the answer to that question was "I no longer like myself!" This time of my life really feels like chaos, a real struggle, and I feel a deep sadness.

—Jodie A.

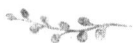

If you were born female, there's likely a lot about your body that no one has explicitly taught you. It's been this way for generations.

My middle school biology teacher tried her best, but there were limits to what she was allowed to cover. To supplement my "education," when I was near puberty, my mom handed me a set of life-cycle books, then ran into the other room. The books had anatomical pictures of both men and women, and I took them to school and showed them to my girlfriends in the hallways so we could giggle. Younger generations don't have much more robust school curriculum and have swapped books for the internet and social media, downloading what they can in private.

Before my own daughters got their periods, I had elaborate plans for celebrating this milestone—I hoped to whisk them away from school and take them shopping and out to lunch; I wanted it to be a big deal. Of course, they had other plans. One initially hid it from me as she did *not* want to make it "a big deal," and the other was at a sleepover with friends when she started. She told me she didn't need anything from me as her friends cheered and celebrated her and told her what to do.

When I was forty-eight and realized I was menopausal, I was *not* greeted by a group of celebrating friends. In fact, I don't ever remember my girlfriends talking about it at all. Certainly, I talked about it clinically as an OB-GYN, but in my friend group no one had discussed menopause, let alone perimenopause. And my mother had never murmured a word.

There are a lot of reasons for the absence of these conversations. Historically, there have been stigma and shame around anything involving female reproductive organs, especially menstruation. And misinformation! To wit, in the nineteenth century, people believed that the presence of a menstruating woman could kill plants, destroy bee populations, and scare away lightning. Even though we have largely moved on from such extreme superstitions, echoes of the perception of women's power and mysterious nature remain, reinforcing the obligation to be secretive around menstruation and, later, menopause. (If you've ever concealed a tampon box under a loaf of bread in the grocery checkout line, you know what I mean.)

A lack of knowledge about how the menstrual cycle works isn't trivial; it has real consequences. It's been found to contribute to the shame and other negative feelings girls and young women have about their reproductive body functions, fueling low self-esteem. I believe the same is true for us later in life when we approach our post-reproductive era, a stage that starts with perimenopause. When you don't understand what is happening in your body during this time, you're more apt to feel stress, confusion, isolation, shame, insecurity, and so much more. Which is why I'm here to fill in the gaps in understanding and blow the doors off secrecy. The more you know, the less lost you will feel.

I'm going to warn you: *A lot* is going on during perimenopause; your body has shifted from a place of relative hormonal stability to one defined by so much fluctuation that it's been branded the zone of hormonal chaos. There's no way to explain this zone other than to get into the scientific detail. In the chapter ahead, you may find yourself saying, "You know, I don't need *this* much knowledge," but I encourage you to stick with it. You might be surprised by how empowering it feels to understand the endocrinological changes that are occurring in your body. By removing the mystery, you create room for greater clarity and an improved connection with yourself and others around you. You might even discuss what you learn with your friends.

How Many Eggs Does a Woman Have?

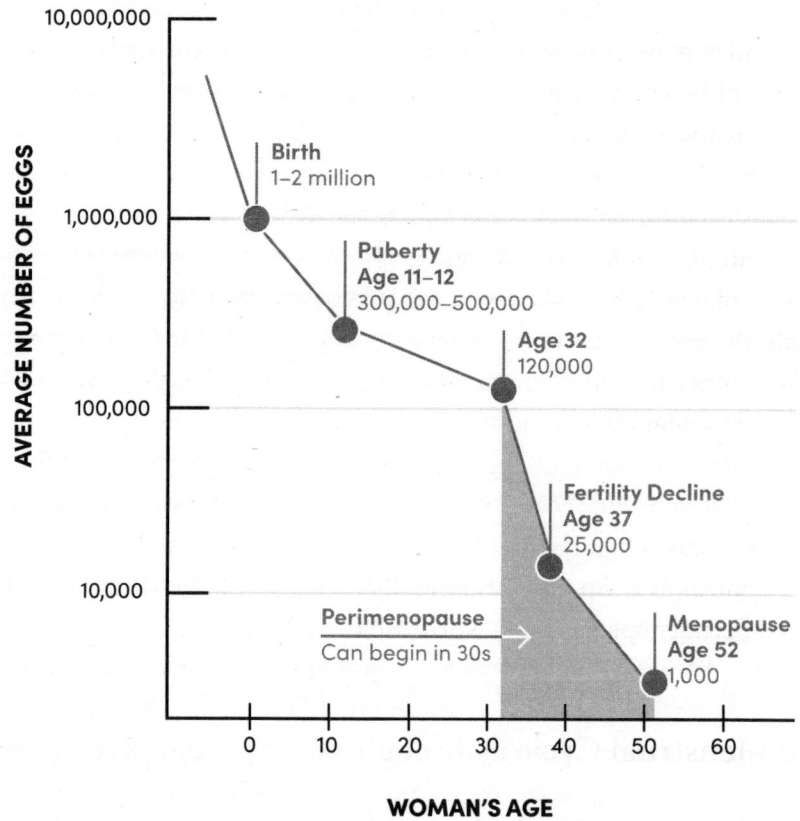

Adapted from illustration by Bailey Mariner featured in "How many eggs does a woman have?" written by Rachel Ann Tee-Melegrito and published by *Medical News Today*

When you're born, your reproductive organs already contain the potential to reproduce your genetic uniqueness. In females, this potential is packaged in cells called oocytes, which are immature eggs that hold your DNA. To reproduce, oocytes need to mature and then be fertilized by sperm cells, but on their own, oocytes possess nearly all the molecules needed for human development.

At birth, you have one to two million oocytes, which means you'll have only that number of eggs throughout your life. That sounds like a lot, but by the time puberty hits, the number will have dropped to between three- and five hundred thousand. This loss occurs by way of a process called atresia, which works sort of like natural selection for your egg supply and will continue to cause a drop-off in oocytes throughout your reproductive life.

The end of puberty is marked by the arrival of your menstrual cycle, the sequence of hormone-driven events that will ready and release a mature egg for possible pregnancy every twenty-eight days or so (in a healthy female). This monthly process of egg recruitment sacrifices up to one thousand eggs each time and combines with atresia to reveal a shocking stat: Only about *four hundred* of the one to two million eggs you started with will be ovulated. This makes sense when you consider that, in a healthy woman, the menstrual cycle will repeat reliably (except for during pregnancy or other hormonal disruptions) for around thirty-three years, or just about four hundred months.

Most women understand the menstrual cycle on the surface, but I want to familiarize you with the details of how a cycle works when it's operating at its prime and is highly predictable. This will help ensure that you have proper context to grasp the disruption that comes with the hormonal volatility of perimenopause. Don't worry, I'll be your guide.

The Menstrual Cycle as It Begins—and Begins to End

Let's rewind to the moment when you had just started your period and your egg supply was about five hundred thousand. At this time, key hormones had been recently activated to initiate the pattern of your menstrual cycle. The hormones most influential to the cycle include estrogen and progesterone, which are released by the ovaries, and luteinizing hormone (LH) and follicle-stimulating hormone (FSH), produced by the pituitary gland in the brain. Throughout the month, levels of estrogen, progesterone, LH, and FSH rise and fall to trigger changes in your reproductive organs. The main agenda is to mature one oocyte from your egg supply, readying it for ovulation and fertilization.

There are four phases of this cycle: menses, follicular, ovulation, and luteal. When we break down the menstrual cycle by phase, we can see clearly the hormonal ebb and flow that drives all the action.

The Menstrual Cycle

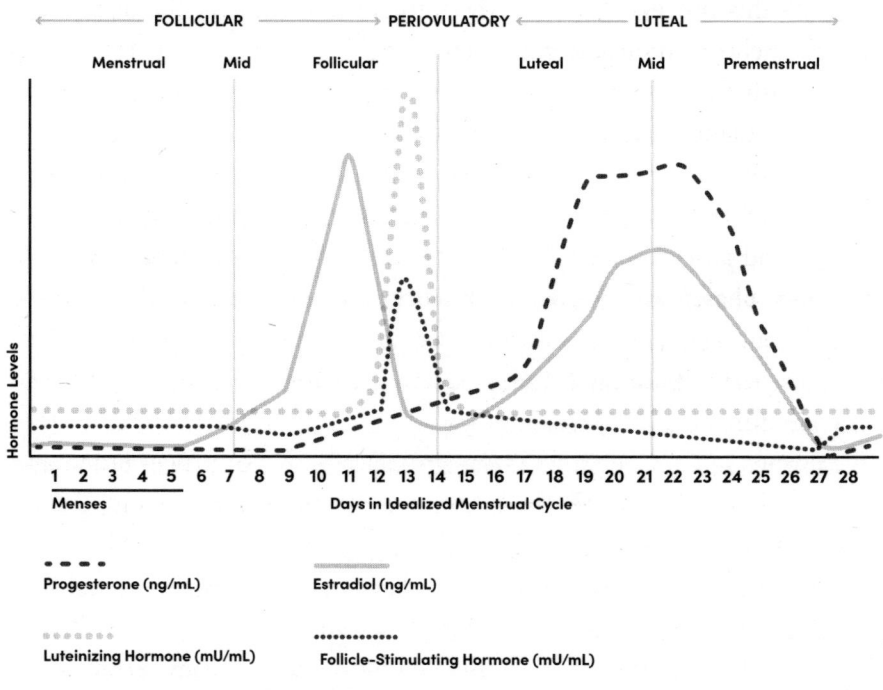

nature.com/articles/s41598-018-32647-0

Menses phase/days 1–5: The menstrual cycle begins with the shedding of your uterine lining, which is made up of tissue, blood, and mucus. Menstruation indicates that last month's ovulation hasn't resulted in pregnancy and signals that estrogen and progesterone are no longer needed. During these first five or so days of your cycle, estrogen and progesterone levels are at the lowest they will be throughout the month.

Follicular phase/days 6–13: The hypothalamus in the brain detects low estrogen levels and signals to the pituitary gland that it's time to release LH and FSH. LH and FSH trigger the ovaries to release progesterone and estradiol, a form of estrogen, and activate growth in your follicles, the small sacs within your ovaries that each contain a single immature egg. As the follicles grow, they produce increasing amounts of estradiol, which causes the uterine lining to thicken in preparation for a potential pregnancy.

Every menstrual cycle will recruit a certain group of follicles to grow, and just one (unless twins are in order) will emerge as the dominant follicle. The dominant follicle will continue to grow into an ovum, or mature egg. It's this process of follicle recruitment that leads to the loss of approximately one thousand eggs each month.

Ovulation/day 14 or so: The pituitary gland produces a surge of LH to trigger ovulation, the process of your dominant follicle releasing the mature egg into a fallopian tube. The empty follicle will then collapse in on itself and form a corpus luteum, a temporary gland that will produce estrogen and progesterone to further the thickening of the uterine lining.

Luteal phase/days 15–28: The mature egg continues its path through one of your fallopian tubes and travels to the uterus, where it may be fertilized by sperm. If the egg is fertilized and implants in the sticky and thickened uterine wall, you become pregnant. If this doesn't happen, the cells of the corpus luteum begin to disintegrate and levels of progesterone and estrogen drop to allow for the thinning of the uterine lining and, shortly hereafter, the menses phase again. The lowering of hormones at this time can produce symptoms of premenstrual syndrome (PMS).

This cycle is repeated month after month *until we reach perimenopause* and the reliable pattern of hormonal cuing starts to become erratic. The reason for this isn't that your hormones are randomly changing—*it's that your egg supply has changed in quantity and quality and increasing levels of brain hormones are needed to stimulate the release of an egg.* The levels of LH and FSH that for so long worked to grow your follicles and produce ovulation are no longer effective. So, what does your brain do in this case? It starts sending higher and higher levels of these stimulating hormones in order to force ovulation. The ovaries strain to respond, and ovulation is delayed, which has a ripple effect and disrupts the delicate hormonal equilibrium of the entire menstrual cycle. A new normal is established; you have now entered the zone of chaos.

The Zone of Chaos Up Close

It may seem dramatic to use a phrase like *the zone of chaos* to describe your hormones during perimenopause, but I don't believe a more appropriate description exists. When you look at this side-by-side comparison of the hormone cycles before, during, and after perimenopause, I think you will agree with me.

In premenopause, we have a predictable ebb and flow of hormones that presents an EKG-like pattern. During perimenopause, this pattern is disrupted. In addition to higher levels and more intense bursts of LH and FSH, which occur as the ovaries' ability to respond declines, you can see fluctuations in estradiol and progesterone. The surges of LH and FSH and the erratic spikes in estradiol combined with lagging progesterone are the hormonal hallmarks of perimenopause.

I used to believe that there's a slow and gentle decline into this transitional hormonal zone that leads up to menopause. But my understanding of what is happening endocrinologically changed when I read Dr. Nanette Santoro's incredible study "Characterization of Reproductive Hormonal Dynamics in the Perimenopause." Even though this research was published in *The Journal of Clinical Endocrinology & Metabolism* in 1996, I had never read it—and it certainly had never been required reading in medical school (or for continuing medical education). The study revealed that the hormonal shift into perimenopause is anything but slow and gentle; it's sudden and tumultuous. This revelation helped reconcile a disconnect between my clinical experience—filled with women with regular periods reporting brain fog, mental health changes, weight gain, sleep disruptions, and generally not feeling like themselves—and my medical school education, which denied the existence of such symptoms.

A myriad of symptoms can occur because of this underlying hormonal havoc. To help you better understand why and how these symptoms develop, I want to talk a little more about what could be considered the two command centers of the chaos: the brain and the ovaries.

Changes in Hormone Level Patterns over Six Months

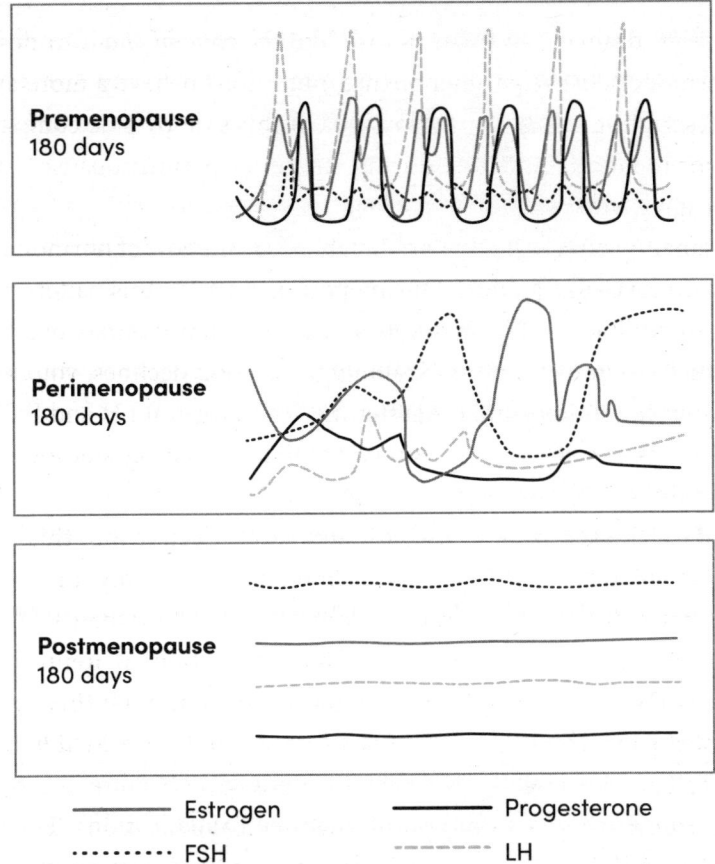

The routine hormonal pattern of premenopause shifts to chaos in perimenopause. Postmenopause introduces the chronic elevation of brain hormones and an absence of ovarian-derived sex hormones, which lead to distinct challenges and changes that are significant enough to warrant their own book.

Harvard Women's Health Watch 1999

The Brain: Where Perimenopause Begins

In chapter 1, I mentioned that in perimenopause the brain is often the first organ to recognize that something is changing within the reproductive system. Indeed, the brain's observation of and response to these changes happen *before the menstrual cycle is disrupted.* Essentially, long before the menstrual cycle becomes irregular, LH and FSH begin to pulsate in a new, disrupted pattern. This shift occurs internally and invisibly; a woman's brain is already registering changes, but there are no immediate outward signs—no skipped periods or other obvious warning signals.

The result? Confusion. Women begin to experience subtle yet profound changes in how they feel, physically, emotionally, and cognitively, without any clear explanation. They may sense that something is off, but when they seek medical advice, they often encounter dismissal.

Unfortunately, many doctors still operate from the status quo of using the menstrual cycle to define perimenopause; you know you have a doctor like this if you've ever heard "Your periods are regular; it can't be perimenopause." I'm familiar with this dialogue because it's a line that I used in the past. I'm not proud to admit this, even though my response was derived directly from the medical guidelines at the time and was the standard of practice.

Thankfully, there are others who have dedicated themselves to the pursuit of the kind of scientific insight that will help overhaul the standards of practice. And an adjacent group—of which I'm proud to now be a member—of passionate menopause clinicians and educators who are ready to broadcast this insight across their platforms so millions of others may learn.

What studies have revealed is that the majority of women will experience neurological symptoms during perimenopause. These may be changes in cognitive function, such as diminished verbal learning and memory and reduced processing speed, attention, and working memory. You may experience this as brain fog and find it difficult to concentrate, recall words, or make decisions. Depression, sleep problems, and vasomotor symptoms (hot flashes and hot flashes that occur at night, a.k.a. night sweats), which often prohibit restorative rest, are also more likely to emerge in perimenopause, all of which may intensify the feeling that you are operating from within a sort of dark cognitive cloud.

When we look at the brain in perimenopause, we can see disruptions in neural mechanisms, which can contribute to the increase in cognitive symptoms. The LH and FSH surges are an indication that the brain isn't getting what it needs: more estrogen and progesterone from the ovaries. And insufficient estrogen and progesterone signal that the entire feedback loop is beginning to break down, causing a chain reaction of missed connections:

- As estrogen levels decline, glucose metabolism in the brain begins to slow and it has to search for other sources of fuel to keep running properly, often catabolizing its own white matter to generate ketones.

- Decreases in progesterone alter the ability of the neurotransmitter GABA to calm the nervous system, making you more sensitive to stress and more likely to experience sleep disruptions.

- Estrogen withdrawal interferes with serotonin, dopamine, and norepinephrine pathways, which can result in disturbed sleep cycles, mood instability, and greater risk of anxiety or depression, reduced feelings of pleasure, lost motivation, compromised ability to learn, and difficulty with decision-making.

My goal in sharing this information is to empower you, not scare you. I want to make it unequivocally known that if you feel different or off or unlike yourself (also known as NFLM; see the introduction) in perimenopause despite no noticeable changes to your menstrual cycle, you aren't imagining it—even if a doctor suggests that you are. You've got some neurological remodeling in progress, and like all remodels, it may come with hidden costs and take far longer than you'd like—but it *is* happening, and this fact shouldn't be kept a secret.

In chapter 4, I'll discuss more on the brain in perimenopause, including taking you through a detailed look at the mental health changes that can occur. I'll also address the timeline of cognitive changes, neurological symptoms for which you should consider seeing a doctor, and supportive strategies that can help. In clinical practice, my colleagues and I are seeing that many of our patients who began menopause hormone therapy (MHT) in perimenopause are reporting generalized improvements in perimenopausal cognitive deficits. But before we can recommend MHT broadly as a treatment, more research is needed.

The Ovaries: They Are Doing Their Best

In perimenopause, the ovaries begin to struggle to produce viable eggs, which, as I've explained, creates fluctuations in estrogen and progesterone. What we start to see are out-of-sync increases and an overall downward trend in estrogen levels and sharp, unpredictable drop-offs in progesterone, much like a free fall on a roller coaster. We don't have an exact egg count that triggers this shift, and it likely varies by individual, but the average age of entering perimenopause is forty-three and a half.

I want to really lean into the definition of perimenopause as a *transition,* one that lasts an average of four years and can go on as long as ten. The shift into hormonal chaos happens rather suddenly, and egg count and quality decline faster than in your premenopausal years; however, it's not as though one day you have eggs and the next day you don't. You were born with a finite supply and are heading toward the day when this supply will run out and your ovaries will retire.

Before this time, you will see disruptions in ovarian-produced hormones throughout the menstrual cycle. If we return to the phases of the cycle, the disruptions appear to begin in the follicular phase. During this phase, one of your ovaries is actively recruiting follicles to advance to the next round. While we don't fully understand the specifics of this process, we can imagine it essentially shopping around for a group of follicles to which it can say, "Hey, you've got potential—here are some hormones to start growing."

In perimenopause, the selection pool has been reduced in quality and quantity and the ovary has to work harder to find an acceptable cohort of new recruits. These issues of quality control stall the entire cycle, and meanwhile, countless cells throughout the body are left eagerly waiting for the estrogen and progesterone that they're used to receiving. This period of ovarian inactivity, hormonally speaking, contributes to the variations in cycle length that some women start to experience in perimenopause.

Estrogen Dominance

Rarely a day goes by without my having a patient or someone on social media say that a functional medicine practitioner has diagnosed them with "estrogen dominance." The problem with this is that estrogen dominance is not an actual diagnosis; it is a description of a hormonal snapshot taken when estrogen is active and progesterone is missing. And while the picture may be entirely accurate one moment, it can be equally inaccurate the next.

In clinical practice, we would define elevated estrogen with low to no progesterone as unopposed estrogen. Estrogen and progesterone work together to regulate the menstrual cycle and support whole body health. The body produces progesterone only after ovulation, so if ovulation doesn't occur, progesterone never rises. And estrogen is left alone without its physiological partner.

What we need to be asking of this hormonal state is: *Why is estrogen unopposed?* Unopposed estrogen is a consequence of missing ovulation, not a standalone condition. We see it occurring as a result of:

- Perimenopause, as ovulation becomes sporadic due to fluctuating signals from the brain

- Polycystic ovary syndrome (PCOS), where ovulation is often suppressed

- Postpartum, before ovulatory cycles resume

- Any anovulatory cycle, regardless of age

Telling someone they have "estrogen dominance" often sounds definitive, like a diagnosis that explains everything. But it usually stops the conversation instead of advancing it. I've seen it used in place of real investigation, which should be driven by questions such as:

- Why isn't this woman ovulating consistently?
- What is her age and cycle history?
- Is this early perimenopause?
- Is PCOS present but undiagnosed?
- Is there thyroid dysfunction or hypothalamic-pituitary-ovarian axis disruption?
- Is she experiencing chronic stress, underfueling, or sleep disruption?

If we stop at "estrogen dominance," we miss the chance to get curious, dig deeper, and treat the whole picture.

When an approved group of follicles emerges, the cycle will resume and a dominant follicle will grow, further secreting estrogen and progesterone. As the follicle quality diminishes, however, the growth and hormone production become less robust and reliable. And even if the cycle stays on track, it may fail to result in ovulation or become what's referred to as an anovulatory cycle. Anovulatory cycles occur at greater frequency during the last two or so years prior to the final period and are identified by increased levels of FSH and low levels of estrogen.

Estrogen: Everywhere All at Once

It's remarkable to think about the scale on which all this is happening. If you can imagine it, all this biochemical activity and these microchanges are taking place in something the size of a small almond! If we zoom out a bit, we can see the entirety of the female reproductive system: the ovaries sitting at the ends of the fallopian tube "arms," which are extended from the top of the inverted triangle that holds the uterus, cervix, and vagina.

Estrogen and Health: The Organs That Feel the Loss

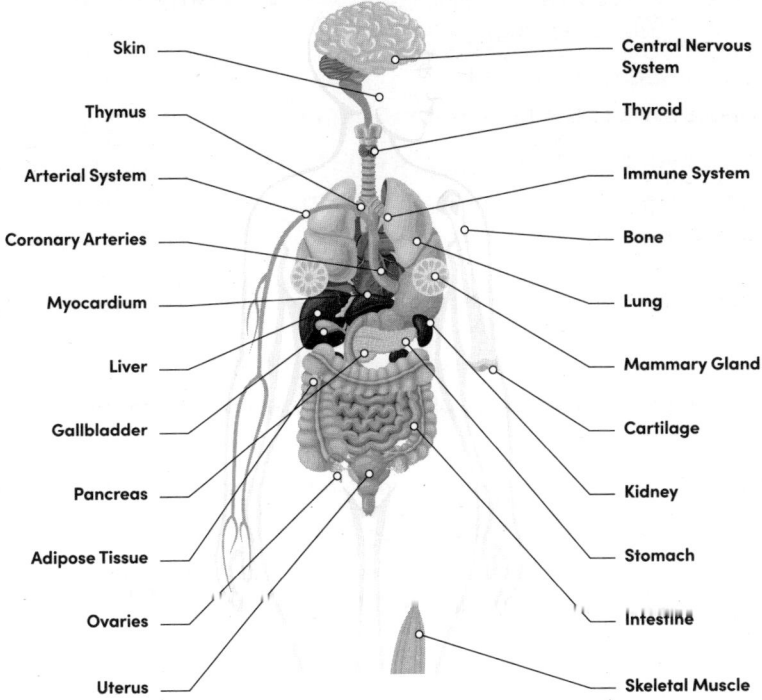

Location of Estrogen Receptors in the Human Body

Keep this vision in your mind because it represents what most people think of when they think of women's health. (For the sake of accuracy, I'll acknowledge that the breasts are often considered as well, but this exercise works better if we stay in the pelvic region.)

Now, I have another image to share with you.

This is an image of the female body that shows *all the organs and tissues that rely on estrogen for optimal function. This* is what we *should* be looking at when we talk about women's health, especially as we move through the hormonal transition of perimenopause.

Your body has estrogen receptors in almost every cell and organ, so when hormone levels begin to change, it affects so much more than the day on which your period falls or whether or not you have a period at all. Yes, the downward trends in estrogen you will experience in perimenopause can contribute to hot flashes, mood swings, and vaginal dryness. But these are frankly just as cliché and myopic as the inverted triangle vision of women's health. Changes in estrogen can also lessen elasticity in the blood vessels and reduce blood flow to the heart, lead to increased bone breakdown and less bone building, and allow for a pro-inflammatory environment in the brain and the rest of the body.

By expanding our view to include the full body, we can see that multiple organ systems are affected by diminishing levels of estrogen. And this big-picture view reveals the information that matters most: When the ovaries transition into the zone of chaos, this can introduce an acceleration toward diseases such as heart disease, osteoporosis, and Alzheimer's, which preferentially affect women as they age. This is the view that I'm using to drive the way I practice women's health. I'm going to help you use this information to your advantage.

Here at the end of this chapter, I hope you feel more informed about what is going on inside your body as your hormones change in perimenopause. What comes next is what you can do about it.

CHAPTER 3

The Troubling Pattern of Misdiagnosis (and Gaslighting)

I was a practicing board-certified OB-GYN who began experiencing rapid weight gain, anxiety, depression, loss of interest in things, sleep disturbances, balance issues, brain fog, memory recall difficulty, forgetfulness, worsening of ADHD symptoms, shortness of breath, heart palpitations, skin changes, and worsening of dry eyes all in my early thirties. I was evaluated by cardiologists, pulmonologists, primary care physicians, neurologists, psychiatrists, and fellow OB-GYNs. They all said it was too early for perimenopause and that I was just experiencing stress from work. I became more fatigued during twenty-four-hour calls and weekend calls. Then came the hot flashes and night sweats in my late thirties. Again, all my labs were normal, and I was told I couldn't be perimenopausal. Then at age forty-two, I started having daily hot flashes . . . up to twelve a day, affecting my work and my life. Finally, my labs were consistent with menopause. I had a diagnosis. I suffered for a decade unnecessarily. No woman should suffer like I did.

—Shelly C.

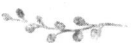

As I outlined earlier, a history of severely underfunded women's health, a stubborn attachment to outdated medical guidelines, and the absence of a robust and standardized diagnostic framework for perimenopause has led to a population of practicing clinicians who struggle to fully support or validate women as they begin to report disruptive perimenopausal symptoms. And the inevitable consequence of this inadequate care is one of two scenarios: women having their symptoms dismissed or women having their symptoms misdiagnosed.

It may seem like dismissal and misdiagnosis are very different scenarios, but the result can be nearly identical: real women being left stranded in perpetual symptomatic limbo without meaningful relief. This doesn't have to be you. In this chapter we'll look closely at some of the most common misdiagnoses in perimenopausal women and the research and insight both patients and providers can use to introduce an essential question: Is it possible that hormones are involved?

DIAGNOSIS: "This is normal."
BUT IT COULD BE: Perimenopause

If you visit a doctor and express symptoms like noticeable changes in your ability to focus, an unfamiliar sort of deep fatigue, and an unrelenting and simmering degree of irritation or dissatisfaction with your life, the first thing you might encounter is *a diagnosis of dismissal*. This is usually expressed through a variety of phrases, including these examples (to which I've added my own two cents):

"It's just a phase—ride it out."
Translation: Your suffering doesn't need my attention or support.

"Welcome to aging!"
As if you should simply accept it and stop complaining. Normalizing suffering doesn't make it acceptable.

"It's all in your head."
One of the most harmful things a woman can hear when she's seeking real answers.

"You're too young for menopause."
Perimenopause can begin as early as your mid-thirties and still be normal. Using age as the only determining factor delays diagnosis and care.

"Try yoga or a glass of wine—it helps me."
Reduces complex hormonal changes to a self-care cliché.

"Everyone goes through it—tough it out."
Implies that struggling is a badge of honor rather than a medical issue worth treating.

"Have you tried losing some weight?"
Blaming the patient instead of addressing the underlying hormonal shifts.

"You're probably just stressed."
Stress may play a role in many perimenopausal symptoms, but this statement ignores the biological root of them.

"Maybe you need antidepressants."
Prescription mood medications are often the first thing a doctor will suggest instead of investigating the hormonal causes of your mood changes.

The common denominator in all these statements is that your pain—and, yes, to have your quality of life upended without a known cause is to experience a form of pain—is insignificant and unworthy of serious clinical attention and effort. This is medical gaslighting.

Medical gaslighting may be a new term, but the experience isn't. The concerns of female patients, perimenopausal or otherwise, frankly, have long been written off as emotional in nature, in part because of the de-prioritization of women's health in research and in medical school curriculum but also because of a professional passing along of bias. I remember throughout my medical training being taught, implicitly and explicitly, that women somaticize, or exaggerate their symptoms, or tend to simply be unhappy. The message was clear: Women complain more. Women are more dramatic. Women are emotional. Women are difficult. Women are unreliable historians. Women are anxious. Women are just looking for attention. These biases were woven into the fabric of my education, shaping the way even I—a female doctor!—viewed my patients and reinforcing the very stereotypes that have long undermined women's health.

These biases aren't coincidental, they are *inevitable consequences of defining medical care and constructing medical systems without women in the room*. This isn't a radical claim; it's simply the truth. There is ample research showing that female patients are often subject to clinical treatment that falls short in the areas of support and validation. What they get instead is a combination of skepticism and a downplaying of symptom severity. For example, a study published in the *Journal of the American Heart Association* in 2022 found that women who visited the emergency room with chest pain experienced a 29 percent longer wait time for potential heart attack evaluation compared with their male counterparts. These women were also less likely to be given an EKG, be admitted to the hospital, and be prescribed medications to manage acute coronary syndrome.

In 2021, the British government launched a survey of nearly one hundred thousand women to help assess the state of women's healthcare in their country. Eighty-four percent of respondents reported that they hadn't been listened to by healthcare professionals, which meant that they felt their symptoms had not been taken seriously. They had to persistently advocate for themselves, sometimes for *years,* to secure a diagnosis for their symptoms, and even when provided with a diagnosis, they found that they were given few opportunities to discuss treatment options and that their preferences were often ignored.

In this same study, if a woman's symptoms appeared to be related to menstrual health, the treatment quality dropped even lower. Women who had severe pain from fibroids or endometriosis were told it was all in their heads, and those who saw a doctor for heavy and irregular periods were told it was just part of being a woman.

Another survey, also conducted in the UK, found that it took an average of nine years for women with endometriosis to receive a diagnosis, with most respondents saying that they had to visit the doctor more than five times and that their pain had been severe enough to send them to the emergency room.

So, what do we do about this unacceptable and infuriating pattern? I'm going to do my part by continuing to work to disentangle perimenopause and menopause diagnoses from the menstrual cycle because they affect so much more than just your period. This isn't to say menstrual issues shouldn't be taken seriously—they absolutely should—but we need to separate out the complexities of women's health to conquer the inequities in care. As I mentioned in the first chapter, it's likely that your OB-GYN isn't set up to successfully treat you through perimenopause and menopause—these really should be their own specialty within medicine.

The Bottom Line: Unlike for many other conditions and diseases, there is no diagnostic algorithm to help your physician solve the puzzle of the symptoms you report. This leaves many healthcare providers feeling ill prepared and potentially defensive, which is itself yet another reason that your concerns get dismissed. Unfortunately, you may find that even a doctor who has provided the absolute best treatment for other areas of your health disappoints you in perimenopause—they haven't been given the resources or training to treat you.

This isn't to excuse the reality that women are being offered little more than dismissive condolences for their symptoms, and clearly a lot of work needs to be done to elevate healthcare standards for women, both broadly and as it applies specifically to the care offered to women in perimenopause and beyond.

The Take-to-Your-Doctor Message: The good news is that I have seen firsthand the exponential growth of interest in providing perimenopausal- and menopausal-informed care—clinicians *want* to learn and to be able to fully support patients as they enter a new hormonal landscape. And many have worked hard to make it known that they have put in this effort. Some, however, might need a push. *Ask them* if they have recently received perimenopausal or menopausal education. If they haven't and if they aren't interested in doing so, you will want to find someone who *can* meet your needs. To find out if a perimenopause-educated clinician is available in your area, I encourage you to check out the clinicians list on my website, thepauselife.com. This list includes providers who have been referred to us by their previous patients.

DIAGNOSIS: Fibromyalgia
BUT IT COULD BE: The Musculoskeletal Syndrome of Menopause

Fibromyalgia (FM) is a disorder that is predominantly diagnosed in women, with a notable uptick in new diagnoses during the perimenopausal transition. The clinical presentation of FM—fatigue, sleep disturbances, muscle aches, brain fog, mood fluctuations—mirrors common symptoms of perimenopause. Several studies have observed that these symptoms often begin or intensify during perimenopause, suggesting that if fibromyalgia is present, hormonal shifts can amplify symptom severity. It's also possible that fluctuating hormones are the true and only origin of these symptoms.

The overlap of FM and perimenopause has created a diagnostic gray zone. I have heard from many women about life in this gray zone, and they describe it as exhausting, frustrating, and humiliating. The emotional toll is compounded by the fact that many doctors, when confronted with a collection of symptoms that matches the one I detailed in the previous paragraph, will try to explain away or minimize the pain by suggesting it's merely psychosomatic or stress induced. I'm going to explain it a bit differently: If you are at least thirty-five and have been given a diagnosis of fibromyalgia by a doctor *without* the topic of hormones being discussed, you may want to consider seeing a physician who is perimenopause-educated. I'll tell you why.

Estrogen plays a key role in pain modulation. When levels of estrogen begin to fluctuate and decline, the central nervous system's regulation of pain, mood, and sleep is affected and you may begin to experience heightened pain sensitivity, increased anxiety, low mood, and disrupted sleep. These are core features of both fibromyalgia *and* the menopause transition. Yet women in this case are more likely to be misdiagnosed with depression or anxiety, while their underlying hormonal chaos and musculoskeletal symptoms go unrecognized and untreated.

This misdiagnosis commonly leads a patient down a path to polypharmacy—that is, the reliance on multiple medications to treat health issues. It's easy to see how this happens. You might take NSAIDs for pain, Ambien for sleep, a benzodiazepine for anxiety, and so on. Once you are taking a few or more medications, it can become tough to isolate and identify the root cause of your symptoms. The problem here is that doctors haven't been taught to peel back the proverbial onion of complex pain to see if changes in estrogen are a contributing factor; instead, it gets chopped up into pieces, and many tears have been and will continue to be shed until we implement a new diagnostic framework.

Emerging research shows that there are metabolic consequences when menopause intersects with fibromyalgia. A 2024 study published by researchers in Spain found that the convergence of the two conditions may disrupt amino acid homeostasis, potentially increasing the risk of metabolic disorders such as type 2 diabetes, high blood pressure, and high cholesterol. This disruption is more pronounced than in menopause or fibromyalgia alone, highlighting the compounded effect of these conditions on metabolic health. Another study found that women with FM had significantly higher body fat and reduced lean muscle mass compared with controls, a deleterious by-product of the sedentary lifestyle often forced on women living with chronic pain.

In the years to come, we may see an overhaul of the diagnosis of fibromyalgia altogether. Groundbreaking work led by Dr. Vonda Wright and published in 2024 introduced the concept of the musculoskeletal syndrome of menopause (MSM), defined as declines in muscle mass, strength, joint integrity, and overall physical function brought on by the loss of estrogen. This symptomatic pattern strongly overlaps with the one we see in fibromyalgia. Their work urges clinicians to consider perimenopause as a critical factor in musculoskeletal complaints, rather than defaulting to chronic pain or mood disorder diagnoses. As MSM gains clinical legitimacy and as awareness of it increases, I suspect we may see its diagnostic numbers rise as cases of fibromyalgia fall.

The Bottom Line: The relationship between fibromyalgia and perimenopause is characterized by a complex interplay of hormonal, psychological, and physiological factors. The decline in estrogen during menopause appears to exacerbate FM symptoms, while the shared symptoms of both conditions suggest a potential interdependence. Understanding this relationship is crucial for developing effective management strategies for women experiencing both FM and menopause.

We need more research to clarify the mechanisms underlying this relationship—and to reduce frustrating diagnostic delays, prevent inappropriate psychiatric labeling, and guide effective, evidence-based interventions that address the root causes of symptoms.

The Take-to-Your-Doctor Message: Estrogen influences multiple systems, including the musculoskeletal, neurological, and endocrine axes. When women in midlife present with widespread pain, cognitive fog, fatigue, and mood shifts, it's essential to consider hormonal status as a primary diagnostic lens—not an afterthought. You can even consider sharing a copy of Dr. Wright's study "The Musculoskeletal Syndrome of Menopause" with your doctor. See the appendix for more information.

> DIAGNOSIS: Interstitial Cystitis (Bladder Pain Syndrome)
> BUT IT COULD BE: The Genitourinary Syndrome of Menopause

Interstitial cystitis (IC), also referred to as bladder pain syndrome (BPS), is an often painful and frustrating bladder condition diagnosed in many perimenopausal women. Noticeable symptoms may include urinary urgency and frequency, nocturia (excessive urination at night), pelvic discomfort, dyspareunia (painful intercourse), and bladder pain. But these same symptoms are also indicative of the genitourinary syndrome of menopause (GSM), making diagnosis of one or the other difficult—particularly in women in their forties and early fifties who haven't been clinically identified as perimenopausal.

There is, however, a key distinction between IC and GSM: Interstitial cystitis is a chronic pain syndrome without a known cause, whereas the genitourinary syndrome of menopause is a well-defined consequence of estrogen deficiency. Research has shown that fluctuations in estrogen can have a significant impact on the genital and urinary organs:

- A 2021 study found that estrogen receptors are abundant in what's known as the bladder trigone: the base of the urinary bladder and urethral tissues. The same study also noted that declining estrogen levels can lead to thinning of the lining of the urogenital area, increasing sensitivity and vulnerability to irritation.

- Additional studies have found that the loss of estrogen affects microbial diversity and epithelial defenses, altering the urinary microbiome during perimenopause and potentially contributing to IC-like symptoms, increased urinary tract infections (UTIs), and overall bladder irritation.

Other research has revealed that the prevalence of IC symptoms increases in midlife, with a notable peak in women aged forty to fifty-nine—

coinciding with the perimenopausal transition. Unfortunately, few clinicians consider the hormone-initiated GSM before interstitial cystitis in perimenopausal women—especially those who still menstruate. As a result, many women are placed on long-term bladder-centric IC treatments, including dietary changes, bladder instillations, or medications, when their symptoms may be better addressed by GSM treatment.

When GSM is the root cause, local estrogen therapy can dramatically improve urinary frequency, urgency, and pain. Research published in the *American Journal of Obstetrics & Gynecology* in 2020 reported that vaginal estrogen acts locally on the tissues and significantly improves urogenital symptoms and overall quality of life in perimenopausal and postmenopausal women.

The Bottom Line: If you are thirty-five or older and you make an appointment with your doctor to discuss urinary urgency and frequency, nocturia, pelvic discomfort, dyspareunia, and bladder pain, GSM should be considered.

The Take-to-Your-Doctor Message: To better understand the root causes of symptoms and possible treatment, talk to your clinician about the following:

- **Assessing menopausal status**—even if you have regular periods.

- **Examining the vulvovaginal tissues** for signs of atrophy, loss of elasticity, or pallor—these are hallmarks of GSM.

- **Using symptom questionnaires** that screen for both bladder pain and genitourinary atrophy.

- **A trial of local estrogen therapy,** particularly when pelvic pain coexists with vaginal dryness, dyspareunia, or urinary symptoms.

For more information, you can also refer your clinician to the most recent statement from the American Urological Association (AUA) on the management of GSM. See chapter 11 for this language.

DIAGNOSIS: Long COVID
BUT IT COULD BE: Perimenopause

A relatively new diagnosis resulting from the pandemic, long COVID is a condition characterized by prolonged, multisystem symptoms following SARS-CoV-2 infection. Its symptoms of fatigue, brain fog, and muscle pain have a striking overlap with those that may be seen in perimenopause. Long COVID is real and debilitating, but this symptom overlap has created a clinical blind spot in post-pandemic care. The good news is that researchers have been collecting data to introduce greater clinical clarity and reduce patient and provider frustration.

In one study, researchers who looked at female patients at three long-COVID clinics in England found that perimenopausal symptoms were highly prevalent among those ages forty to fifty-four—the demographic most likely to be in the perimenopausal transition. This suggests that a significant number of women presenting to long-COVID clinics may be experiencing the consequences of unrecognized perimenopause, or more likely, there is an interplay present between the prolonged viral impact of COVID and hormonal disruption.

This research is observational, which means that it doesn't prove causation. However, it does tell us to pay closer attention to symptoms that are present in women post COVID infection. If you have fatigue, sleep disruption, palpitations, mood swings, joint and muscle pain, and cognitive difficulties, long COVID is certainly possible but shouldn't be assumed. Instead, it should be considered alongside the potential contributing factor of perimenopause.

The overlap of symptoms between these two conditions raises critical questions we should be asking clinically: Is it possible that some women are being misdiagnosed with long COVID when they are actually in perimenopause—or vice versa? And more importantly, are they being treated effectively, or are they being referred down symptom-specific pathways that ignore the hormonal component altogether?

The Bottom Line: Long COVID and perimenopause have a shared pathophysiology of neuroinflammation, mitochondrial dysfunction, and autonomic dysregulation. But the reality is that women presenting to long-COVID clinics aren't being screened for perimenopausal status and are often placed on treatment protocols that focus exclusively on viral recovery, rehabilitation, or psychiatric support, without ever addressing estrogen loss as a potential root contributor to their symptoms.

Not only is introducing perimenopause into the diagnostic picture of long COVID in women clinically responsible, it may also reduce diagnostic delays, unnecessary referrals, and inappropriate treatments. In some cases, hormone therapy may improve symptoms mistakenly attributed to long COVID, and in others, a combined strategy addressing both viral and hormonal factors may be needed to produce the best outcome.

The Take-to-Your-Doctor Message: It's clear that a more integrated, hormone-aware approach to post-viral care is urgently needed; and in some cases, the onus may fall on you, the patient, to bring the awareness to the table. If you've experienced prolonged (lasting three or more months) symptoms post COVID infection, you may want to ask of yourself: Am I in the perimenopausal age range (anywhere from your mid-thirties to your early fifties), and/or have I noticed any menstrual changes, vasomotor symptoms, or mood shifts? If the answer is yes to one or both of these questions, it is worth asking your doctor if hormonal decline, independently of or synergistically with viral consequences could be contributing to your symptoms.

DIAGNOSIS: Adrenal Fatigue
BUT IT COULD BE: Perimenopause

Among the most common "diagnoses" I see in clinical practice, particularly among women in their forties and early fifties, is adrenal fatigue. Patients will come to me after their clinician has told them that their symptoms are the result of chronically depleted adrenal glands because of prolonged stress. Here's the problem with adrenal fatigue: Despite its prevalence in popular health culture, it's not recognized by the broader medical community; that is, it's not a validated clinical diagnosis, in large part because it's not supported by robust, peer-reviewed evidence.

When we examine the symptoms most often attributed to adrenal fatigue—brain fog, sleep disturbances, fatigue, irritability, low libido, and inability to handle stress, we see that these closely mirror those of perimenopause. When we zoom in a bit more, we see that the adrenal glands *do* play a role in the manifestation of these symptoms but it's not because they are "tired," it's because perimenopausal fluctuations in estradiol can disrupt the hypothalamic-pituitary-adrenal (HPA) axis. The HPA axis is our neuroendocrine system that regulates the body's response to stress by controlling the release of cortisol and other stress-related hormones.

There's ample research showing that the hormonal chaos of perimenopause can bring about disruptions in HPA axis function. Researchers from Vanderbilt University Medical Center in Nashville, Tennessee, reported that estradiol volatility was linked to altered cortisol patterns and increased vulnerability to stress, particularly in women with a history of mood disorders. Decreases in estradiol were similarly tied to elevated morning cortisol levels and increased negative mood, especially in those who may be experiencing perimenopausal depression. These changes in cortisol secretion are often misunderstood as "adrenal exhaustion" when in fact they reflect a dysregulated HPA axis because of hormone withdrawal.

Estrogen withdrawal also appears capable of causing a blunted cortisol awakening response (CAR). This is the sharp increase in cortisol levels observed immediately after you wake up; when it's altered, you are more likely to feel morning fatigue and a general lack of energy. In women experiencing severe vasomotor symptoms (like hot flashes), we see a significantly diminished CAR. These women aren't experiencing acute adrenal failure; they are likely in perimenopause.

It's important to point out that there is such a thing as true adrenal insufficiency, which happens when the adrenal glands don't make enough cortisol. Adrenal insufficiency, also known as Addison's disease, is distinct from adrenal fatigue and warrants evaluation by an endocrinologist. Symptoms of Addison's disease can include weakness, fatigue, dizziness, low blood pressure, lack of appetite, and irregular or absent menstrual periods.

The Bottom Line: In perimenopausal women, the symptoms commonly labeled as adrenal fatigue are often more accurately explained by HPA axis dysregulation brought on by estradiol fluctuations. The misdiagnosis of adrenal fatigue delays appropriate treatment, fosters fear, and often leads to costly and ineffective supplement regimens.

The Take-to-Your-Doctor Message: You can avoid this unnecessary and expensive detour by encouraging your clinician to adopt a hormone-informed lens. This lens would include taking into consideration the following:

- Cortisol dysregulation is often secondary to estradiol instability (in other words, it happens in response to changes in estradiol).

- Mood changes and fatigue may signal neuroendocrine transition, not burnout.

- Interventions like hormone therapy, lifestyle support, and cognitive tools can often restore equilibrium more effectively than adrenal-targeted supplements.

The End of Misdiagnosis in Perimenopause: Hormones Have to Matter

A laundry list of symptoms might land you in your doctor's office during perimenopause, hoping for help. But instead of help, your symptoms get dismissed. Or you receive a misdiagnosis for a condition that has similar symptoms, and you are given a treatment protocol. If this protocol isn't entirely effective, it could be because the hormonal influence hasn't been considered and addressed.

Now, this doesn't mean that perimenopause is to blame for every instance of fatigue, unexplained weight gain, brain fog, low libido, and complex pain. It's essential to have your clinician rule out overlapping conditions, such as lupus, hypothyroidism, Hashimoto's disease, low iron storage, clinical deficiencies in vitamins or other nutrients, or chronic inflammation. Each of these can exacerbate symptoms of perimenopause or initiate symptoms all on its own, which is why I test all my patients for these before assuming that any changes to their health status are solely based on hormone fluctuations. I encourage you to find a menopause-educated clinician who can help you navigate the path of perimenopause and to share any of the scientific resources in this chapter (and book) with a clinician who may want to learn and grow alongside you.

Part Two

A WINDOW OF VULNERABILITY

CHAPTER 4

This Is Your Brain on Perimenopause

> When I hit forty, I started to have balance problems and dizziness, which I noticed in yoga class and when driving a car. After that, anxiety showed up in a big way. I was diagnosed with agoraphobia and prescribed an SSRI.... I was so anxious that I couldn't go shopping or have a social life; I was a broken woman lying in bed most of the time. Then I started to have vision changes, dry skin, low libido, and joint pain. I had never heard of the word *perimenopause*. Then on social media I found Dr. Haver talking about perimenopause and hormone therapy. I decided to try it myself, and after four months, my anxiety and depression are gone. And my cognitive function is soaring. For me, it has been a life changer.
>
> —Petra M.

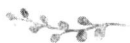

Let's get right to the point: Things shift in your brain during perimenopause. In fact, as I mentioned in chapters 1 and 2, when your hormones enter the zone of chaos, the brain is often the first to respond, bringing about emotional, psychological, and cognitive symptoms that most women never expect. These symptoms can range from mildly bothersome to majorly, even catastrophically, disruptive. You may notice increased anxiety, loss of libido, depression, irritability, or anger or feel that your thinking, processing, and multitasking abilities have stalled and that you're moving through dense fog. You may even find yourself wondering where your mind has gone and worrying if you will ever feel like yourself again.

This may be of little consolation, but if you've experienced any of these changes, *you are not alone*. The hormonal shifts in perimenopause bring about a neurological remodeling that alters the entire neurotransmitter network—the locus of control for both your mental health and your cognition. While not every woman in perimenopause will experience disruptions across all these brain-maintained functions, surveys have shown that most women—*70 percent*—report some noticeable change in mood or cognitive abilities during this transition. Again, you are not alone. Far from it.

Chapters 5 and 6 will dig deeply into mental health and cognition respectively and offer you detailed information about symptoms and useful strategies that may help improve brain health and function. I will also let you know how to identify when changes to your mood, mental health, or cognitive function may warrant seeing a specialist.

Before we get to those important topics, however, I think it will be helpful to provide you with an overview of how the brain responds on a neurological level to the sex hormones* undergoing the biggest changes: estrogen, progesterone, and testosterone. This chapter won't be an exhaustive examination of the brain's inner workings, but it will offer up enough intel for you to grasp the deep connection between your central nervous system (controlled by your brain) and your endocrine system.

The Three Key Sex Hormones and How They Shape Your Brain

We don't often take the time to acknowledge the marvel that is the human brain. I'm not a neuroscientist, but when I start digging into brain science, I can't help but feel an immense sense of awe and amazement. To use an unavoidable pun, it's *mind-blowing* to try to grasp all that is going on neurologically as we breathe, react, talk, and cope with our lives.

---

* Because the hormones estrogen and progesterone are produced by the ovaries and are essential to all things reproductive, they've long been defined as reproductive hormones. Yet the more we learn about the pivotal roles they fill *outside* reproduction, the more we realize the need for a rebranding. Dr. Lisa Mosconi, a neuroscientist who is also the director of the Weill Cornell Women's Brain Initiative and an author, defines estrogen and progesterone as sex hormones, and I'm going to use this definition, too.

An interesting fact about the brain is that it doesn't operate in isolation—that is, it's not simply a command center that sends out one-way orders to the rest of the body. It's instead a masterful network manager that keeps vital mechanisms running through its relationships with other cellular networks in the body.

For our purposes, we are looking closely at the relationship of the brain with the endocrine system. These two are so interconnected that an entire branch of medicine, called neuroendocrinology, is dedicated to the study of how they affect each other. A neuroendocrinologist studies how the nervous system controls hormone secretion and how, in turn, hormones affect the nervous system.

When hormones and their metabolites interact with the brain, they are classified as neurosteroids. Neurosteroids are highly influential in the brain, where they activate and organize essential neurotransmitter pathways to such an extent that they are said to be capable of restructuring the nervous system. As neurosteroids, estrogen, progesterone, and testosterone help regulate functions related to mood, behavior, and cognition. To put it plainly, your sex hormones have immense power in shaping how you feel each day.

The work of estrogen, progesterone, and testosterone is made possible thanks to hormone receptors that are housed within your brain cells and cell membranes. These receptors anticipate the delivery of these hormones and then bind to them, triggering a cascade of cellular responses. You might think of the receptors as runners in a relay race, awaiting the hormone "batons" so that they can then blast off and signal the next cellular action to take place.

Some of the actions triggered by the arrival of your sex hormones wholly transform nervous system functions. Among other critical actions, sex hormones cue receptors to promote neural pruning, which is the removal of unused or weak synapses to allow for more efficient communication between nerve cells, and myelination, which is the process of insulating critical nerve "cables" in a fatty coating to speed up connections. Let's explore a little more about the distinct role each sex hormone and its receptors play in your brain.

Estrogen

Estrogen has two main types of receptors in the brain called ERα (alpha) and ERβ (beta). Through its interaction with these receptors, estrogen plays a key role in several neural mechanisms, including:

Neurotransmitter activity. Estrogen helps regulate the release and metabolism of important neurotransmitters. Neurotransmitters are key brain chemicals that facilitate communication between nerve cells and enable functions related to movement, emotion, and more. The neurotransmitters that rely on estrogen include . . .

- **Dopamine:** Often called the "feel good" chemical, it plays a role in pleasure and reward.

- **Serotonin:** A mood-boosting chemical that influences emotional stability, sleep, and appetite.

- **Acetylcholine:** Important for learning and memory.

- **Beta-endorphin:** A natural painkiller that also improves mood.

Neuroprotection. Estrogen has several neuroprotective effects. It influences cerebral blood flow, helping ensure that vital nutrients reach the brain; assists in reducing neuroinflammation in part by increasing activity of antioxidant enzymes; and supports the growth, survival, and repair of brain cells and nerve connections. Estrogen also helps prevent neurodegeneration, which is the breakdown and loss of brain cells that can lead to negative changes in memory, cognition, and mood.

Brain energy metabolism. Estrogen increases the absorption and use of glucose, the brain's preferred fuel source, and helps the brain receive sufficient energy to support its functions.

If you glossed over the last few paragraphs, I'll sum it up for you like this: Estrogen is a big deal to your brain. It has a significant effect on brain functions that involve memory, emotional regulation, information integration, sensory processing, and higher-level cognitive functions, such as decision-making, language use, and reasoning.

Progesterone

Like estrogen, progesterone has two primary brain-based receptors, simply called PR-A and PR-B. Also like estrogen, progesterone has proven neuroprotective effects. It consistently supports the generation of new brain cells and the formation of new blood vessels that deliver vital oxygen to the brain.

While there is overlap in how estrogen and progesterone influence brain function, progesterone on its own is a powerful neurosteroid that affects multiple neurotransmitter systems related to mood, anxiety, cognitive function, and neuronal excitability. Here are some of the key neurotransmitters affected by progesterone.

GABA. Progesterone (along with its by-product allopregnanolone) enhances GABA-A receptor activity and delivers significant antidepressant, anti-anxiety, and sedative effects. This explains why some women feel calmer during phases of their cycle when progesterone is higher, such as during the luteal phase, and why progesterone therapy may benefit mood disorders in perimenopause and menopause.

Glutamate. While estrogen (estradiol to be more specific in this case) increases activity of the excitatory neurotransmitter glutamate, progesterone helps counterbalance this excitability, which may protect against mood swings, anxiety, and neuroinflammation.

Noradrenaline. This neurotransmitter plays a big role in stress and mood regulation. Progesterone reduces noradrenaline levels in the brain, which may explain why hormonal fluctuations affect mood stability.

Acetylcholine. Progesterone modulates acetylcholine signaling, which is critical for memory and learning. An increase in brain fog during perimenopause may be in response to diminishing levels of progesterone.

Testosterone

Testosterone is an androgen, which is a type of steroid hormone that is primarily associated with male reproductive development and function. Because of the association with male reproduction, testosterone has historically been labeled a male sex hormone, but it performs essential roles related to brain health in both sexes. It's also critical to metabolism, bone health, and liver function. Like estrogen and progesterone, it deserves and demands to be considered beyond its limited association with reproduction.

In perimenopause, testosterone levels don't surge and dip (excluding it from the zone of chaos). But they do follow a slow and steady decline that can begin as early as your mid-twenties. From that point forward, levels decrease by about 1 to 2 percent each year. This gradual downward slope is very similar to what happens in men, except women just start at a lower absolute level. By the time we are in our late forties and early fifties, we may have lost more than half our peak testosterone levels.

In my clinical practice, patients usually don't even have testosterone on their radar and are more likely to attribute their symptoms solely to estrogen loss. I explain to them that the impact of diminishing levels of testosterone can be profound, even though it has a much slower rate of attrition. The symptomatic response to testosterone loss isn't typically as severe as what we see in response to fluctuations in estrogen and progesterone but may be noticeable in the areas of motivation, cognition, emotional energy, muscle mass, and sexual desire.

In the female brain, testosterone acts primarily through androgen receptors (ARs) but can also be converted in the brain into estradiol, allowing it to activate estrogen receptors (ERs). This dual mechanism is what gives testosterone such wide-reaching effects across brain structure and function. Testosterone influences brain health and behavior in several ways.

Nerve protection. One of testosterone's critical roles is stimulating myelination, which is the formation and maintenance of the insulating sheath around neurons. Myelination is crucial for efficient nerve conduction and nerve protection, and less myelination has been linked to accelerated cognitive decline.

Neurogenesis. Testosterone promotes the generation of neurons in the adult brain—called neurogenesis—by enhancing the survival of new neurons in the hippocampus. Testosterone also stimulates the growth of other cells and aids in recovery after injury.

Emotional regulation. Emotional regulation may not sound critical, but when translated to real life, this can mean the difference between having an overblown, wrecking-ball response to a situation and reacting with calm and reason. Testosterone influences emotional regulation by acting on brain regions such as the limbic system. Not only does the limbic system play a critical role in basic emotions, such as anger and fear; it also affects memory, motivation, sexual stimulation, learning, and even your sense of smell.

Sexual motivation. Testosterone influences sexual motivation through direct action on reward pathways in the brain and modulates neurotransmitters critical for arousal and pleasure. The conversion of testosterone to estradiol in the brain may also affect our sexual motivation, but the exact importance of this chemical conversion remains under study.

Testosterone: Can It Bring Back Your Lost Libido?

Even though circulating testosterone levels in women only moderately correlate with desire, many women ask me about the role of testosterone in the treatment of low sexual desire. The short answer I can give is that carefully prescribed transdermal testosterone therapy has indeed been shown to improve sexual desire, arousal, and satisfaction in women with hypoactive sexual desire disorder (HSDD).

My patients' experience largely matches that of the research data, with most experiencing notable increases in libido. They have also reported improvements in brain fog, self-confidence, self-image, motivation, and emotional connectedness. All that said, dosing is highly important and needs to be managed by a menopause-trained physician.

It's also important to point out that testosterone isn't a panacea. Desire in women is complex and often intertwined with emotional, relational, and psychological factors. Hormones lay the foundation—but they are only part of the full architecture of sexual health. We will cover this topic in more detail in chapter 11.

Ultimately, testosterone acts as an under-the-radar architect of a woman's midlife health by shaping brain structure, influencing cognition and emotion, and supporting sexual vitality. When we pay attention to testosterone's unique trajectory and effects, it allows us to treat the whole woman, not just the parts that have been deemed appropriately female. Evaluating testosterone levels with your clinician can shine a light on an overlooked component of your well-being.

Effects of Estrogen, Progesterone, and Testosterone in Brain Function

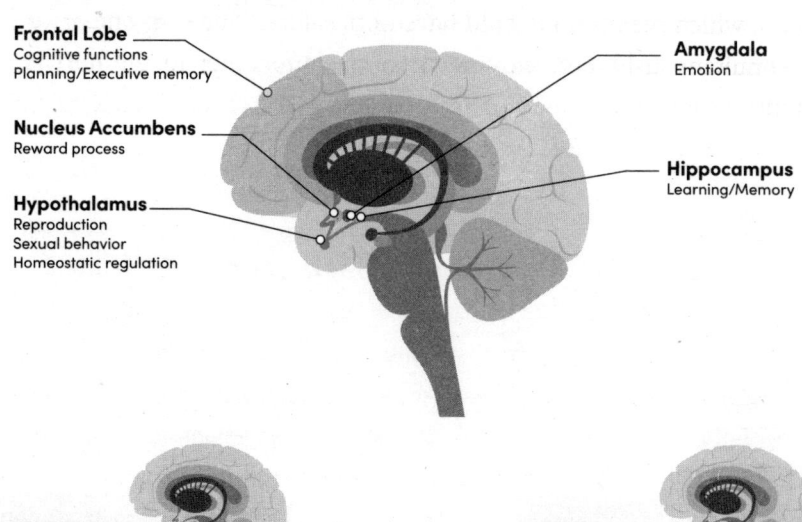

The figure shows areas of the brain regulated by steroid hormones (top), and some of the effects on the prefrontal cortex when a normal or abnormal balance between estrogen and progesterone is present (bottom).

frontiersin.org/journals/public-health/articles/10.3389/fpubh.2018.00141/full

Reproductive Hormones *Are* Brain Hormones

When you realize the crucial roles estrogen, progesterone, and testosterone play in brain health and function, it becomes abundantly clear that these hormones influence so much more than your reproductive health. Understanding the neural mechanisms that rely on estrogen, progesterone, and testosterone also helps us appreciate how hormonal changes during perimenopause can introduce mental health and cognitive changes. The altered brain mechanisms that we start to see in perimenopause involve the same set of neurons that influence mental health and cognitive function, which means you could have noticeable changes in one or both areas simultaneously. Let's explore these more together in the next two chapters.

CHAPTER 5

The Mental Health Changes You May Notice

> My experience started with extreme anxiety. I've always suffered with a bit of anxiety and depression, but this was next level. My ability to handle stress just fell through the floor. I accepted it at first due to my history. It wasn't until the drenching night sweats started that I thought things weren't right. I was now a bit scared that something was really wrong! Then came the insomnia and the weird electric shock feelings. In response to these symptoms, my doctor just upped my antidepressant dose. I'm lucky enough to have a bit of medical knowledge from my previous career as a nurse, so I asked if it may be perimenopause, and the doctor said, "You're still very young. It's not likely." I was forty-two at the time. I ended up making an appointment with a menopause-specific doctor, and that one-hour call literally saved my life. I was at the point where my mental health was a real risk. She ran blood tests to rule out anything else, and since then, I've been on hormones. It has been a lifesaver.
>
> —Jane B.

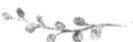

When I started working on this book, I found myself unexpectedly thinking about my mother's perimenopause. For a long time, I had tucked those memories away; I was busy with my own life, my own medical training, my own transitions. But as I began to understand just how destabilizing perimenopause can be, something surfaced—the name of a medication she used to take in her forties to help her "relax": Butisol. I remember thinking of it as "Mama's little helper." I also remembered her holding those pills in her hand like a talisman, as if they were the only thing tethering her to calm. She was running a restaurant, raising eight children, grieving the loss of one child to cancer, supporting another who had just come out as gay, and desperately trying to manage the chaos of a family that was deeply loving but also stretched thin. She often seemed to be struggling with anxiety, sleeplessness, mood swings, and feelings of overwhelm.

It wasn't until I was studying pharmacology in medical school that I learned that Butisol is a barbiturate. My mother had been prescribed a central nervous system depressant to manage her grief and what were in hindsight no doubt symptoms of her perimenopause. As far as I know, no one ever talked to her about hormones. No one ever said the word *estrogen*. Her mental health was pathologized, medicated, and quite literally suppressed; barbiturates deaden nerve impulses and impair cognitive function.

Now, decades later, I'm appalled to think about what she endured and how little the field of medicine understood or even cared about women in midlife then. The image of her fingers curled around that bottle has never left me. It reminds me that what we call "mental health" in perimenopause is often deeply hormonal, deeply contextual, and profoundly misunderstood. And it reminds me why this chapter matters. We must stop drugging women into silence and start listening to what their bodies are trying to say.

Biological Shifts Beget Psychological Symptoms

The emotional and psychological symptoms of perimenopause have long been chalked up to personality flaws or excessive stress or waved off based on the medical bias that women are just . . . unhappy, unnecessarily complicated, dealing with unresolved trauma, or even unintelligent. I know this because I was trained in the medical system that taught this brand of bias and characteristic dismissiveness. We learned that women tended to somaticize their emotions, that they were more likely to complain, and that midlife unhappiness was almost a psychological inevitability. It took years to untangle this bias in myself, and much of medicine is still working on doing the same.

Thankfully, we finally have science, often the only lever strong enough to shift long-standing trends in clinical practice on our side. Research now confirms what many women have long known intuitively: The mood-related symptoms that emerge during perimenopause are often biological, not purely psychological. Indeed, we now have clear evidence that the hormonal fluctuations of perimenopause can profoundly affect mental health. And when you step back and look at the full picture, this shouldn't be surprising. We've already recognized the hormonal roots of postpartum depression, driven by the dramatic withdrawal of estrogen and progesterone after birth. Similarly, we accept that premenstrual dysphoric disorder (PMDD) is triggered by sensitivity to hormonal changes in the luteal phase of the monthly cycle. What's happening in perimenopause is more of the same: hormone-driven mood dysregulation—only now it's happening in the context of erratic and sustained endocrine disruption. It may be too soon to call this a watershed moment, but it's a significant shift in how we understand women's mental health in midlife. And it's long overdue.

Mental health changes in perimenopause may start out as only vaguely noticeable. You may feel a sort of emotional dullness or start to experience joy to a lesser degree; you may remark that you're just not feeling like yourself (as I wrote about in the introduction, "not feeling like myself" is an acknowledged symptom of perimenopause). For some women, the trajectory of mental health changes in perimenopause will stop there; for others, it will continue on to more acute or intense symptoms, giving rise to increases in anxiety, depression, and/or intense feelings of irritability or anger.

Whether your symptoms are subtle or severe, research and data have shown that mood changes in perimenopause are widespread. In a 2025 study titled "Mental Well-Being in Menopause," researchers noted that up to 50 percent of women may experience heightened depressive symptoms during this period and about 25 percent may develop major depressive disorder (MDD). Data provided by one hundred thousand women and analyzed by telehealth provider Evernow revealed that 70 percent reported mood swings, anxiety, or depression. In my own community survey, 82 percent of women in perimenopause reported anxiety, depression, or panic attacks.

What this information is telling us is that in perimenopause women are vulnerable to disruptive mental health disorders and we must be vigilant about paying attention. Clinicians should be building their patient approach around this reality. It's important to note that a vulnerability is *not* an inevitability; not all women in perimenopause will experience disruptive mood changes. But all women will likely know someone who does, and we will all be better served by understanding a bit more about what our sisters, daughters, granddaughters, and friends may be going through. It's also critical that we recognize and respect the research we have now that demonstrates a clear link between hormone-driven changes in brain chemistry during perimenopause and disruptions to a woman's mental health. To overlook this connection in clinical care is to ignore a growing body of evidence and to risk leaving patients feeling misunderstood, dismissed, and inadequately supported.

Almost every day, I see patients who tell of the painfully disruptive nature of changes to their mood and emotional state. Most of them don't know they are in perimenopause, because a doctor has yet to suggest it as a possible explanation for their symptoms. While validation doesn't solve everything, I always start there: *There's nothing wrong with you* and *There's a reason you're feeling this way,* I explain. These phrases never fail to offer at least some relief. Someone has finally said it. Someone has finally removed the mystery, a force multiplier of misery for many women who may be struggling at this time of their lives. And I'll say it now to you, too: *There's nothing wrong with you.*

Now, let's remove the mystery around what mental health changes may happen in perimenopause.

Now Entering: Anxiety, Depression, and Irritability

One of the most common and consequential misdiagnoses in perimenopausal women is the attribution of emotional distress to primary psychiatric disorders, such as generalized anxiety disorder (GAD) or clinical depression. These misdiagnoses fail to acknowledge or address an underlying hormonal instability, leading to treatments like antidepressants that may suppress symptoms but ignore the contributing or causal factor of neuroendocrine dysregulation. As a clinician, I'm continually shocked by the number of women in midlife who are reflexively offered SSRIs or anti-anxiety medications when they report mood changes, irritability, or anxiety without any discussion of the potential role of hormonal shifts taking place.

Studies have shown that there is a marked increase in feelings of despair, mood swings, and anxiety in perimenopausal women. In one recent hospital-based observational study of 108 perimenopausal women with no prior psychiatric diagnoses, nearly one in three met the clinical criteria for a depressive disorder. An additional 7 percent were diagnosed with anxiety, and 5 percent experienced depression with anxiety. What's more, the study found that women in the *late stages* of perimenopause were significantly more likely to struggle with mood symptoms. Risk was also higher in women with a later onset of menarche (your first period), a family history of psychiatric illness, lower educational attainment, or rural residence, underscoring how biological and social factors intersect.

Even if you don't have a history of depression, perimenopause *quadruples* your risk of developing a first episode of major depression. This isn't theoretical. In clinical practice, I've seen this play out time and time again. High-functioning women who are CEOs, teachers, caregivers, physicians, and more, come to me in tears, unable to sleep, anxious, short-tempered, or profoundly sad, often for the first time in their lives. These symptoms aren't "just stress" or "just aging." They are rooted in biology—in the neurohormonal chaos of perimenopause.

And if you do have a history of depression? You're at an even higher risk of relapse. A large-scale study found that 57 percent of women with previously diagnosed depression suffered a relapse during perimenopause, often with more intense and harder-to-treat symptoms.

Symptoms such as excessive worry, restlessness, fatigue, difficulty concentrating, sleep disturbances, increased heart rate, and sweating are common in perimenopause. And they can land you with a diagnosis of an anxiety or panic disorder that doesn't acknowledge the real culprit: hormone-triggered dysregulation of the stress system. Women experiencing fluctuating sex hormones in perimenopause often exhibit increased reactivity to stressors as a result of altered neural pathways that manage our response to external stimuli. This can happen when the hypothalamic-pituitary-adrenal axis, or HPA axis, crucial to regulating the stress response, develops heightened sensitivity and cortisol becomes poorly controlled. This dysregulation occurs in part as a response to molecular alterations to neurotransmitter function, and neurotransmitters, as you learned in the previous chapter, are responsible for so much of your emotional well-being.

There is evidence that disruptions to the balance of neurotransmitters like serotonin, dopamine, and GABA, brought on by fluctuating hormones, can precipitate a unique, hormone-sensitive depression and anxiety phenotype. What this means is that the kind of depression or anxiety you might experience in perimenopause is distinct from MDD or GAD. Despite this evidence, *there is no DSM-5 diagnostic category for perimenopause- or menopause-related depression.* That absence sends a dangerous message: That this isn't real. That it's not worthy of clinical recognition. That you're supposed to just ride it out, or take your prescription for an antidepressant or anti-anxiety medication and be on your way.

The depressive symptoms of perimenopause rarely exist in isolation. They're deeply entwined with fatigue, brain fog, irritability, changes in libido, sleep disruption, and, yes, vasomotor symptoms like hot flashes and night sweats. Expressions of these symptoms are highly individual; that is, some women may have only a little of one symptom and a lot of another; others may have a little of all or a lot of all. (Yes, we each get our own little perimenopausal snowflake that we wish would dissolve just as easily as one.)

Irritability is considered a bridge symptom linking anxiety and depression and should be treated with the same seriousness as any other mood disorder. On its own, it's a clinically distinct mood state—and I want to really emphasize this distinction because, out of all the symptoms of perimenopause, irritability can be one of the most detrimental.

A study published in the journal *Psychoneuroendocrinology* in 2021 revealed that irritability, defined as a low threshold for experiencing frustration or anger, is prevalent during perimenopause; perimenopausal women experience 41 percent more irritability when compared with premenopausal women. In my own case, I noticed a new lower-than-low tolerance for the sounds of my husband eating and breathing, sounds I had been around for more than thirty years without agitation!

Irritability can worsen depressive symptoms and lessen quality of life, and it often intensifies isolation because—let's face it—other people don't usually want to approach an irritable person with kindness and compassion, or try to console you as they might if you were expressing more sadness than normal. We aren't even kind to ourselves when we are irritable; we are more likely to become self-critical and feel guilty when we are easily frustrated or constantly feeling on edge. Yet irritability in perimenopause isn't indicative of having developed an unwelcome or unbecoming character trait; it can be a sign of neurochemical chaos and altered neurotransmitter function.

What we need to accept is the fact that noticeable increases in irritability, anger, mood swings, anxiety, feelings of despair, and sadness in perimenopause are a common experience and normal part of the transition. It's also key to remember that some women may be more sensitive than others to the hormonal chaos because of genetics, prior mood disorders, or life stressors. By accepting this reality, we make room for acknowledgment and action.

Mental Health in Perimenopause: Hormones *Must* Matter

Multiple studies have proved that perimenopausal women who report symptoms of depression and anxiety to their doctors tend to be underevaluated for hormonal factors *even when* they present with co-occurring vasomotor symptoms such as hot flashes and genitourinary symptoms such as vaginal dryness or pain with intercourse. This disconnect is the result of a nonexistent diagnostic framework for perimenopause and often leads to the overprescription of antidepressants, while hormone therapy is overlooked as a viable and evidence-based treatment option.

Despite their widespread use, SSRIs and SNRIs don't address the hormonal basis of perimenopausal mood disorders. While they may offer partial relief—particularly in cases where chronic stress, insomnia, or long-standing mood disorders are present alongside hormonal fluctuations—they fail to target the root cause: erratic and declining estrogen levels. When I began researching this book, much of the older literature I found still listed antidepressants, anti-anxiety medications, and psychotherapy as the primary treatment strategies for women experiencing anxiety and depression in midlife. Hormonal fluctuations were rarely mentioned, and if they were, they were framed as peripheral. But more recent and more nuanced studies are beginning to correct that oversight.

We now understand that the mental health challenges of perimenopause are unique, both in their symptom profile and in their physiological triggers. Estrogen plays a critical role in the regulation of mood, neurotransmitter activity, and stress reactivity. As levels begin to swing and fall, mood stability often unravels. Emerging evidence suggests that the benefits of SSRIs and other antidepressants during perimenopause are modest at best, especially for new-onset depression or anxiety (antidepressants are often prescribed for symptoms of anxiety) that clearly tracks with hormonal disruption. In fact, several studies now indicate that hormone therapy may be more effective than SSRIs for treating mood disorders that begin in perimenopause and that estrogen should be considered a first-line therapy, either on its own or added to an existing psychiatric regimen that's no longer effective during this hormonal transition. It's time we stop pathologizing women's distress without addressing the biological reality driving it.

In my clinical practice, I have witnessed how transdermal estradiol, delivered through a patch, gel, or spray, can dramatically improve mood symptoms for women in perimenopause. Unlike oral estrogen, transdermal estradiol bypasses the liver, delivering more consistent blood levels and avoiding the spikes and valleys that can worsen emotional instability. Numerous studies support the use of transdermal estradiol in reducing depressive symptoms in perimenopausal women, particularly those with high sensitivity to hormonal fluctuation.

Here are the key things we now know about the effects of estradiol from research and clinical use:

- **Direct mood effects:** Estradiol regulates serotonin, dopamine, and norepinephrine—the same neurotransmitters many antidepressants target.

- **Brain-calming effects:** Estradiol regulates activity in the amygdala, hippocampus, and hypothalamus, reducing over-reactivity to stress.

- **Effective in early perimenopause:** Transdermal estradiol is particularly effective for women who are still menstruating but irregularly and who report emotional or cognitive symptoms.

- **Synergy with antidepressants:** In some cases, estradiol works even better when combined with SSRIs or SNRIs—especially for women who haven't responded to antidepressants alone.

- **Improved safety profile:** Because it bypasses the liver, transdermal estradiol has no increased risk of blood clots and stroke versus oral formulations.

Despite this mounting scientific and anecdotal evidence, the medical establishment remains reluctant to embrace the use of hormone therapy for perimenopausal depression and other mental health challenges women may face at this time of their lives. This act of withholding, while largely unintentional, represents a continuation of the larger historical trend of minimizing women's health concerns. It's not just a matter of limiting pharmaceutical options for patients. Offering antidepressants without considering or even mentioning hormonal therapies reinforces the idea that these symptoms are "just psychological" or "all in your head" rather than a manifestation of the profound hormonal changes occurring during this life stage. Until we integrate hormone literacy into the treatment matrix of perimenopausal mental healthcare, we will continue to see misdiagnosis and the misuse of medications.

What I have seen work best is an approach that considers the interconnected nature of our hormones and our mental health (and physical health, but I will get to more on that later). This approach often results in an integration of strategies that can include hormone therapy, targeted pharmacological treatments, and lifestyle modifications. Perimenopausal women can be transformed by this type of tailored care, and I think they should be offered nothing less.

What to Do for Mental Health Changes in Perimenopause

First off, if you're struggling emotionally in midlife, I want to remind you that you're not alone—and you're not broken. You're experiencing a predictable, well-documented biological transition that can profoundly affect mental well-being. I hope hearing this can help at the very least remove some of the mystery and lessen the frustration that comes with feeling unseen and misunderstood.

Next, I want you to keep in mind that the most effective strategies for feeling better are going to vary based on the individual, and that finding what works best for you will require some trial and error. In an ideal scenario, you'll be able to find a menopause-educated practitioner (search the clinicians list on thepauselife.com for one near you) who can support you through this trial-and-error process and modify treatment protocols as necessary. If you don't have access to a local menopause-educated practitioner, you may be able to use a telehealth provider.

Above all else, it's essential to become your own best advocate. Being an advocate means paying attention to your symptoms and responding to them with the appropriate degree of seriousness. Mental health changes in perimenopause can be more than just debilitating; they can be life-threatening. If you have unaddressed trauma, it's important to note that hormone-driven changes to brain chemistry seem to have an uncanny ability to conjure up suppressed, even painful, issues. And unfortunately, you can't medicate trauma (I've tried; it doesn't work). Therapy and especially cognitive behavioral therapy will likely be necessary—and incredibly beneficial—for you, alongside any other treatment modalities. Help is available, and so many resources can be accessed online.

I've noted the research-supported use of MHT in perimenopause, but hormone therapy isn't medically appropriate for everyone (see chapter 14 for contraindications), and you'll need to discuss with your doctor whether the benefits for you outweigh the risks. Other types of treatments, such as acupuncture, have proved to be effective at reducing symptoms of anxiety in perimenopausal women. In chapter 15, you'll find a detailed look at the lifestyle modifications that can play an essential role in supporting mood stabilization. Here are some of the most effective and evidence-based strategies:

- **Exercise:** Regular physical activity enhances mood by increasing endorphins and reducing inflammation.

- **A brain-targeted eating pattern:** Diets rich in phytoestrogens (from soy, chickpeas, and other plant-based foods), omega-3 fatty acids (found in fatty fish, walnuts, and flaxseeds), and antioxidants (from fruits and vegetables) support hormonal balance and brain health.

- **Sleep hygiene:** Improving sleep quality through consistent routines and addressing menopause-related disturbances are essential for emotional regulation.

- **Stress management:** Practices like mindfulness, yoga, and meditation help reduce the impact of stress on mood and cognition.

- **Social connections:** Building a strong support network can alleviate feelings of isolation and foster emotional resilience.

Many of my patients who are on the other side of their most severe perimenopausal mental health symptoms have shared with me their biggest regret: *I wish I had started putting myself first sooner.* I hope what you've learned in this chapter inspires you to prioritize your mental health starting right now.

Clinical Questions and Considerations

Since there is no definitive diagnostic test for perimenopause, I rely heavily on patient input when evaluating them for evidence of what may be hormone-based changes in well-being. Below are some of the questions I use during these evaluations. Clinicians may want to consider a similar line of questioning when investigating mood disorders in midlife women.

- Is the onset of mood symptoms coinciding with changes in menstrual regularity, vasomotor symptoms, or cognitive complaints?
- Does the patient report cyclical mood worsening, especially mid-cycle or premenstrually?
- Does the patient report a history of postpartum depression or anxiety?
- Have traditional antidepressants been ineffective or poorly tolerated?
- Would a trial of transdermal estradiol be appropriate based on the patient's symptom profile and risk factors?

CHAPTER 6

Strange Cognition: The Rise of Brain Fog and ADHD-Like Symptoms

I am forty-eight and an OB-GYN sonographer. A few years ago, I started having deep leg aches/hip pains, heart palpitations, itchy ears, and clogged tear ducts, which resulted in constant and embarrassing eye watering. But the symptoms I detest the most are brain fog and feeling like I have ADD. I can't get words out or remember simple things, and I can't concentrate—I was scared I had early-onset dementia. I had always been known as the friend who remembered people's life stories, kids' names, and other details. But suddenly I felt like I had a head full of cotton.

—Amanda N.

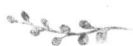

"I feel like I'm losing my mind."
"I'm struggling at work."
"I'm embarrassed in meetings."
"I've never been like this."

I hear these reports of symptoms related to brain fog over and over again from a large number of my patients. Often what has inspired them to utter these phrases is an experience more alarming than a hot flash or a missed period. It may be a moment or recurring moments of forgetting words mid-sentence or walking into a room and struggling to recall the reason they did so. It might be needing to reread the same paragraph three or more times and still not feeling like they've absorbed the meaning . . . or putting the car keys in odd places, like the fridge (me), or not remembering the name of someone they've known for years (also me). Others tell me about missed appointments, driving to the wrong location to pick up their kids, or frantically searching the house for glasses that sit just out of sight atop their head. These memory missteps are understandably disturbing—and the concern only increases if the lapses start to occur more regularly. Like Amanda, whom I quoted above, many women describing these experiences begin to fear they may be developing early-onset dementia or premature cognitive decline.

I see another group of patients whose expressions reveal a different type of cognitive struggle. These women say things like . . .

"I am always so disorganized."
"I feel like I don't measure up and never will."
"I feel like a failure."

They go on to share details about difficulties with time management (often called "time blindness"), organization, and self-esteem. They are plagued by feelings of inadequacy and have difficulty prioritizing tasks and managing their workload. In a lot of ways, their symptoms mirror those seen in attention deficit hyperactivity disorder (ADHD), but despite these similarities, in most cases it's not an exact diagnostic match.

While the symptomatic experience of women in each of these patient groups may be different, what is usually very much the same is the underlying hormonal environment. Yes, hormonal chaos can derail cognitive capabilities across a wide spectrum of brain functions, initiating both brain fog and brain disorganization. These issues are so commonly reported in perimenopause—indeed, 85 percent of women in perimenopause report some experience with these distressing symptoms—that I feel it's important to offer some insight into how symptoms may present in daily life and how disruptive, even destructive for some, these symptoms may be.

The Basics of Brain Fog

What is brain fog exactly? I think it's important to note that it's not a clinical diagnosis—that is, your doctor will never diagnose you with brain fog. The term itself is said to have grown out of two phrases—*clouding of consciousness* and *fogging the light of reason*—which were used by a German physician in the early nineteenth century to describe cognitive changes associated with delirium. Decades later, in the 1990s, use of the phrase *brain fog* increased as people with chronic fatigue syndrome and fibromyalgia adopted it to describe an aspect of their symptomatic experience. It became popular again during the COVID-19 pandemic when, after acute COVID infection, some were plagued by enduring cognitive difficulties. These difficulties came to be referred to as "COVID brain fog" and are considered a component of long COVID (see chapter 3 for more on long COVID's overlap with perimenopause).

What this short history lesson tells us is that, as a descriptive phrase, *brain fog* is here to stay. It also tells us that it has been around long enough that when you use it to describe your symptoms, most clinicians will know what you mean. When patients use it in my office, I understand it to represent a constellation of cognitive symptoms that can include memory lapses, concentration issues, slowed thinking, and mental fatigue. Some also detail a component of brain fog that feels existentially disruptive; they describe feeling off or not like themselves. I've seen patients brought to tears over the severity of these changes. These are women who are managing careers, parenting, aging parents, and households. They're highly capable and organized. And they're now grappling with a brain that doesn't feel like their own.

This isn't just anecdotal. Research shows small but consistent declines in memory performance and executive function during the menopausal transition. A 2024 study highlighted how retrieval-based memory functions, in particular, are affected during perimenopause. The study reported that women in this stage may feel like they know something but struggle to access it quickly—what we often call tip-of-the-tongue moments. While these changes typically remain within the normal cognitive range, the distress they cause is real and deserves to be acknowledged.

Additional research is tying altered cognitive function directly to hormonal fluctuations, especially the sharp changes in estrogen levels that characterize perimenopause.

How Hormone Changes Disrupt Cognition

As I've explained, we now know that estrogen plays a vital role in brain health and function. We know this thanks to the many neuroscientists who have been hard at work over the last couple of decades trying to glean meaningful insight into how hormones affect the brain. Their work has produced evidence that our sex hormones, especially estrogen, have deep and significant neurological influence that extends well beyond reproductive function. In the 2015 study "Perimenopause as a Neurological Transition State," researchers defined estrogen as "a master regulator" of function in the female brain because its reach extends to so many neural processes.

In chapter 4, we discussed in detail the mechanisms that rely on estrogen, but I'll recap here briefly. We know that estrogen enhances cerebral blood flow, ensuring that the brain receives an adequate supply of oxygen and nutrients necessary for optimal function. It acts as an anti-inflammatory agent, protecting neural pathways from damage and reducing the risk of neurodegenerative conditions. It also enhances synaptic activity, which is essential for communication between neurons, and affects production of neurotransmitters such as dopamine, serotonin, and acetylcholine. Last but certainly not least, it supports the energy-production systems within brain cells (mitochondria).

It's clear that the brain is heavily influenced by estrogen. And neuroscientists have found that brain regions that are deeply involved in memory, focus, emotional regulation, and executive function, namely the hippocampus, prefrontal cortex, and amygdala, are densely packed with estrogen receptors—hence the heightened sensitivity. As estrogen levels fluctuate and begin a downward trend in perimenopause, the unreliable delivery of this essential hormone disrupts neurological processes, resulting in a sort of cognitive impairment. The symptomatic expression of this altered neurological state includes all the complaints expressed by my patients above: memory lapses, challenges in executive function such as planning and multitasking, mental sluggishness, and even mood disturbances. When we consider what's happening on a molecular level in the perimenopausal brain, we begin to understand why these symptoms are so common and why they shouldn't come as a surprise.

Interestingly, the brain does try to adapt to changing estrogen levels. Dr. Lisa Mosconi, director of the Weill Cornell Women's Brain Initiative, and her team have produced advanced imaging studies that compare the female brain through various stages of hormonal changes. These images have revealed that women's brains exhibit progressively higher numbers of estrogen receptors as we go from premenopause to postmenopause. What this tells us is that as our estrogen levels decline, our brains build more and more receptors to try to connect with as much of it as possible. Dr. Mosconi's research also found that higher estrogen receptor density was associated with increased presence of neurological symptoms such as mood changes and memory complaints.

One of the most brilliant aspects of this work is that it was designed to reveal the effects of endocrine aging separate from chronological aging. This is critical, and the results powerfully underscore the importance of recognizing brain fog as a biologically driven phenomenon rather than allowing it to be dismissed as a psychological issue or a normal part of aging. We must acknowledge the cognitive changes for what they are—a reflection of the complex interplay between hormones and brain function—and let them serve as a reminder of how deeply connected our reproductive and neurological systems are. Understanding this relationship empowers women to approach perimenopause with greater knowledge and confidence, armed with strategies to support their cognitive health.

Is There a "Menopause Penalty" in the Workplace?

It's been estimated that nearly eight out of ten women will go through perimenopause (and likely into postmenopause) while they're still at work. This means enduring potentially debilitating symptoms while still trying to get your job done—something that can be increasingly difficult if your cognitive processes begin to diminish. The most frustrating aspect of such changes can be the fact that even if your professional performance starts to suffer, your intelligence hasn't changed at all. Many women struggle to reconcile this disconnect, and few find the support they need at work, which could lessen the stress they feel over their changing capabilities.

Studies are just starting to reveal the true cost of being a working woman while approaching menopause. Research published in 2025 by CESifo, a global, independent research network of prominent economists, found that there is a significant decline in earnings among menopausal women. They reported that women who visited a healthcare provider with menopause-related symptoms were found to have reduced their earnings by 10 percent four years later because they either cut back on their work hours or quit altogether. The effects were especially severe for women with lower socioeconomic status and who work manual or routine-intensive jobs.

There is much work to be done at the systemic level to correct unequal pay and discriminatory practices against women at all stages of life. When it comes to the stages of perimenopause and menopause, I believe we have only begun to see what's really lost as a result of trying to work through cognitive and other disruptive symptoms. We don't have to wait for more research to know that women need more support as they strive to work through this stage of their lives. We need companies to offer access to information on perimenopause and to menopause-related healthcare; we need for it to not be taboo to bring up brain fog with a boss; we need flexible work schedules; and we need mental healthcare to be prioritized.

As economists tie individual losses to corporate ones, I suspect we will see more businesses interested in supporting workers, because there will be a financial incentive to do so. We already have some such evidence from Mayo Clinic: Their 2023 study "Impact of Menopause Symptoms on Women in the Workplace" noted that menopause symptoms lead to an estimated $1.8 billion in lost work time per year ($26.6 billion annually when medical expenses are added) in the United States alone. It seems that some companies, such as Adobe, Bank of America, and Bristol Myers Squibb, have been paying attention to these numbers, as they are now offering menopause-specific benefits to employees. Let's hope other companies soon follow suit.

The Trajectory of Cognitive Changes in Perimenopause

Cognitive changes that begin in perimenopause are real and can be highly disruptive. Thankfully, they are usually temporary. As the hormonal chaos of perimenopause settles into the steadier low-estrogen environment of postmenopause, many women report a return to baseline mental clarity. This may not mean you'll enjoy a return to your premenopausal cognitive capabilities, but most of us can expect a relatively stable brain state in postmenopause that is reliably functional and recognizable—that is, you'll no longer find yourself needing to trudge through the foreign land of brain fog to complete a simple task.

For some women, perimenopause will mark the start of a cognitive decline that may eventually lead to the diagnosis of dementia or Alzheimer's disease, the most common form of dementia. This decline is more likely in women who have a first-degree relative with Alzheimer's or who carry the APOE4 gene; in these groups, perimenopause appears to activate the accumulation of amyloid plaques, which are a hallmark feature of Alzheimer's. Early-onset types of dementia and Alzheimer's disease, defined as occurring in people under sixty-five, are relatively rare, but they are a recognized and significant subset of cases (as of 2015, about 3.8 percent of all Alzheimer's cases in the United States were considered to be early onset). If your brain fog is accompanied by a retreat from friends and family and difficulties with everyday tasks such as paying bills and managing household chores, you may want to consider seeing a mental health professional or consulting your primary care doctor about the need for a neurologic evaluation.

Many women reading this book might be tempted to skip over talk of dementia, Alzheimer's disease, and brain-healthy habits, assuming these are concerns for much later in life. That's understandable—we've been culturally conditioned to associate cognitive decline with "old age," something to worry about when you're doing crosswords over tea in your seventies or eighties. But for women, cognitive vulnerability starts much earlier, even if symptoms don't show up for decades. One key reason? Hormones. The hormonal fluctuations of perimenopause affect the brain in real time, and it's been theorized that this is why nearly two-thirds of all clinically diagnosed cases of Alzheimer's disease are in women. That's not a small difference. That's nearly seven out of ten, even if most aren't early onset.

We still have much to learn about why this happens, and that's exactly why more research is urgently needed. Dr. Lisa Mosconi is one of the few leading the way in this area. Her groundbreaking work explores how the menopause transition may play a critical role in the development of Alzheimer's disease, and her book *The XX Brain* breaks down more than a dozen modifiable factors that influence your brain health and what you can do about them. Your brain deserves care now, not just later. Prioritize sleep. Connect with friends. Laugh more. Reduce your stress. Eat antioxidant-rich foods. These aren't luxury habits, they're neuroprotective acts of self-preservation, and your future self will thank you.

If you are experiencing lapses in cognitive function and want to understand more about them—that is, how often these lapses are occurring and any trends in the type of cognitive change—you can talk to your doctor about the Everyday Memory Questionnaire—Revised (EMQ-R). The EMQ-R is a thirteen-item questionnaire used in both clinical and nonclinical populations to screen for perceived memory and attention difficulties in menopausal women. Its use was validated by Australian researchers in a 2023 study that marked an important shift: EMQ-R became the first established tool to help measure memory and attention symptoms, or brain fog, in menopause. Historically, this form of cognitive testing has been designed and used only to detect dementia and to answer the question, Does this person have it or not? But that model doesn't allow for measuring the subtler cognitive changes many women experience during the menopause transition.

The EMQ-R asks about common, relatable lapses: forgetting words mid-sentence, losing track of conversations, walking into a room and forgetting why. These may sound minor, but they can be deeply distressing and are often dismissed. The EMQ-R allows us to capture and quantify these experiences in a simple, validated way. In many ways, this is a breakthrough. For the first time, we have a low-barrier, research-backed tool that helps women and clinicians alike see cognitive shifts that were previously invisible to the medical system and frequently brushed off entirely. If your clinician refers you to a neurologist for reported memory issues, the neurologist will likely have you complete this type of questionnaire.

Many times when patients are dealing with brain fog, I find what complicates it is the ways in which it overlaps with other perimenopausal symptoms—poor sleep, anxiety, and mood shifts, all of which exacerbate cognitive strain. Sleep disturbances in particular reduce memory consolidation and increase daytime cognitive fatigue. This is why it's so important to address brain fog with a combination of evidence-based lifestyle interventions (see the list of brain-supportive strategies at the end of this chapter). More than one approach may be needed to help women restore mental clarity and quality of life during perimenopause and beyond.

Hormone therapy, *especially transdermal estradiol,* has emerged as a potential intervention to mitigate the cognitive decline associated with perimenopause. Estrogen therapy (ET) has been shown to improve executive function and memory, and women who start ET closer to the onset of menopause may experience more pronounced cognitive benefits compared with those who begin treatment later. The higher treatment response to hormone therapy in early perimenopause is believed to occur because it has been introduced before the neuroendocrine system has adapted to prolonged estrogen deficiency.

It's important to note that the effectiveness of hormone therapy can vary based on a woman's unique symptoms, health history, and risk factors. This is why it's so critical for a clinician to take a personalized approach to each patient to ensure the treatment is tailored to individual needs.

When Guidelines Are Behind the Times

It's important to talk honestly about guidelines, those heavily referenced, rarely questioned rules that shape what clinicians are "allowed" to do. Current guidelines don't recommend hormone therapy solely for cognitive symptoms, citing inconsistent evidence and the need for more robust trials. But here's my frustration: These guidelines often reflect studies that excluded perimenopausal women, used non-bioidentical hormones like synthetic progestins or conjugated equine estrogens, and applied protocols that don't resemble modern clinical care.

In other words, they weren't testing *what we actually use today:* bioidentical estradiol and progesterone, transdermal routes, individualized risk assessment. Yet those outdated studies are still the foundation for our current recommendations. It's like judging 2025 medicine with data from the 1990s.

And more troubling is *the underlying mindset many of these guidelines still carry*—the idea that cognitive complaints during menopause are exaggerated or imagined. This is the persistent "it's all in her head" bias that exists in how we study and treat women's brains. The burden of proof still lies with the patient: Prove your suffering is real; prove your symptoms matter; prove they're not just emotional.

Yes, guidelines are meant to protect patients. But they can also protect outdated thinking. They're slow to evolve, often written by committees far removed from day-to-day patient care, and deeply influenced by research that was never designed to ask the right questions about women in midlife.

So no, current guidelines don't recommend hormone therapy for cognitive function alone. But that doesn't mean that we doctors shouldn't listen to women. It means that we need to demand better research and smarter questions and that we need to challenge what's long been accepted, because the women we serve deserve nothing less.

The Perimenopausal Brain and Its Link to ADHD

I mentioned above another group of patients who experience a different brand of cognitive symptoms. These patients have difficulty with time management and organization, and they may also experience . . .

- emotional dysregulation (e.g., mood swings, anxiety, depression)
- social difficulties and relationship problems
- low self-esteem and/or feelings of inadequacy
- difficulty prioritizing tasks and managing workload

Many of these women come to me wondering if they have adult-onset attention deficit hyperactivity disorder (ADHD). What I typically say is that, first, I'm not the one to diagnose ADHD. That assessment needs to be done by a psychologist, psychiatrist, or primary care doctor with training in neurodevelopment. Second, I'm quick to say, it's *possible* you have ADHD but it's likely that you are in perimenopause and experiencing hormone-driven cognitive symptoms that closely mimic ADHD.

ADHD is a neurodevelopmental condition traditionally characterized by persistent patterns of inattention, hyperactivity, and/or impulsivity. For several decades, clinicians have been using this definition to diagnose ADHD in children, with boys being two to three times more likely than girls to receive a diagnosis. In recent years, there has been an increase in adult cases, especially in women ages thirty to forty-nine, and the diagnosis of ADHD in this group nearly doubled between 2020 and 2022.

Symptoms of ADHD often present differently in girls than in boys. Girls are more likely to struggle with focus, organization, and time management; they might seem unmotivated or get upset easily and have difficulty completing projects. Boys, on the other hand, demonstrate more traditional symptoms of ADHD. They may be hyperactive and impulsive and take excessive risks. (There can, of course, be overlap between the symptoms and genders.) So, is it possible that underdiagnosis of ADHD in girls has led to the jump in adult ADHD diagnosis in women? Again, yes, it's possible, but we simply can't rule out the influence of perimenopause.

As I explained earlier, perimenopause is an inflection point for cognitive functions that rely on reliable estrogen delivery. Estrogen plays a vital role in modulating dopamine transmission in the prefrontal cortex, the brain's hub for executive function, attention, and working memory. During perimenopause, estradiol levels fluctuate unpredictably, leading to dysregulation of these neural circuits. This can result in what many women experience as brain fog but what may clinically resemble or amplify ADHD symptoms.

Determining a Diagnosis

There are three possible explanations for what could be going on when you are in perimenopause (whether you know it or not) and experiencing disruptive symptoms such as time blindness, disorganization, restlessness, and emotional dysregulation:

1. **Pre-existing ADHD (diagnosed or undiagnosed) has gotten worse:** Women with pre-existing ADHD often report a worsening of core symptoms—inattention, distractibility, disorganization, time blindness, emotional dysregulation, and memory lapses—during perimenopause. These issues aren't simply a matter of perception. As estrogen declines, so too does its regulatory influence on dopamine, a neurotransmitter essential for attention, motivation, and executive function.

    These neurochemical changes can amplify cognitive dysfunction to the point of causing significant distress and impairment, leading some women to seek evaluation for the first time in their forties or early fifties. For these women, perimenopause becomes the lens through which long-standing, subclinical ADHD is finally recognized.

2. **Undiagnosed perimenopause:** You're likely well aware by now that perimenopause itself is associated with cognitive shifts—particularly in attention, working memory, and executive functioning. These changes, often referred to as "menopause brain,"

overlap with ADHD symptomatology, creating a diagnostic gray zone. In the absence of training on cognitive aging in women, clinicians may be quick to assign a psychiatric diagnosis without fully considering the neuroendocrine root of these symptoms.

3. **Incorrectly diagnosed ADHD:** In some cases, women with true ADHD are misdiagnosed with depression, anxiety, or "just aging," leading to unneeded prescription medication or untreated impairment.

Despite the diagnostic ambiguity and challenges surrounding the interplay of ADHD and perimenopause, there *are* viable approaches to symptom management. Some effective options pair pharmacology with cognitive strategies and lifestyle interventions. If you have any cognitive symptoms suggestive of ADHD, it's critical for your hormonal status to be considered to create a full diagnostic picture. Failing to consider the hormonal milieu and its impact on cognitive symptoms can lead to inappropriate or incomplete treatment.

Cognitive Restoration May Require an Integrated Approach

When we look at the research on treatment strategies for symptoms related to attention and memory in perimenopausal women, we see that some ADHD medications and hormone therapy have proved to be effective. Here's some of the science:

- In a randomized trial, *atomoxetine,* a non-stimulant norepinephrine reuptake inhibitor, was associated with improvements in subjective attention and memory in both perimenopausal and postmenopausal women.
- Similarly, *lisdexamfetamine,* a stimulant commonly used in ADHD treatment, improved executive functioning and working memory in midlife women with new-onset difficulties. In both studies, the

medications were found to be beneficial regardless of whether the women had a formal ADHD diagnosis or not.

- In clinical trials, women receiving *estrogen therapy* reported improvements in verbal memory, sustained attention, and cognitive flexibility, especially when started before the brain had fully adapted to prolonged hormone deprivation. Though MHT isn't specifically designed for ADHD, these outcomes suggest that MHT may help stabilize cognitive functions that become compromised in perimenopause and that closely resemble or intensify ADHD symptoms.

While pharmacologic treatments such as atomoxetine and lisdexamfetamine have demonstrated benefits for cognitive function in midlife women, MHT may serve as a foundational intervention, particularly in women experiencing broader perimenopausal symptoms such as vasomotor instability (hot flashes), sleep disruption, mood swings, and musculoskeletal pain. In these cases, targeted hormone therapy, either systemic estrogen or combination estrogen-progestogen (progestogen is the general term for any hormone, natural or synthetic, that shows similar effects as progesterone) for those with a uterus, can improve cognitive clarity and reduce the need for polypharmacy.

However, this bears repeating: It's essential to screen carefully for contraindications to MHT and to tailor treatment based on individual symptomatology, risk profile, and cognitive burden.

Clinical Questions and Considerations

If you saw yourself in the list of ADHD-like symptoms and you are in search of clinical support, you will want to find a clinician who takes an informed, nuanced approach that includes evaluating your hormonal status, considering a trial of MHT (if you are eligible), and monitoring your cognitive response. This framework validates the neuroendocrine basis of perimenopausal cognitive changes, and works to address the root cause rather than to merely suppress symptoms. These are the questions a skilled clinician should be asking:

- Is this pre-existing but previously undiagnosed ADHD that has gotten worse?

- Is it ADHD that has been masked by coping mechanisms and/or the neurotransmitter support offered by premenopausal estrogen levels?

- Or is this cognitive dysfunction rooted entirely in perimenopausal neuroendocrine shifts (that is, not true ADHD, but presenting with overlapping symptoms)?

Each scenario demands a distinct treatment approach, and all require a menopause-informed diagnostic framework.

Habits Can Shape Your Brain Health, Too

Although brain fog and ADHD-like symptoms are rooted in hormonal changes, lifestyle plays a significant role in managing their impact. Research suggests that adopting specific behaviors can support cognitive health during perimenopause and beyond (you'll notice significant overlap between these and the habits that may benefit mental health):

- **Exercise:** Aerobic activity increases blood flow to the brain and supports the release of brain-derived neurotrophic factor (BDNF), which improves neuroplasticity.

- **Nutrition:** A diet rich in omega-3 fatty acids, antioxidants, and phytoestrogens can reduce inflammation and protect brain function.

- **Sleep hygiene:** Sleep disturbances are common in perimenopause, but addressing them is critical for memory consolidation and overall cognitive performance. Strategies such as maintaining a consistent sleep schedule, reducing caffeine intake, and creating a relaxing bedtime routine can improve your sleep quality.

- **Stress management:** Chronic stress exacerbates cognitive symptoms by increasing inflammation and disrupting the HPA axis. Practices like mindfulness, yoga, meditation, or simply taking time to relax can significantly reduce stress and its effects on the brain.

- **Cognitive training:** Brain games, reading, and learning new skills maintain neuroplasticity and may slow cognitive decline.

Women navigating the menopause transition deserve better than being labeled as inattentive or disorganized and sent off with a prescription for stimulant medication. They deserve a nuanced evaluation that considers hormonal status, life stage, and neurochemical balance, as well as compassion for the invisible cognitive load they're carrying.

CHAPTER 7

Perimenopause and Metabolic Syndrome

I have been a vascular surgeon for more than twenty years, and I am a single mom in my early fifties. I have always considered myself high functioning, up until about eight months ago when I developed symptoms I attributed to "stress" that progressively worsened. I came across Dr. Haver's work and realized I was not actually "going crazy" but rather experiencing significant perimenopause symptoms. My symptoms included severe exhaustion (where I could barely get through my day), waking up in the middle of the night, night sweats, anxiety with palpitations (particularly in the morning), brain fog, and weight gain (despite no changes in diet/exercise). When my primary care physician drew labs, they reflected signs of perimenopause: elevated LDL/total cholesterol (despite being vegetarian with prior low LDL/total cholesterol) with normal HDL and triglycerides. I also had elevated cortisol. I have recently started hormonal therapy and am starting to feel "normal" again. This has been life changing.

—Stephanie S.

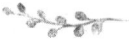

I was blindsided by my own labs. I was in my late forties, and on routine yearly wellness exam blood work, I was shocked to find my LDL had shot up. I was eating well, exercising regularly, and maintaining what most would consider a healthy lifestyle, but my LDL levels had gone way up, well beyond anything I'd seen before. My blood pressure had crept higher, too. There had been no drastic changes in my habits, no obvious red flags. But something fundamental had shifted.

I wasn't alone. In my clinic, I started seeing more and more midlife women walk through the door with similar stories. They came in disheartened, holding lab reports that showed rising cholesterol, prediabetes, or new-onset hypertension, even when they hadn't changed a thing. They felt betrayed by their bodies.

The only response most of these patients received from their doctor was a prescription for a statin or an antihypertensive (blood pressure medication). Many were also told to eat better and exercise more, despite having explained that they had made no modifications to their daily habits (if anything, they had been eating fewer calories and working out more to try to address the abdominal weight gain that had also recently appeared). There was no discussion of what might be driving these changes, no effort to explore if there might be an underlying metabolic component that could be contributing to their symptoms.

The cluster of interrelated risk factors my patients were presenting with put them dangerously close to a diagnosis of metabolic syndrome, which is a group of conditions that includes . . .

- abdominal obesity (waist circumference more than thirty-five inches)
- elevated triglycerides ($\geq$150 mg/dL)
- low HDL cholesterol (<50 mg/dL)
- elevated fasting glucose ($\geq$100 mg/dL)
- high blood pressure ($\geq$130/85 mmHg)

Having three or more of these factors increases a woman's risk of cardiovascular disease, fatal heart attack, stroke, type 2 diabetes, and even some cancers. Recent statistics have estimated that patients with metabolic syndrome have double the risk of developing atherosclerotic cardiovascular diseases (those caused by plaque buildup in the arterial walls) and five times the risk of type 2 diabetes when compared with the general population. Metabolic syndrome can also put you in the position of developing these diseases prematurely.

If you look at the risk factors for metabolic syndrome, you will see that "being past menopause" is on the list (it's at the bottom of the list, but still, we got a spot, ladies). I think we've found the elephant in the room. Recent research confirms what many of us in the Menoposse have long suspected: Menopause itself, regardless of age, is a major and independent factor in the health shifts that put us on the fast track to developing metabolic syndrome. In perimenopause, it's important to understand that these shifts can begin quietly before our periods stop and before anyone thinks to investigate. And they can trigger profound but largely invisible (except for belly fat, which likes to make itself very apparent) changes in your body.

While metabolic syndrome has long been dismissed as a lifestyle disease—blamed on poor diet, inactivity, and "bad choices"—it can absolutely develop in a perfectly healthy woman with no changes to her eating or exercise habits, underscoring the powerful biology of menopause itself.

What my labs and the labs of countless patients revealed was a clear, consistent pattern: rising risk factors for metabolic syndrome that couldn't be brushed off as random. This wasn't a coincidence or just bad luck. The biased old guard will shrug and say, "Well, that's just aging." The fitness bros will smirk and tell us that we've let ourselves go, that we're lazy now, not hitting the gym hard enough. And the wellness influencers? They'll chalk it up to "adrenal fatigue" and offer up detox teas or a new supplement bundle as if a hormone-driven metabolic shift could be fixed with a smoothie and some affirmations.

Let me be clear: No supplement resurrects ovarian function. Nothing over the counter replaces estrogen's metabolic role once it declines. Yet that's the physiological shift at the center of what we're seeing. The data doesn't lie. Women deserve science, not scapegoats.

Before perimenopause, our estrogen enables protections across many systems that regulate inflammation, glucose (blood sugar) metabolism, and blood pressure, and this puts us in better health generally than men of our same age. But as we enter perimenopause, all of this begins to change—and we have practically no clinical acknowledgment of this reality. We don't have any established efforts focused on early recognition and targeted intervention for women, and this leaves us vulnerable at precisely the moment our risk skyrockets.

But here's the deeper issue: *This isn't just about biology; it's about bias.* Women in midlife are structurally underserved. Gender disparities in research and clinical practice mean that women with metabolic syndrome often go undiagnosed, undertreated, and misunderstood. Prevention strategies are rarely tailored to the hormonal realities of the menopausal transition. Drug trials that inform standard care protocols were built on male physiology. And the "watchful waiting" approach too often leaves women in the lurch until disease has already taken hold.

Our entire model of metabolic health wasn't designed for women, and it shows. But it doesn't have to be this way. *Perimenopause should be seen as a critical window for prevention and metabolic recalibration, not as an inevitable slide into decline.* With the right tools—education, diagnostic strategies, lifestyle support, and, when appropriate, hormone therapy—we can shift the trajectory of women's health.

The goal is not just to normalize what happens in menopause but to use our knowledge to optimize it. Because when women are informed, supported, and treated based on evidence that reflects *their* physiology, they don't just survive this transition; they reclaim their power.

The Metabolic Syndrome of Menopause

I believe that in order to bring attention to what's really going on inside women's bodies during perimenopause, menopause, and postmenopause, we need to give this pattern of metabolic dysfunction a distinct diagnostic name. And this is what a team of researchers and I have recently done; we've introduced a new concept called *the metabolic syndrome of menopause* and written a paper (and presented it as a poster at the Endocrine Society meeting in July 2025) based on robust scientific evidence that identifies and details the characteristics of this syndrome. It's currently under review for publication. The idea is simple and long overdue: When estrogen levels drop during the menopause transition, a very specific set of health changes can follow, and they're often overlooked or misunderstood.

You likely understand all too well by now that estrogen isn't just relevant to reproduction; it's a whole-body hormone with radical reach, and it has a profound influence on how your metabolism functions and begins to dysfunction. When estrogen declines, it throws off how efficiently our tissues store and use fuel to keep essential systems running. During this time, many women start to experience what's called *preferential* weight gain (though, of course, it's not preferred at all!) in the abdominal region, not because they've changed how they eat or move, but because their metabolism has fundamentally shifted. Researchers writing in the journal *Gynecological and Reproductive Endocrinology & Metabolism* put it succinctly: "Things drastically change as we approach the menopausal transition. As a matter of fact, many women suffer weight gain and an increase in central adiposity in the years preceding the menopause." This increase in belly fat, also known as visceral fat, isn't just frustrating; it's dangerous. It raises the risk for insulin resistance, type 2 diabetes, and metabolic dysfunction-associated steatotic liver disease (MASLD), a chronic liver condition that can progress to serious liver damage and is becoming more common in postmenopausal women.

In addition to shifts in fat storage, women approaching menopause are also likely to see levels of LDL (the "bad" cholesterol) and triglycerides go up and levels of HDL (the "good" cholesterol) lower. We begin to see a loss of muscle tissue, too, which decelerates metabolic function. Despite maintaining a status quo in routine as it relates to patterns of eating and exercise, the number on the scale keeps creeping up. And the combined effect of all these changes raises the risk for heart disease, which is the number one killer of women.

For too long, the rise in metabolic risk factors in midlife women has been blamed on "just getting older" or even personal failure like poor diet, inactivity, and "bad choices." But it's time we start treating it for what it is: a biological shift.

By calling it the metabolic syndrome of menopause, we're not just naming a problem; we're giving it an identity. And there's power in that. Medical systems, governing bodies, and clinicians respond to definitions. They need names to build frameworks around: for screening protocols, diagnostic criteria, early-intervention strategies, and treatment guidelines. Without a name, it's easy to ignore. With one, we can begin to shift clinical practice.

It's time to stop minimizing the metabolic reality of menopause and start treating it like the serious health issue it is. If we want real progress, we need more than vague acknowledgments. We need clear definitions that demand action: better screening, earlier detection, and targeted, sex-specific treatments that reflect the unique hormonal changes women experience during the menopause transition.

Why It's Not Just About Age and Lifestyle: The Hormonal Piece We're Missing

Age and lifestyle are relevant to metabolic function. Diet, exercise, and body weight all matter a great deal when we talk about metabolic syndrome. But here's the truth: If we focus *only* on those things and ignore the powerful role of hormones, *especially estrogen,* we're missing the full picture of what's really happening in women's bodies in perimenopause and menopause.

Estrogen has a protective effect on metabolism. All the work estrogen does is accomplished by way of estrogen receptors, specifically ERα (alpha) and ERβ (beta). Your metabolic tissues, like fat, muscle, the liver, the pancreas, and even the brain, are packed with these tiny hormone-sensing switches that get activated upon estrogen's arrival. When estrogen binds to these receptors, it helps keep the entire metabolic system in balance.

ERα is especially important when it comes to metabolism. It helps regulate how and where fat is stored, how sensitive our cells are to insulin, how much energy we burn, and how much inflammation we carry in our fat tissue. When estrogen is present and ERα is activated, the system runs more smoothly. But when estrogen levels drop during menopause, ERα signaling drops, and this can lead to bigger fat cells (especially around the waist), increased inflammation, insulin resistance, and muscle loss.

ERβ is still being studied, but it's also present in many of the same tissues and may play a protective role, especially in skeletal muscle and the liver. What *is* known is that the balance between ERα and ERβ matters and that menopause throws that balance off.

These changes happen in both subcutaneous fat (the kind just under the skin) and visceral fat (the kind that wraps around your organs and raises your risk for serious disease). And as the fat cells change shape and function, the body becomes more prone to storing metabolically harmful fat.

Bottom line: Estrogen doesn't just disappear quietly. It takes a whole set of protective mechanisms with it. Understanding the role of estrogen receptors helps explain *why* perimenopause so often coincides with weight gain, insulin resistance, high cholesterol, and rising cardiovascular risk. And it reinforces why women in midlife need care strategies that go beyond calories and treadmills; they need solutions that take their hormones into account.

Risk Factors for Metabolic Syndrome

I want to isolate and expand on some of the risk factors and their markers that we see rise during perimenopause. Some of these, such as weight gain, may be externally observable. But most will remain invisible until they show up on your labs, like they did for me and many of my patients.

Visceral Fat

WHY BELLY FAT BECOMES A BIGGER PROBLEM IN PERIMENOPAUSE

One of the first signs that something was changing in my own body during perimenopause was a slow but relentless accumulation of fat around my midsection. I hadn't changed my diet. I hadn't stopped exercising. But my shape was changing, and nothing I did seemed to reverse it. Like many of my patients, I felt confused and frustrated. For someone who had always been in control of my health, this shift felt like a betrayal, and I knew I wasn't alone.

Women in my clinic were telling me the same story: "I'm doing everything right, but my belly keeps growing." These were women who had taken care of themselves for years by eating mindfully, staying active, and managing stress, and suddenly they were seeing fat collect in ways that felt foreign and, in many cases, deeply discouraging. They often assumed they were to blame or, worse, were told by their doctors that it was just "part of getting older."

But the truth is, this isn't about lack of discipline. Again, this is about hormones, specifically estrogen.

Before menopause, estrogen plays a powerful role in fat distribution. It encourages fat storage in the hips, thighs, and buttocks—areas rich in subcutaneous fat, which lies just beneath the skin and is relatively metabolically harmless. Estrogen also promotes fat cell hyperplasia, meaning new fat cells are created in smaller sizes with better blood supply and less inflammation. This pattern helps maintain metabolic health.

But during perimenopause and after, as estrogen levels begin to fluctuate and decline, that protective fat distribution breaks down. The body starts to favor hypertrophy: enlarging existing fat cells instead of creating new ones. Blood flow decreases, inflammation increases, and fat begins to shift inward to the abdominal cavity.

This is visceral fat. It wraps around your internal organs—your liver, intestines, and pancreas—and adds up quickly. Research shows that visceral fat can increase significantly during the menopause transition. In premenopausal women, it typically accounts for about 5 to 8 percent of total body weight. But after menopause, that number can rise to 15 to 20 percent. For a woman who weighs 150 pounds, that's a jump from 7.5 to 12 pounds of visceral fat to as much as 22.5 to 30 pounds, all without a single change in eating or exercise habits.

Why does this shift in body composition matter? Because visceral fat isn't just about the number on the scale. Visceral fat contributes to metabolic dysfunction. It increases the risk of insulin resistance and type 2 diabetes. It's linked to higher cholesterol and cardiovascular disease. And unlike subcutaneous fat, visceral fat acts like a toxin factory, pumping out hormones and other substances that create the kind of chronic low-grade inflammation that can damage the cells of the body over time.

Estrogen, through its interaction with estrogen receptors, is a quiet protector, not only helping keep visceral fat in check but also assisting in regulating how your immune system responds to stress and injury and toning down the release of cytokines like IL-6, TNF-α, and IL-1β, signaling proteins that help control inflammation. An excess of cytokines is associated with everything from insulin resistance to cardiovascular disease. Estrogen also inhibits something called the inflammasome, a molecular switch that activates inflammation inside cells.

As estrogen levels fluctuate and decline during perimenopause, that control mechanism weakens and the inflammasome switch is more likely to turn on, revving up inflammatory signals. In my clinical practice, I often see this show up symptomatically as achy joints, fatigue, unexplained weight gain, or even a rise in blood sugar and cholesterol. Things women (and their doctors) often chalk up to aging, when in fact they may be tied to increases in visceral fat that can initiate a silent shift in the body's inflammatory balance. Chronic low-grade inflammation is a major contributor to the diseases we associate with midlife and beyond: heart disease, diabetes, fatty liver, and even certain types of cancer.

To make matters more complicated, after menopause women experience a decrease in resting energy expenditure (REE), which is a slowing down of metabolism that is driven in part by a decline in muscle mass (see chapter 9 for more on muscle loss). So even if you are eating the same and staying active, your body is burning fewer calories at rest. That, too, adds fuel to the fire when it comes to visceral fat accumulation.

This shift in fat storage is another powerful example of how estrogen and other hormones protect our health. Losing that protection as we make our way toward menopause dramatically raises the stakes, making midlife a critical time for targeted prevention and care.

Know Your Risks: If you are in perimenopause and your estrogen levels have begun a downward trend, this alone puts you at increased risk of preferential visceral fat gain. You are also more likely to gain intra-abdominal fat because of genetic factors; consistent poor sleep; a pattern of higher caloric intake relative to energy expenditure; routine consumption of high-calorie, low-quality ultra-processed foods; low physical activity; and prolonged periods of high stress. Smoking and heavy alcohol intake are additional risk factors for visceral fat gain.

Know Your Numbers: We can't monitor visceral fat on the scale, which in some ways I view as a positive thing. I spent too many decades of my life focused on what the scale said, and I personally don't want to rely anymore on those numbers as the key arbiter of my health. I've been encour-

Perimenopause and Metabolic Syndrome

aging my patients, too, to move away from weight as the be-all-and-end-all indicator of wellness. That being said, there is value in assessing and monitoring your visceral fat mass, because it's so intricately linked with metabolic mayhem.

You can assess your visceral fat percentage one of two ways:

- **Get a DEXA scan.** A DEXA scan is an imaging test that measures body composition and bone density. I'll discuss more on its important role in assessing your risk for osteoporosis in chapter 8, but it can also be a valuable tool that allows you to get a baseline reading of your body composition. The scan gives you a percentage breakdown of fat and muscle tissue. In most cases, women under sixty-five won't be able to get a DEXA scan covered by insurance (I hope this will change), but you can pay out of pocket for one. They run between one hundred and three hundred dollars. In my clinic, we rely on a tool called the InBody scan to help determine a patient's body composition. Some health clubs or gyms also have InBody devices, and the company makes scales for home use, too. If you have one done professionally, make sure you also have access to someone who is trained to understand the readings and can help you do the same.

- **Calculate your waist-to-hip ratio.** The easiest and most affordable way to get an approximation of visceral fat is to use a tape measure to measure your waist and hips and then calculate your waist-to-hip ratio:

1. Measure your waist just above your belly button; this is your *waist circumference*.

2. Measure the largest part of your hips; this is your *hip circumference*.

3. Divide your waist circumference by your hip circumference; this is your *waist-to-hip ratio*.

4. Use this chart to help you determine if you have a measurement of abdominal obesity that may put you at increased health risk:

HEALTH RISK	WAIST-TO-HIP RATIO
Low	0.80 or lower
Moderate	0.81-0.85
High	0.86 or higher

Separate from visceral fat, your practitioner can run labs to check levels of inflammation. In our clinic, we use high-sensitivity CRP and sedimentation rate as inflammatory markers. It's important to note, though, that these markers are non-specific—they don't tell us exactly where inflammation is coming from or what's causing it. A mildly elevated result could reflect anything from recent exercise to a hidden infection to ongoing metabolic changes. In clinical practice, I interpret these values as part of a broader picture: not as a diagnosis on their own, but as signals that prompt me to dig deeper, looking at symptoms, lifestyle, hormonal status, and other labs to understand what's really driving the inflammation.

The Role of MHT: Hormone therapy isn't prescribed for weight loss, but some research has shown that it can be helpful in establishing a healthier distribution of fat—that is, it can result in abdominal fat being relocated to the peripheral areas of your body, where it's less likely to be harmful to your health. However, this benefit seems to disappear quickly after stopping MHT, making it clear that we need to optimize other strategies to protect against visceral fat gain.

GLP-1s and Perimenopause: What You Need to Know

In my clinical practice, I've seen firsthand how visceral fat gain and rising cardiometabolic risk in midlife women are too often met with shame and blame. But these aren't moral failings. For many of my patients and for myself, these changes were the biological consequences of hormonal decline, especially the loss of estrogen during perimenopause. (My most trusted source on the specifics of endocrinological influences on obesity and body composition is Dr. Rocio Salas-Whalen, who is triple board-certified in obesity medicine, internal medicine, and endocrinology. Her book, *Weightless,* is an excellent resource in this area.)

The good news is, we now understand this shift more clearly than ever before. And with that understanding comes access to more supportive, evidence-based therapies such as GLP-1 receptor agonists (GLP-1s).

While lifestyle changes and hormone therapy are foundational in restoring and maintaining healthy metabolic function, these strategies alone aren't always enough. For some women, particularly those with long-standing metabolic risk driven by elevated visceral fat, we've seen remarkable results with GLP-1s such as semaglutide, liraglutide, and the emerging utreglutide. Originally developed for diabetes, these medications improve insulin sensitivity, reduce appetite, promote weight loss, and lower inflammation, and they're showing real promise in supporting women's metabolic health during and after perimenopause.

These medications aren't a magic bullet, and they're certainly not for everyone. But for patients who haven't responded to traditional interventions, they can be a powerful part of a comprehensive, evidence-based approach to care.

Emerging research is showing that GLP-1s may work synergistically with estrogen.

In animal models simulating postmenopause, GLP-1s not only improved glucose metabolism but also enhanced fat breakdown and shifted metabolic gene expression. This suggests a unique interplay between GLP-1 and estrogen pathways.

In a recent study on utreglutide, postmenopausal women saw significant reductions in body weight, blood pressure, and lipids, alongside improved glucose regulation. These effects target the very risks, such as cardiovascular disease and type 2 diabetes, that rise sharply in perimenopause.

GLP-1s are generally well tolerated in women, with most side effects being mild and gastrointestinal, and these symptoms often improve over time or with dose adjustments. When used thoughtfully, alongside strength training, high-quality nutrition, and hormone therapy where appropriate, GLP-1s offer us a new tool to address an old problem with the nuance it deserves.

This is the future of menopause care: personalized, science backed, and shame-free.

Insulin Resistance

THE HIDDEN LINK BETWEEN HORMONES AND BLOOD SUGAR

One of the less obvious but incredibly important changes that happen during perimenopause is a rising resistance to insulin, the hormone that helps move sugar (in the form of glucose) from your bloodstream into your cells. This phenomenon, known as *insulin resistance,* is a core feature of metabolic syndrome and a major risk factor for developing type 2 diabetes. And yes, estrogen plays a central role here, too.

Estrogen helps protect women from insulin resistance by supporting glucose metabolism and contributing to keeping inflammation levels low. In addition to moderating cytokine levels, estrogen interacts with receptors within immune cells, such as macrophages and monocytes, that influence inflammation. When women are in the premenopausal stage of life, we appear to have a protection plan against insulin resistance that is ensured in part by the presence of estrogen. As estrogen levels fall during perimenopause, immune cells become more active in ways that promote chronic low-grade inflammation, and this inflammation disrupts how well your cells respond to insulin.

The result? Blood sugar becomes harder to regulate. Elevated blood sugar is considered a gateway to metabolic syndrome because it contributes to the larger cardiometabolic dysregulation that correlates with increased risk of heart attack, stroke, and fatty liver disease. What's happening here is that the body doesn't respond as efficiently to insulin's signals and more glucose lingers in the bloodstream. Over time, the loitering presence of glucose in your blood vessels raises the risk of developing prediabetes and eventually type 2 diabetes. And when I write "over time," I mean it—signs of abnormal glucose metabolism can be seen *thirteen years* before a type 2 diabetes diagnosis.

This is why insulin resistance is such a critical piece of the metabolic puzzle during perimenopause. There is an under-the-surface hormonal shift driving your metabolism toward insulin impairment regardless of your dietary and lifestyle habits. When we acknowledge these metabolic changes as biological, hormonal, and reversible, we introduce the empowering potential for action. With the right support, it's possible to improve insulin sensitivity, reduce inflammation, and lower the risk of type 2 diabetes and heart disease during this critical phase of life. I'll review some supportive strategies at the end of this chapter.

Know Your Risks: Risk factors for developing insulin resistance include . . .

- being age forty-five and over
- a family history of type 2 diabetes
- obesity, especially abdominal obesity (visceral fat)
- being physically inactive
- high blood pressure and/or high cholesterol
- polycystic ovary syndrome (PCOS)
- sleep apnea
- fatty liver disease
- use of certain blood pressure medications, steroids, or medications used to treat psychiatric disorders or HIV
- Cushing's disease
- hypothyroidism

Know Your Numbers: Since there are no early signs of insulin resistance, it's important to use lab results to establish a baseline that you and your practitioner can monitor as you progress through perimenopause.

You will want to make sure to test fasting glucose and hemoglobin A1C (HbA1c), the latter of which measures your average blood sugar over the last two to three months. The higher your HbA1c, the greater your risk for developing type 2 diabetes. Both fasting glucose and HbA1c are standard on annual physical panels, but you will want to confirm that they're being checked.

I recommend also asking for the homeostatic model assessment for insulin resistance (HOMA-IR) to be done if you have any of the risk factors noted above. This test generates a HOMA-IR score, which is based on a ratio involving fasting glucose and fasting insulin. A HOMA-IR score allows a practitioner to assess how responsive you are to insulin and is considered a better predictor of developing insulin resistance.

The Role of MHT: While the research in this area is still developing, studies have shown that hormone therapy can help reestablish some of the protections against insulin resistance introduced by endogenous (produced in the body) estrogen. We have seen randomized trials show that hormone therapy use in menopausal women can significantly reduce the risk of prediabetes developing into type 2 diabetes. However, we don't know for certain its broader role in supporting glucose metabolism in perimenopausal women. For women in the menopause transition, lifestyle strategies that focus on nutrition and exercise can be highly effective.

High Blood Pressure

THE BLOOD PRESSURE SPIKE NO ONE TALKS ABOUT

We tend to think of high blood pressure, or hypertension, as a health concern that affects more men than women. It's true that more men than women under the age of sixty have high blood pressure, but after sixty, rates of hypertension are higher among women. The primary reason for this shift is the loss of estrogen, which before menopause protects against unhealthy increases in blood pressure. This is why in perimenopause we see many women suddenly diagnosed with hypertension even if they've never had blood pressure issues before.

And if you experience surgical menopause (such as after a bilateral oophorectomy—surgical removal of the ovaries), the change can be even more dramatic. Research has shown that the sudden loss of estrogen from ovary removal is linked to a higher risk of hypertension, heart disease, and stroke.

Estrogen plays an important role in supporting cardiovascular health through its direct impact on your vascular system. We take for granted the functionality of the vascular system, which consists of an astounding sixty thousand miles of blood vessels that are responsible for the transport of oxygen-rich blood throughout your body. It is, to put it mildly, a crucial component of your health.

Cells within the endothelium, which lines all your blood vessels and arteries, contain estrogen receptors. When estrogen reaches these receptors, it enhances the release of nitric oxide, and this encourages vasodilation, the process by which your blood vessels relax and widen. This effect of estrogen helps maintain healthy blood flow and pressure.

What we see happening in perimenopause is that as estrogen levels begin to decline, blood vessels become less flexible and narrower, leading to an increase in blood pressure. The body also becomes more sensitive to internal chemical stressors, like angiotensin II, a hormone that narrows blood vessels and raises blood pressure. (ERα, in particular, has been shown to play a major role in defending against this kind of hypertension.)

All of this points to an important reality: Perimenopause changes the way a woman's cardiovascular system functions. It increases the risk for high blood pressure, which in turn raises the risk for heart attacks, strokes, and other serious complications.

The good news is that understanding this connection can lead to better, more personalized care. For some women, hormone therapy may be part of that picture. For others, it may mean earlier screening and lifestyle interventions. Either way, it's time we stop thinking of high blood pressure as an inevitable part of aging and start recognizing it as a clear signal of hormonal change.

Know Your Risks: Risk factors that increase your chances of high blood pressure include . . .

- race—Black women have the highest rates of high blood pressure and will want to be highly responsive to any notable increases
- family history of high blood pressure
- type 2 diabetes
- having had gestational hypertension or preeclampsia
- polycystic ovary syndrome, lupus, or rheumatoid arthritis
- use of oral contraceptives—some medications may affect your blood vessels and blood pressure
- lifestyle factors, such as high salt intake, tobacco use, routine daily alcohol use of one or more drinks, or binge drinking

Know Your Numbers: These are healthy and unhealthy blood pressure ranges, according to the American Heart Association:

BLOOD PRESSURE CATEGORY	SYSTOLIC MMHG (UPPER NUMBER)	AND/OR	DIASTOLIC MMHG (LOWER NUMBER)
Normal	less than 120	and	less than 80
Elevated	120-29	and	less than 80
High Blood Pressure (Hypertension) Stage 1	130-39	or	80-89
High Blood Pressure (Hypertension) Stage 2	140 or higher	or	90 or higher
Hypertensive Crisis (consult your doctor immediately)	higher than 180	and/or	higher than 120

The Role of MHT: If you and your practitioner decide that a trial of hormone therapy is right for you, a critical part of their job will be determining the appropriate formulation based on your personal health status and relevant risk factors. When your doctor is considering the safest formulation of estrogen, it's extremely important that they look especially close at your risk factors for high blood pressure. The reason for this is that oral estrogen, delivered in a pill that you swallow, is metabolized in the liver and this process can lead to higher levels of certain proteins in the blood and create a procoagulant state in the bloodstream. The combined effect can lead to elevated blood pressure and increases risk of blood clot formation. If you have a personal or genetic history of clotting disorders or high blood pressure, this is an unwelcome risk.

Non-oral forms of systemic estrogen, such as skin patches, gels, or vaginal rings, bypass the liver and therefore don't carry the same risks. A study of more than one hundred thousand women, ages forty-five and older, taking oral estrogen hormone therapy for menopause found that estrogen ingested in pill form may be associated with an increased risk of high blood pressure compared with systemic transdermal and local vaginal estrogen.

Cholesterol

ABNORMAL LIPID METABOLISM

As women move through perimenopause and into postmenopause, many are surprised to hear their doctor say for the first time, "Your cholesterol is creeping up." In a lot of cases, they've been eating generally the same diet and following the same exercise routine, yet the numbers in their lipid panel begin to shift upward.

In my own clinical practice, I've seen this happen again and again. Women in their forties and early fifties come in for routine labs only to discover that their LDL cholesterol has suddenly spiked. I was one of these women when at the age of forty-eight my own cholesterol levels jumped unexpectedly. At the time, my reaction was the same as my patients': *This doesn't make any sense.* It wasn't until I dove into the research that I discovered estrogen plays a crucial role in regulating lipids, and we were all perimenopausal women with estrogen levels in flux. Abnormal lipid metabolism as a consequence made perfect sense. I only wished I had been taught about the correlation in medical school.

We do know that there is a relationship between estrogen and cholesterol—evidence has shown that cholesterol levels rise and fall slightly during the monthly menstrual cycle as estrogen levels change. A closer look at lipid function reveals that estrogen helps regulate how your body handles fats and works in ways that lower LDL and raise HDL. Estrogen acts as an antioxidant, too, so when it declines in menopause, LDL particles can more freely oxidize and become damaging to your arteries.

When estrogen declines, either gradually through perimenopause or suddenly through surgical menopause, you lose that protective balancing effect. The impact on the cholesterol levels you see reported in your lab work can be swift and dramatic.

Research has confirmed what I've seen in my patients: LDL cholesterol can increase by nearly 18.6 percent during the perimenopausal transition. That's not a small shift, it's a clinically meaningful one. One study published in the journal *Frontiers in Endocrinology* in 2025 found that a specific type of LDL called small dense low-density lipoprotein cholesterol (sdLDL-C) may serve as a reliable marker of shifting hormones in women. The researchers observed that sdLDL-C levels presented "a gradually and significantly upward trend in premenopause, perimenopause, and postmenopause women." The association was strong enough that we may one day be able to use sdLDL-C levels as a biomarker of perimenopause.

SWAN (the Study of Women's Health Across the Nation) confirmed, too, that, within just one year after the final menstrual period, LDL levels can rise significantly, no matter your age, race, or background. This study reported that postmenopausal women typically have an abnormal lipid profile across the board:

- higher total cholesterol
- higher LDL
- higher triglycerides
- often lower HDL

These changes directly raise your chances of developing heart disease, the number one killer of women. I've had patients who've never had an abnormal lab suddenly face a statin prescription. They're understandably confused and frustrated; no one warned them that perimenopause could do this.

This is why I've been working hard to promote the message that perimenopause is a *metabolic event*, not just a reproductive milestone. If we're not looking at the whole picture—including cholesterol, inflammation, blood sugar, and fat distribution—we're missing key opportunities to protect women's health.

AMH and Cholesterol

Emerging data shows that anti-Mullerian hormone (AMH), long used as a marker of ovarian reserve (the number and quality of eggs available), also holds important clues about a woman's long-term cardiometabolic health. In one of the most comprehensive longitudinal studies to date—SWAN—researchers followed more than 1,400 women from premenopause through postmenopause to examine how changes in AMH and estradiol affected their lipids and lipoproteins. What they found reinforces something I see every day in clinical practice: The hormonal shifts of midlife don't just influence symptoms; they also directly affect cardiovascular risk.

The decline in estradiol was associated with a distinctly more atherogenic lipid profile, including higher triglycerides, higher apolipoprotein B (a marker of artery-clogging lipoproteins), lower HDL cholesterol, and higher LDL cholesterol. In plain terms, as estradiol drops, the risk factors for heart disease increase. AMH, on the other hand, told a more complicated story. Women with lower AMH before menopause and those who experienced greater declines tended to have higher HDL cholesterol and apolipoprotein A-1, markers that have traditionally been viewed as protective. But we now understand that HDL cholesterol may become dysfunctional after menopause, losing its anti-inflammatory and cardioprotective effects. So what once looked like a positive signal may not be so simple.

The big picture is this: Both estradiol and AMH are shaping our metabolic landscape long before we hit menopause. The changes they can bring about are measurable, meaningful, and predictive of future risk. Once again, it becomes clear that perimenopause isn't just a hormonal nuisance; it's a window of opportunity for smarter screening, early intervention, and prevention that could change the entire trajectory of a woman's health.

Know Your Risks: You are at increased risk for high cholesterol if you have type 2 diabetes or familial hypercholesterolemia (FH), an inherited condition that causes very high levels of LDL, or if you are obese. Lifestyle factors, such as a diet high in red and processed meats and/or ultra-processed foods, low levels of physical activity, and smoking, will also put you at higher risk of having an abnormal lipid panel.

Know Your Numbers: Knowing your numbers is essential. I encourage every woman in perimenopause to get baseline labs and track changes over time. A standard lipid panel will check levels of total cholesterol, LDL cholesterol, HDL cholesterol, and triglycerides. Along with those tests, I recommend asking your practitioner to check apolipoprotein B (ApoB) and lipoprotein(a), referred to as Lp(a), as these are more specific for assessing risk of coronary artery disease.

The Role of MHT: If your levels of unhealthy cholesterol have increased, targeted lifestyle changes may be enough to lower them (see chapter 15 for effective strategies). If these efforts prove to be ineffective, hormone therapy or cholesterol-lowering medications may be appropriate. Women on menopause hormone therapy have been shown in research to experience, on average, a 12 percent reduction in LDL; if you are a candidate for MHT, it may be worth exploring this option. There is no one-size-fits-all approach, but there is power in being informed.

As a physician who's walked this road with thousands of patients and as a woman who's experienced it myself, I can tell you that your symptoms, your labs, and your instincts all matter. And when it comes to cardiovascular health, timing matters, too. Midlife isn't the time to look away. It's the time to pay close attention to yourself and, when needed, take action.

Liver Health

WHAT PERIMENOPAUSE HAS TO DO WITH LIVER HEALTH

The topic of liver health rarely comes up when we talk about perimenopause. But it should. The impact of estrogen loss on liver health can be significant and serious, and it can lead to increased risk of a condition called metabolic dysfunction–associated steatotic liver disease (MASLD) and its more severe form, metabolic dysfunction–associated steatohepatitis (MASH). These were formerly known as non-alcoholic fatty liver disease (NAFLD) and non-alcoholic steatohepatitis (NASH) but were renamed to reflect the systemic metabolic dysregulation and to focus on what the disease is versus what it is not.

Traditionally, MASLD has been considered a lifestyle-related condition associated with obesity and insulin resistance, but it's now increasingly being recognized as a hormonally influenced condition, particularly in perimenopausal and postmenopausal women.

Multiple studies have demonstrated that postmenopausal women are at significantly higher risk for MASLD than other subgroups. A review study published in the journal *Endocrinology* evaluated 541 people with biopsy-confirmed MASH and found that postmenopausal women had the highest rates of advanced liver fibrosis, more than men and more than premenopausal women. Even when researchers adjusted for age, ethnicity, and inflammation, the risk remained. Women over fifty were nearly twice as likely to have advanced fibrosis. This correlation is strongest in women who haven't received hormone therapy, underscoring the liver-protecting effects of estrogen.

An interesting aspect of the research was the fact that even lean postmenopausal women had a higher risk than lean premenopausal women, suggesting this isn't just about body fat; *it's about hormones.* I've seen evidence of this in my own clinic, where postmenopausal patients who are lean and active have come to see me with labs showing abnormal liver enzymes or imaging studies that reveal fatty liver. Many are shocked because they had never heard that menopause could affect their liver health.

Emerging evidence supports the idea that MASLD in women should be considered, at least in part, a hormone-sensitive condition, similar to osteoporosis or the genitourinary syndrome of menopause. In a 2021 review published in the journal *Maturitas*, researchers highlighted how estrogen deficiency, insulin resistance, dyslipidemia (high blood lipids), and sarcopenia (loss of muscle mass and strength) converge in postmenopausal women to increase MASLD risk and severity.

Estrogen plays a protective role in hepatic (taking place within the liver) lipid metabolism, insulin sensitivity, and inflammation control. The decline in circulating estradiol in perimenopause can lead to an increased accumulation of intrahepatic fat (fatty liver), promoting progression to MASLD and, in some cases, MASH.

Other factors that influence liver health in women include body fat distribution, reproductive history, age at first menstruation, and hormonal conditions like Turner's syndrome and PCOS. Women with PCOS continue to face a heightened risk for MASLD as they transition into menopause, independent of BMI, perhaps because they are already more likely to exhibit insulin resistance and androgen excess. There is a complex, sex-specific web of factors influencing liver health that we've only begun to untangle.

It has also been determined that gut microbiome alterations from estrogen loss may contribute to the development of MASLD. This is because estrogen deficiency can decrease levels of short-chain fatty acids (SCFAs) like butyrate, which are crucial for maintaining gut barrier integrity and regulating metabolic functions in the liver.

All this is to say that we have some compelling scientific evidence supporting the link between your hormones and liver health. Yet many women presenting with elevated liver enzymes, abdominal weight gain, or imaging evidence of fatty liver are diagnosed with MASLD without any consideration of hormonal status. More often than not, women in this case are given a default prescription of weight loss and lifestyle changes, which, while important, are frankly insufficient for women whose disease is driven by estrogen withdrawal, not just caloric excess or low levels of physical activity. In my clinical experience, women in perimenopause frequently present with normal weight or modest weight gain yet show significant accumulation of fat in the liver. They are often frustrated by the lack of progress despite their dietary diligence, because, again, the missing variable is hormonal regulation.

Adding to the seemingly never-ending supply of frustration and fury, there are no FDA-approved medications for MASLD. Right now, the main approach is managing the underlying metabolic risks, like insulin resistance, high cholesterol, and visceral fat. But there's a glaring gap: There are no sex-specific guidelines for MASLD, even though outcomes and risk factors differ significantly for women.

As clinicians, we must stop treating women as though their physiology simply mirrors that of men. And as women, we need more awareness, better screening, and personalized care. We deserve to know that perimenopause doesn't just change our hormones; it can change our liver, too.

Know Your Risks: Women who undergo early menopause—whether naturally or through oophorectomy (surgical removal of the ovaries)—have significantly increased risk of developing MASLD. If menopause happens before age forty, the risk of severe liver fibrosis increases by 90 percent compared with women who go through menopause later.

Other risk factors for MASLD include . . .

- family history of fatty liver disease or obesity

- high cholesterol or high triglycerides

- insulin resistance

- obesity, especially abdominal obesity

- polycystic ovary syndrome (PCOS)

- type 2 diabetes

- hypothyroidism

Know Your Numbers: Liver function tests measure enzymes and proteins in the blood to assess your liver health. The table below from the National Institutes of Health lists common liver function tests along with their normal ranges in adults, using conventional units (note: normal reference ranges vary between males and females and may be higher for those with a higher body mass index). These markers are typically checked as part of a comprehensive metabolic panel (CMP), which is usually ordered during an annual wellness exam.

TEST (FULL NAME)	NORMAL RANGE
Alanine transaminase	4 to 36 IU/L
Aspartate transaminase	5 to 30 IU/L
Alkaline phosphatase	30 to 120 IU/L
Gamma-glutamyltransferase	6 to 50 IU/L
Bilirubin	2 to 17 μmol/L
Direct bilirubin	0 to 6 μmol/L
Prothrombin time	10.9 to 12.5 seconds
Albumin	35 to 50 g/L
Total protein	60 to 80 g/L
Lactate dehydrogenase	50 to 150 IU/L
Note: Reference ranges may vary slightly among laboratories and can differ for men, women, and children. (Units—IU/L: international units per liter; μmol/L: micromoles per liter; g/L: grams per liter.)	

The Role of MHT: Lifestyle interventions remain foundational for MASLD management. However, in estrogen-deficient women, these lifestyle changes may not be fully effective unless the underlying hormonal imbalance is also addressed.

Evidence suggests that menopause hormone therapy may have a protective role in MASLD prevention and progression. In one study, women on estrogen therapy showed lower liver fat and improved insulin sensitivity. Additionally, phytoestrogens have been explored as an alternative for those who can't or don't want to use MHT, though results remain preliminary.

MHT shouldn't be prescribed to women in perimenopause solely for liver health, but if you are already considering hormone therapy for relief of vasomotor or genitourinary symptoms or to improve your mental health, the hepatic benefit may serve as an additional incentive to do a trial of hormone therapy.

How We Can Use Insight to Create Action

Understanding the metabolic syndrome of menopause is about more than naming a phenomenon. It's about changing how we care for women during one of the most vulnerable metabolic transitions of their lives. As a physician, I've seen the devastating consequences of missing this window and I've also seen the power of catching these changes early. The truth is, we're not screening women often enough or thoroughly enough for the metabolic shifts that happen in perimenopause and beyond.

Risk assessment is the first and most essential step. Too often metabolic issues like dyslipidemia or insulin resistance aren't picked up until they've already progressed to disease. It doesn't have to—nor should it continue—to be this way. The early signs are there long before a diagnosis of type 2 diabetes or cardiovascular disease is made. As I see it, clinicians and patients can get ahead of disease progression by monitoring metabolic markers and taking strategic action to prevent—and treat as needed—metabolic dysfunction.

Key Metabolic Markers to Monitor: Throughout this chapter, I've identified key markers of metabolic health that women entering perimenopause will want to monitor, and I'll summarize these here. Each year, aim to get . . .

- a comprehensive metabolic panel including fasting glucose, HbA1c, and liver function tests

- a HOMA-IR score to assess for early insulin resistance (optional but ideal)

- a body composition measurement—this is not just weight or BMI but a waist-to-hip ratio or a DEXA scan that can reveal levels of visceral fat present

- high-sensitivity CRP and sedimentation rate tests

- a blood pressure test

- a full lipid panel including LDL, ApoB, and Lp(a)

Strategic Actions to Prevent and Treat Metabolic Dysfunction: Some of the most powerful tools in supporting blood sugar and lipid metabolism and protecting arterial and heart health are lifestyle related. You can accomplish a lot of good by creating behavioral patterns that include regular exercise and nutrient-dense foods.

Physical activity, especially resistance training, is one of the most potent interventions we have. It can help preserve muscle mass, reduce chronic inflammation, improve insulin sensitivity, and counteract a shift toward visceral fat accumulation. I always tell my patients that lifting weights is one of the best things you can do for your metabolism in midlife, and that engaging in at least 150 minutes of moderate-intensity or 75 minutes of high-intensity cardio per week is also essential. We have, thankfully and finally, moved into an era in which women are encouraged to lift weights, and heavy weights at that, but routine cardio remains vital to your vascular system and can also help relieve stress.

Nutrition also plays a foundational role. Anti-inflammatory dietary patterns, which are rich in fiber, healthy fats, lean proteins, and phytoestrogens, can support metabolic health and ease the transition. Supplements like omega-3 fatty acids, vitamin D, magnesium, and flaxseeds have shown promise in both research and clinical practice.

These routine habits may seem humdrum, but let me tell you, my own dedication to these humble stalwarts of self-care has been transformative. I've never felt better since I started prioritizing strength building, cardiovascular exercise, and anti-inflammatory eating.

If you have lab work that reveals the metabolic syndrome of menopause, your strategic approach will shift from prevention to treatment and management. While physical activity and nutrition will remain critical, you will also need to create in partnership with your clinician a multifaceted and individualized approach. I will share what I've seen in the research and what has been effective in my patients.

Menopause hormone therapy: Beyond treating classic menopausal symptoms like hot flashes and night sweats, estrogen therapy has been shown to reduce inflammation, improve lipid profiles, and enhance insulin sensitivity. In fact, studies have demonstrated that estradiol can reverse the elevation of pro-inflammatory markers commonly seen after perimenopause, restoring balance to immune pathways that estrogen once kept in check. One randomized controlled trial published in *Atherosclerosis* showed that 17β-estradiol significantly improved both endothelial function and inflammatory profiles in postmenopausal women. These studies reinforce the value of MHT as a form of metabolic therapy and not just a symptom reliever. They also tell us that if we see metabolic markers jump in perimenopause, hormone therapy may be a component of correcting dysfunction before it progresses to more serious disease states. It's time we view metabolic syndrome not just through the lens of lifestyle (because this lens is often clouded over with judgment and bias) and see it clearly as dysregulation that can occur in response to the hormonal shifts that begin in perimenopause.

Of course, hormone therapy isn't appropriate for everyone, and it's not the only option.

GLP-1s: For women with more significant metabolic challenges, we now have emerging pharmaceutical options like incretin-based therapies (e.g., GLP-1s), which have been shown to reduce insulin resistance, lower inflammation, and, in some cases, produce weight loss of up to 30 percent when combined with lifestyle interventions. These therapies are reshaping how we approach metabolic care in women and may prove especially useful for those experiencing rapid visceral fat gain and declining insulin sensitivity after perimenopause.

It's Time We Recognize the Metabolic Syndrome of Menopause

The metabolic syndrome of menopause isn't a niche concept. It's a missing piece in the broader understanding of women's metabolic health. For decades, metabolic syndrome has been defined and studied largely through a male lens, with little regard for the role sex hormones play in shaping metabolic outcomes. But we can no longer afford to ignore the profound impact that estrogen loss has on fat distribution, glucose regulation, lipid metabolism, and inflammatory balance.

As women transition through menopause, they undergo a series of metabolic shifts that are biologically driven by hormone deprivation. Despite this, medical education continues to downplay or overlook the metabolic consequences of menopause, focusing instead on vasomotor symptoms and bone health. The result? Women with early signs of insulin resistance, dyslipidemia, or fatty liver disease go undiagnosed, untreated, and often blamed for not doing enough to manage their health.

In my clinical work and in my own menopause journey, I've seen how empowering it can be when women finally understand what's really happening in their bodies. When they realize their weight gain, rising cholesterol, or sudden fatigue is not a personal failure but a physiological response to estrogen loss, it changes everything. It opens the door to action, to options, to hope.

But systemic change is needed. Clinicians must be trained to recognize the metabolic shifts of menopause and initiate early screening and intervention. Researchers must prioritize studies that explore the sex-specific mechanisms of metabolic dysfunction, and guidelines must be updated to reflect these differences. We need sex-specific prediction models, precision therapies, and care pathways that consider the full complexity of a woman's hormonal and metabolic environment.

There is so much opportunity here. With early detection, targeted lifestyle interventions, appropriate use of MHT, and newer medications where needed, we can not only manage but also *prevent* much of the downstream disease associated with the metabolic syndrome of menopause. We can reduce cardiovascular events, delay or avoid the onset of diabetes, and otherwise support healthy aging for millions of women.

But first we have to name it. Teach it. Talk about it.

The metabolic syndrome of menopause is real. And it's time we treated it that way.

CHAPTER 8

Osteoporosis: The Debilitating Bone Disease That Starts Sooner Than You Think

After happily staying home with my daughters, I went back to work at forty. A few years in, I began to experience a variety of frustrating symptoms and saw specialists along the way without much improvement. It was very convenient to blame joint pain on sitting at a desk, and heart palpitations on work stress. UTIs were said to be due to female anatomy rather than estrogen loss. Sleep disturbances, weight redistribution, dry eyes, and serious scalp inflammation (leading to scarring hair loss) were blamed on "getting older."

It wasn't until the unexpected osteoporosis diagnosis at fifty-two (I was in menopause) that I really began to put things together. I began to dig deeper in my personal education about menopause. I began to pay more attention, ask more questions, and talk with more women about these things. It took many years for me to get comfortable with the idea of HRT. My doctor didn't push it, but looking back, I almost wish that she had! HRT isn't magic, but it has helped me a great deal!

—Marcie D.

Osteoporosis is the progressive bone disease that leads to thin and brittle bones and puts you at increased risk for fracture. It can be devastating and quite stealthy: It generally doesn't make itself known with pain or other symptoms in the early stages. It creeps in inconspicuously, weakening the architecture of the skeleton until one day a fracture becomes the first sign. And for women in perimenopause, that "one day" may arrive much earlier than anyone expects.

Most of us, including those in the medical field, have been led to believe that osteoporosis is an inevitable disease of old age, something to worry about decades after menopause. But the truth is far more urgent. Accelerated bone loss begins in perimenopause, during the years when women still have periods and often appear hormonally "normal" on lab work. If we're not looking for it, we'll miss it. And we *are* missing it—over and over again.

I've lost count of how many times I've had to deliver an osteoporosis diagnosis to a woman under the age of sixty-five. Almost without exception, the reaction is stunned confusion.

"But I'm active."
"I eat healthy."
"I take calcium and vitamin D."
"I lift weights."
"How is this possible?"

These are women who have done everything they believed they were supposed to do. They show up to their appointments having checked all the boxes—nutrition, exercise, supplements. Yet there it is on the DEXA body composition scan: osteoporosis. Not mild osteopenia. Not borderline findings. But true, high-fracture-risk osteoporosis. And nearly every time, it's discovered years before our current medical guidelines would have ever recommended screening.

As a clinician, these are some of the most difficult conversations I have. I see the disbelief in their eyes as they try to reconcile their commitment to health with a diagnosis that implies something has been silently slipping away beneath the surface. There is fear, grief, and, more than anything else, a sense of betrayal. They ask, "Why didn't anyone tell me to check my bones earlier?" And the honest answer is as frustrating as it is devastating. Our current screening recommendations for osteoporosis don't reflect the biological reality of perimenopause. They are rooted in outdated risk models and economic considerations, not in the lived experiences or emerging data that points to a far more urgent timeline for bone loss and fracture prevention.

The reality is that osteoporosis is far more common than many women are led to believe. For women over the age of fifty, the lifetime risk of sustaining an osteoporotic fracture is estimated to be between 40 and 51 percent. In other words, nearly one in two women in this age group will experience a fracture linked to low bone density during her lifetime. In the United States alone, more than eleven hundred women per one hundred thousand aged fifty-five and older are hospitalized each year for osteoporotic fractures.

These aren't rare or obscure statistics. They are an urgent public health signal. Vertebral (spine) fractures affect approximately 21 percent of postmenopausal women over the age of fifty, and the number climbs to nearly 50 percent in women over seventy-five. Among women who have already sustained a fracture, the risk of a second major osteoporotic fracture within the next five years exceeds 20 percent, with the most common sites being the hip, spine, forearm, and upper arm.

Despite this, many women won't be screened until their mid-sixties, unless they present with a prior fracture, extremely low body weight, or other classic high-risk features. But here's what the guidelines fail to account for: The most rapid loss of bone density often occurs in the years immediately surrounding menopause, when estradiol levels fall and bone resorption sharply increases. Women may lose up to 20 percent of their bone mass during this window. Yet because their calendar age is still considered young, their risk is ignored.

These women are often health conscious, proactive, and highly motivated. And still, the diagnosis comes. Not because they were doing something wrong, but because no one ever told them what to watch for. No one taught them that strength and structure must be preserved, not just for aesthetics or performance, but for survival. No one ever told them how closely bone health is intertwined with hormones. And no one said that prevention can't wait until they reach retirement age.

This is the system failing quietly. And by the time a woman hears her bones have become porous enough to carry a formal diagnosis, it has already failed her.

We must begin earlier. We must talk to women in their forties and early fifties about what is happening to their bones as their hormones shift. We must stop assuming that an active lifestyle is enough to protect against a silent disease that depends so heavily on timing and biology. And we must, once and for all, remove the false comfort that "feeling fine" means the skeleton is holding strong.

Because the truth is this: Osteoporosis is common. It's serious. And it's often preventable, if only we are willing to look for it.

When a Fracture Happens, We're Too Late

This isn't just professional for me. It's personal.

My mother fractured her hip at age eighty-seven and underwent a hip replacement. She never walked again. I was shocked to discover that she had never been screened for osteoporosis. No one had ever talked to her about bone density or warned her she was at risk. She wasn't told—nor were most women in her generation—that she could do something to protect the structural integrity of her bones so they could carry her through the final decades of her life with strength and dignity.

All she was ever told about her health was to eat less, take up less space, and weigh less. In other words, to "stay small."

The system failed her. And it nearly failed me, too.

In all my years of medical training, no one ever said it's critical that you teach your patients to preserve and even increase bone density. No one emphasized how essential it is to instruct women on maintaining muscle mass to avoid sarcopenia, a progressive decline in strength and function that often travels alongside osteoporosis and independently leads to disability.

Strength and function weren't part of the conversation. Frailty and hip fractures were things we were instructed to document, not to prevent. And here's the part that still shocks me: My mother's story isn't unique. It's tragically common.

Osteoporotic hip fractures in adults over sixty-five carry *a high risk of death;* even when surgery is performed, approximately *one-third of patients die within a year.* Surgical intervention does reduce mortality compared with no treatment at all, but outcomes are still heavily influenced by age, sex, co-morbidities, and, most critically, the condition of the bone itself at the time of the fall.

That is why we care. Because this isn't just about broken bones. It's about broken lives. It's about independence lost, pain endured, and futures cut short because we failed to prioritize prevention.

We can do better.

And women deserve better.

The system continues to fail millions of women by focusing on weight instead of strength and on screening timelines that don't allow for proactive intervention. Currently, the U.S. Preventive Services Task Force recommends that unless a woman has specific risk factors, bone density screening should start at age sixty-five. Unfortunately, a devastatingly low percentage of women above sixty-five do get this important scan: Just 26.5 percent, according to a large-scale analysis using data from more than 1.6 million women.* And these guidelines are outdated. They don't account for the accelerated bone loss that occurs during the menopause transition. The results: *Women are often left undiagnosed until after their first fracture,* an event that, in many cases, could have been prevented with earlier intervention.

This is one of the many ripple effects of the misinterpretation of the Women's Health Initiative study. After the early termination of the estrogen and progestin arm of the study in 2002 and flawed media coverage of its findings, the use of hormone therapy plummeted along with its protective effects on bone. Women who could have benefited from estrogen to maintain bone density (more on this later) were instead told to "ride it out," leading to a generation of fractures, surgeries, and lost independence.

We can't continue to rely on fracture as a diagnostic threshold; fractures severely affect quality of life and can create a significant physical, psychological, and economic burden. By the time a woman breaks a bone, the

---

* The same analysis showed that only 21.1 percent of women aged fifty to sixty-four were screened for osteoporosis, and even more concerning, screening rates *declined* by 31.4 percent among women in this age group between 2008 and 2014. Disparities were also significant: Non-Hispanic Black women were the least likely to be screened.

disease has already advanced. Screening must shift earlier and prevention must be reframed as *critical*, not optional.

My message to you in this chapter isn't based on fear; it's instead based on *power*. We now know how to intervene. Hormone therapy, when timed and personalized, can preserve bone density. Resistance training stimulates skeletal and muscular adaptation, with measurable gains even in women who start in midlife. Tools like DEXA scans, early biomarker screening, and weighted vests give us ways to monitor and act.

Yet most women still aren't told this. They're told to accept weakness and fractures as part of the deal. We must rewrite that narrative. The time to act is now in perimenopause, when everything is still so possible. This is your window, and you must not procrastinate on prevention.

The Relationship Between Bone Health and Hormones

Bone is living tissue. It's constantly being broken down and rebuilt in a delicate cycle known as remodeling. Throughout most of a woman's life, this cycle remains in balance, with old bone being resorbed by osteoclasts, the cells responsible for bone breakdown, and new bone being laid down by osteoblasts, the cells that build bone. But this balance depends heavily on estrogen. And during perimenopause, that hormonal anchor becomes less reliable.

Estrogen is a key regulator of the skeletal system. When estrogen levels start to fluctuate and decline as they do unpredictably in perimenopause, bone resorption starts to outpace bone formation. The result? A net loss in bone mass.

This loss isn't uniform throughout the skeleton. The lumbar spine and femoral neck (hip) are hit hardest, particularly because they're rich in trabecular (spongy) bone, which is more metabolically active and more sensitive to hormonal changes than cortical bone. These are also the areas most critical for mobility and the ones most vulnerable to debilitating fractures.

What's especially insidious is that bone loss begins while estradiol levels are still within the so-called normal range. In fact, studies using quantitative computed tomography imaging (QCT) have shown that up to 6.3 percent of trabecular bone density in the lumbar spine can be lost each year during perimenopause—*a rate faster than in early postmenopause.* Yet no standard clinical practice encourages us to check in this window. We're flying blind at the exact moment women need intervention the most.

A growing body of research shows that hormones other than estrogen may contribute to changes in the rate of bone remodeling in perimenopause.

Follicle-stimulating hormone (FSH). According to a review published in the *International Journal of Medical Sciences,* rising levels of FSH may be a cause of perimenopausal bone loss. As you may remember from chapter 2, an increasing amount of FSH is released from the brain as ovarian estradiol production becomes inconsistent in perimenopause. The process is still being unraveled, but it appears that the presence of high FSH may directly stimulate osteoclast formation and compound bone loss during the transition.

Progesterone. Progesterone, too, may ultimately prove to influence bone turnover in a more profound way than we realize. We know that progesterone collaborates with estrogen in bone formation and that there is an association between bone building and ovulation—specifically, that elevated progesterone in the luteal phase (triggered by ovulation) is osteoanabolic, or bone building. What we don't know yet is if progesterone changes in perimenopause lessen this building effect.

Anti-Mullerian hormone (AMH). AMH has emerged as a helpful marker of ovarian aging and bone loss risk. It declines gradually with diminishing ovarian reserve and has been shown to predict skeletal deterioration, even when estradiol is still in the normal range.

There's still so much that's not understood about the mechanisms involved in bone remodeling, and we need more science before these seeds of understanding can be broadly applied in ways that benefit patients in perimenopause and beyond.

The Hidden Architecture of Bone Loss—
and Why We Must Act Sooner

To understand the urgency of preserving bone in midlife, we first must understand when bones are at their strongest. Typically, women reach their maximum bone mineral density (BMD) in their mid-twenties, between ages twenty-two and twenty-six, and from that point on, bone becomes something we maintain rather than build. What we do in our thirties and forties matters because this is the phase of life when the body begins to withdraw from the bone "bank" and the losses accelerate sharply in perimenopause.

One of the most dangerous myths in women's health is that bone loss begins after menopause. It doesn't. As I've explained above, it begins long before most women, or their doctors, are paying attention. Data from longitudinal studies shows that, in early perimenopause, BMD in the lumbar spine declined by about 0.14 percent per year and in the femoral neck (hip) by 0.11 percent per year. But those numbers skyrocket as women approach their final menstrual period. In late perimenopause, bone loss in the spine can reach up to 6.3 percent annually, which is five to ten times the rate of bone loss that may be attributed to aging alone. This is far from subtle erosion.

By the time a woman reaches menopause, she may have already lost 10 to 20 percent of her total bone mass. And if no one told her what was happening or what to do about it, that loss continues into the early postmenopausal years. Eventually, it slows. But by then, the damage is done.

Let's talk about that damage. It's not just low bone density on a report. It's the thinning of your bones' internal scaffolding, which comprises trabecular or spongy bone. The degradation of this interior of your bones is a threat to the very structure that keeps you upright, balanced, and mobile. This is why fractures of the spine and hip steal independence, mobility, and, in some cases, life expectancy. These fractures may happen later in life, but the breakdown begins in perimenopause.

Yes, estrogen therapy after menopause can help. Studies show it can increase spinal BMD by up to 31 percent, preserve bone architecture, and cut fracture risk in half. *But why would we ever allow that bone to disappear in the first place?*

The bottom line is that once estrogen is gone, your body no longer turns up production of new bone cells. If you do nothing, what's left is a silent vulnerability that won't reveal itself until a fracture does.

This is why prevention must replace our current model of reaction. We can't afford to keep waiting until after the fall, after the scan, after the diagnosis. The work of protecting our bones must begin *before the damage is visible*, with strength training, high-quality protein, vitamin D, calcium, and, yes, for many women, hormone therapy started at the right time.

We don't want to rebuild. *We want to not lose it in the first place.*

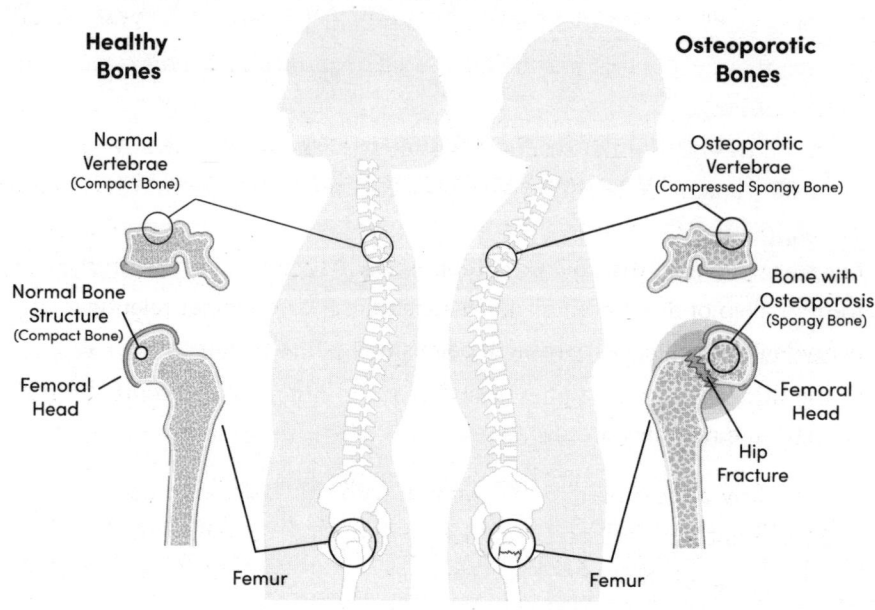

researchgate.net/figure/Comparative-view-of-normal-bone-osteopenia-and-osteoporosis-26-Reproduced-under-the_fig2_340836563

Bone Loss Progression

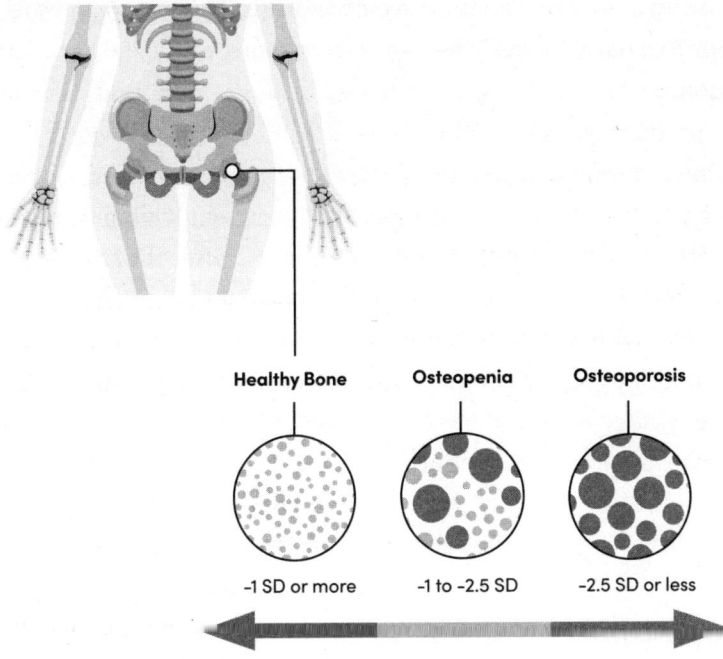

researchgate.net/figure/Comparative-view-of-normal-bone-osteopenia-and-osteoporosis-26-Reproduced-under-the_fig2_340836563

The Hidden Burden: Chronic Back Pain in Women with Osteoporosis

For many women, the pain of osteoporosis may not come first in the form of a hip or arm fracture—it will instead manifest itself as relentless, everyday back pain. Chronic back pain is one of the most common and overlooked symptoms of osteoporosis, especially in postmenopausal women. The numbers are striking:

- In a study of postmenopausal women with spinal osteoporosis, 63 percent reported persistent lumbar back pain and 62 percent reported persistent thoracic back pain.

- Among women aged sixty-five to seventy-five with osteoporosis, 75 percent reported back pain.

- In a rheumatology clinic setting, more than 52 percent of postmenopausal women with osteoporosis and back pain were found to have at least one vertebral fracture, often undiagnosed prior to imaging.

What makes this especially concerning is that pain isn't always explained by visible fractures. Spinal deformities, vertebral microdamage, and loss of mobility can all contribute to chronic discomfort—even when X-rays or DEXA scans don't reveal dramatic bone loss.

But of course, the consequences of chronic back pain in this population go well beyond pain, with documented links to increased fall risk and diminished quality of life. In many cases, it triggers a cascade of inactivity and loss of independence.

As clinicians, we must ask, Are we looking closely enough? Pain shouldn't be written off as "just part of aging." In the context of osteoporosis, it can be a red flag for vertebral fractures and an opportunity to intervene early with imaging, medications, physical therapy, and other support. We need to shift the focus from treating fractures to preventing them.

And this is where most of you reading this book come in—*you* are living in a moment that is rich in opportunity for prevention. It's heartbreaking to look at the number of women affected by osteoporotic back pain, even more so because it's avoidable. I want to do everything in my power to convince you that your only option is to take action now to create a different future for yourself, as pain and disability are not a certain fate. Read on for specifics about doing so.

A Revised Bone Screening Protocol Based on Reality

So, the question isn't if bone loss is occurring in perimenopause; it's how much, how fast, and how long we'll wait to intervene. The sooner we recognize that timeline, the sooner we can rewrite it.

To repeat, despite everything we know about how early and aggressive bone loss begins in perimenopause, our current screening practices remain anchored to a postmenopausal framework. By the time most women are offered a bone density scan at age sixty-five, many have already crossed the threshold into osteopenia or osteoporosis, often without symptoms.

This gap in care leaves many midlife women in a state of diagnostic limbo. We rely on age cutoffs when we should be thinking about hormonal status, symptoms, and physiology. A woman in her late forties with irregular cycles, vasomotor symptoms, and a family history of fractures may already be losing bone at a rapid rate, even if she doesn't yet meet formal screening criteria.

In light of the scientific insight I've sought out on bone health and my own clinical experience, I encourage all my patients to invest in bone density screening at any stage of menopause, starting at perimenopause. It's shocking how many women in their forties and early fifties who are still menstruating and are active, outwardly healthy individuals get diagnosed with low bone density—and these known diagnoses likely represent just the tip of the iceberg when we consider the low rates of screening in this demographic. The benefit of a diagnosis is that it often becomes a powerful motivator. When women can see the numbers, they're far more likely to act, whether that means starting or increasing strength training sessions, improving nutrition, or considering hormone therapy. Knowledge isn't just power; it's prevention.

This is where newer tools show promise. There is potential to use bone turnover markers as indicators of changing bone health. Bone turnover markers, such as serum osteocalcin and urinary N-telopeptide, rise sharply during perimenopause and could offer early insights into accelerated bone remodeling. Using these markers isn't yet standard practice, but in my opinion, it should be. They give us an opportunity to act earlier, to tailor prevention strategies to women before fractures occur, and to shift our approach from reactive to proactive.

A more effective screening paradigm would also consider what we know about variations in bone loss patterns based on genetics, race, and body composition. Research has shown that . . .

- Black women tend to have higher peak bone mass and a slower rate of bone loss, but when fractures do occur, they are more likely to be underdiagnosed and undertreated.

- Asian women often have smaller skeletal frames and lower baseline BMD, which can mask risk until significant loss occurs.

- Latina women may face higher rates of vitamin D deficiency and lower rates of screening.

- Thin women, regardless of race or ethnicity, are at higher risk because lower body weight is associated with less mechanical loading on bones and faster turnover.

Few of these differences are factored into the current osteoporosis guidelines, which recommend screening all women sixty-five and older and women under sixty-five who present one or more of the following risk factors: family history of hip fractures, smoking, excessive alcohol consumption, low body weight, and certain medical conditions or medications.

I think these screening guidelines overlook the long game of prevention we must play to preserve bone, and they most certainly miss the opportunity for early detection in late perimenopausal or early postmenopausal women.

This is why I encourage baseline DEXA scans for women in their late forties or early fifties—especially if they have any of the risk factors mentioned. The goal is to gain information, not find reasons for fear. In my practice, when women see numbers assigned to their bone loss through a DEXA scan, it becomes a powerful motivator because they are no longer dealing with theory; they are dealing with reality. They start lifting weights with intention and prioritizing calcium and vitamin D. They ask about hormone therapy. I witness firsthand how early detection changes their trajectory. These patients are given the opportunity to intervene before irreversible damage occurs. And that, to me, is the definition of good medicine.

What Is FRAX, and Where Does It Fit?

The FRAX (fracture risk assessment) tool was developed to estimate a person's ten-year probability of experiencing a major osteoporotic fracture such as a hip, spine, forearm, or shoulder fracture. The probability is calculated based on a combination of clinical factors, including age, sex, body mass index (BMI), personal and parental fracture history, smoking, alcohol use, glucocorticoid exposure, and other secondary causes of osteoporosis. Bone mineral density (BMD) at the femoral neck can also be added, though it's not required.

FRAX is widely used in clinical practice to help guide treatment decisions and determine when pharmacologic intervention may be appropriate. It's especially useful in cases where a woman's BMD is in the osteopenic range but additional risk factors elevate her fracture likelihood. If you have your bone density results, you can search for a FRAX calculator online and fill out the questionnaire to see your ten-year probability of a major fracture.

It's important to understand that FRAX was designed for and validated primarily in postmenopausal populations. It reflects long-term fracture risk but doesn't account for the hormonal shifts and rapid, short-term bone loss unique to perimenopause. As a result, it may underestimate risk in younger midlife women who are losing bone quickly but don't yet meet traditional criteria for high risk.

In my practice, I use FRAX as part of a broader risk assessment, not as the sole determinant of whether a woman should be treated. For women in perimenopause with concerning symptoms, family history, or early DEXA changes, FRAX can be informative, but it shouldn't be the only voice in the room.

Strategies to Support and Restore Bone Density

Once low bone density is identified, whether through a DEXA scan, bone turnover markers, or clinical history, the next step is decisive action. Bone loss doesn't have to be an inevitability of aging. It's a modifiable, biologically driven process with well-studied interventions. But timing is critical. Intervening during the rapid-loss phase of late perimenopause or early postmenopause offers the greatest opportunity to preserve bone mass and prevent fractures.

Bone isn't static scaffolding. It's dynamic, responsive tissue that is acutely sensitive to hormones, nutrition, and mechanical load. Which is why the most effective approach is layered: hormonal, pharmacologic, and lifestyle interventions working together to stabilize or rebuild bone.

Hormonal Interventions

Estrogen therapy is the most direct way to counteract the hormonal mechanisms driving bone loss. Estrogen suppresses bone breakdown in a couple of ways: It limits the formation of osteoclasts by regulating RANKL, a protein that plays a key role in osteoclast activity and survival, and it reduces cytokines like IL-1β, IL-6, and TNF-α, which promote the breakdown of bone (and are generally inflammatory). Estrogen additionally promotes activity and survival of osteoblasts, your bone-building cells, and improves bone microarchitecture by increasing trabecular bone volume and wall thickness.

Large-scale trials and meta-analyses have confirmed that HRT reduces the risk of vertebral fractures by up to 34 percent and hip fractures by 27 percent when initiated within ten years of menopause. Transdermal estradiol appears especially favorable for bone preservation, as it leads to consistent levels and has a lower risk for blood clots when compared with oral formulations.

In women with persistently low bone density despite estrogen therapy, or in those with symptoms of androgen deficiency such as low libido or fatigue, testosterone may offer additional benefit. Testosterone directly stimulates osteoblast proliferation and enhances bone formation. It also serves as a substrate for aromatization to estradiol, amplifying skeletal protection. Small studies have shown increased lumbar spine BMD in postmenopausal women using combination estrogen-testosterone therapy, though more long-term safety data is needed.

Non-Hormonal Pharmacologic Interventions

When HRT is contraindicated or if you just don't want to take it, several pharmacologic agents offer strong evidence for fracture prevention:

- **Bisphosphonates** (e.g., alendronate, risedronate, zoledronic acid) reduce osteoclast activity and lifespan and are well studied: Data shows 50 to 70 percent reductions in vertebral fractures and 40 to 50 percent reductions in hip fractures in women taking medications within this drug class. Long-term use, however, requires careful monitoring for rare side effects like atypical femur fractures and osteonecrosis of the jaw.

- **Denosumab** is a RANKL inhibitor that prevents osteoclast differentiation and activity. It has been shown to increase BMD more robustly than bisphosphonates and reduce both vertebral and nonvertebral fractures (fractures that occur outside the spine). It's particularly useful in patients with renal impairment or intolerance to oral bisphosphonates.

- **Selective estrogen receptor modulators (SERMs)** like raloxifene act as estrogen agonists (mimicking estrogen) in bone and antagonists (blocking estrogen) in breast and uterine tissue. They increase spinal BMD and reduce vertebral fracture risk but haven't shown significant protection against hip fractures.

- **Calcitonin,** while less potent, may be considered for women with painful vertebral fractures. It inhibits osteoclast function and may provide short-term pain reduction.

- **Anabolic agents** (e.g., teriparatide, abaloparatide) are typically reserved for women with severe osteoporosis or prior fragility fractures. These medications stimulate osteoblast activity and new bone formation but are used in limited durations because of cost and long-term safety concerns.

- **Romosozumab** is a monoclonal antibody that has shown promise as a dual-action drug: increasing bone formation and decreasing resorption. However, cardiovascular safety signals require individualized risk assessment.

Weighted Vests: A Simple Tool with Powerful Effects

Weighted vests may not look like cutting-edge medicine, but the science behind them is compelling. For midlife and postmenopausal women, especially those at risk for osteoporosis, a weighted vest can provide a safe, accessible way to simulate the bone-strengthening benefits of resistance and impact exercise.

The principle is simple: Mechanical loading stimulates bone formation. When you wear a weighted vest during everyday movements—walking, climbing stairs, or body-weight exercises—you increase gravitational stress on the skeleton, prompting osteoblast activity and helping maintain bone mineral density.

Studies support the use of weighted vests:

- A five-year trial found that postmenopausal women who performed jump training while wearing weighted vests maintained hip bone density and significantly reduced their fracture risk.

- A twelve-week intervention combining weighted vests with resistance training showed reductions in bone resorption markers and improvements in muscle strength.

- The INVEST (Incorporating Nutrition, Vests, Education, and Strength Training) trial is currently evaluating whether weighted vests can mitigate bone loss during intentional weight loss in adults ages sixty to eighty-five. The results of this study may provide a scalable and evidence-based approach to pursuing metabolic health *and* maintaining bone strength in midlife as well as old age.

Weighted vests may also improve balance, proprioception, and functional strength, all of which are critical for preventing falls. Studies have shown that women who exercised while wearing a weighted vest demonstrated greater postural stability and lower-extremity strength than those who didn't.

Here are some important considerations if you want to select a weighted vest for yourself:

- Choose a vest with adjustable weights so you can increase the load gradually over time. Most protocols suggest starting with 3 to 5 percent of your body weight and working up to at least 10 percent. However, research in older women shows that bone benefits typically don't appear until the load reaches 10 percent of ideal body weight.

- Use the vest during low-impact activities or strength training, not during high-impact cardio.

- Avoid use if you have spinal compression fractures or a history of fragility fractures, severe balance impairments, or other conditions that limit safe movement.

For many of my patients, this simple tool becomes a daily cue to focus on strength, balance, and bone health. It's low tech but grounded in powerful physiological benefits. In the right context, a weighted vest isn't just gear, it's a strategic tool for prevention. I wear mine during everyday activities like walking on the treadmill while working, taking the dog out, and doing chores. It adds load to movements I'm already doing. But to be clear, I don't use it as a replacement for resistance training. It's a supplement, not a substitute.

Lifestyle Interventions: Foundations of Long-Term Bone Health

Even with the most effective medications, lifestyle strategies are essential and can be particularly effective in midlife when bone remodeling is most active:

- **Weight-bearing and resistance exercises** introduce mechanical loading or force on bones, which stimulates osteogenesis. Wolff's law, an anatomical law developed by German surgeon Julius Wolff in the nineteenth century, tells us that bone adapts to the loads placed on it—and that increased loading is what will cause bones to strengthen. This is why early and consistent resistance training matters, not just for aesthetics, but for survival.

    We tend to think of resistance training as something we do solely for the sake of our muscles, but muscle and bone are intimately connected and often work as one unit. Your bones have rigid levers within them to which muscles attach and apply force. Every time you lift, push, pull, or bear weight, your muscles are placing tension on your bones. This mechanical stress is what signals your bones to maintain and even increase their density.

    Research consistently shows that resistance training is one of the most effective ways to preserve or even improve bone mineral density (BMD)—especially at critical sites like the spine and hips. Programs that include impact loading (such as jumping or heel drops) and progressive resistance training are especially effective and have been shown to increase BMD at these clinically relevant sites. The LIFTMOR trial, for instance, demonstrated significant improvements in lumbar spine and femoral neck BMD in postmenopausal women performing high-intensity resistance and impact training.

- **Calcium and vitamin D** are critical co-factors for bone mineralization. Women aged fifty and older should aim for 1,200 mg of calcium daily, ideally from food sources, and maintain a 25(OH)D level (this is how it will appear on lab work) of at least 30 nanograms/milliliter. Supplementation should be individualized to avoid excess intake, especially in women at risk for kidney stones or vascular calcification.

- **Protein intake** is often overlooked in bone health. Adequate protein supports muscle mass (which provides mechanical loading) and collagen synthesis within bone. Your individual protein needs vary based on your lean muscle mass percentage, a number you can obtain from a body scan. In my clinic, my recommendation to patients varies based on scan results. For women with normal to above average muscle mass, I suggest a daily intake of 1.2 to 1.5 grams of protein per kilogram (0.54 to 0.68 grams per pound) of ideal body weight. For those who have low muscle mass or are even sarcopenic, a higher intake of 1.5 to 1.8 grams of protein for every kilogram of ideal body weight (0.68 to 0.82 grams per pound) is recommended.

- **Avoidance of smoking and moderation of alcohol, along with prioritization of restorative sleep,** are also modifiable lifestyle factors that influence bone turnover and repair.

It's Yours to Protect

We possess the ability to eliminate a considerable number of osteoporosis risk factors and to achieve and maintain normal peak bone mass—yet medicine has historically and consistently failed to provide adequate clinical emphasis on the finite window of bone preservation. Women simply haven't been and are still not being given the message that they must concentrate early-in-life efforts on achieving skeletal security. The result is that we are all left to play a dangerous game of catch-up, with devastating consequences if we lose. The good news is that you don't have to lose—your bone density is yours to keep if you start now on supportive strategies.

CHAPTER 9

Sarcopenia: The Muscle Loss No One Warned You About

When I was thirty-seven, my younger daughter was three and we thought about trying for a third. As I paid attention to my cycle, I realized it was not as regular as it had been in the past. After a few months, my doctor did blood work, which showed I was perimenopausal! I was "hormone therapy averse" at the time and ignored the many symptoms that I now connect to perimenopause: poor sleep, brain fog, poor memory, irritability, fatigue, plus the obvious ones like low libido, vaginal dryness/atrophy, belly fat, and hot flashes. My doctor mentioned prescribing hormone therapy to protect my heart, bones, and brain, but at that age I felt like those things didn't apply to me. Along with dealing with many of the above symptoms all this time, I was diagnosed with osteoporosis at fifty-three. I *finally* started MHT ten months ago to protect my bones, brain, and heart. I had no idea that most of the things I dealt with would have improved—I wish I had paid more attention twenty years ago. My story would be different.

—Wendy C.

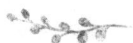

If osteoporosis is the silent thief of our skeleton, sarcopenia is its equally insidious accomplice that steals muscle, strength, and function. Throughout my medical education, I was taught that muscle loss is just part of aging and that it's something gradual yet inevitable that leads to frailty in our seventies or eighties. This narrative couldn't be more wrong. The path to sarcopenia doesn't start in old age. It starts in perimenopause.

You may notice it only in very subtle ways at first. Your clothes might fit a little differently, and things like carrying groceries could start to feel slightly more difficult. Your usual workouts leave you sore for days. And somewhere within this shift, often while you're still trying to manage hot flashes, sleep issues, brain fog, and mental health changes, you realize you feel *weaker*. It's more than just feeling tired or unmotivated; you feel physically less capable than you did just a few years ago.

What I've come to understand, both from the research and from listening to thousands of women in various stages of menopause, is that this loss of strength isn't just aging; it's hormonal. The same hormonal transition (that is, declining levels of estrogen) that erodes bone density also begins to degrade skeletal muscle long before we would ever call it "frailty," which is the medical term a doctor would apply to a state of increased vulnerability defined by muscle weakness and other functional declines.

Yet no one talks about this. We don't routinely measure lean body mass. We don't warn women that muscle is at risk. We don't teach them that muscle isn't just for aesthetics or metabolism; it's foundational to their long-term independence.

Which is why I'm making sure to talk to you about it now with the same sense of excitement and urgency as though I were delivering this message to my own daughters. I want you to know about the science of muscle loss in midlife women, the hormonal and inflammatory pathways involved, and the tools we now have to intervene. Because just like with bone, early awareness and action can change the trajectory. When we talk about aging well (an arc that begins now), we're not just talking about hormones or hot flashes. We're talking about preserving *function*.

And muscle is central to that story.

Estrogen's Muscle Blueprint

Muscle tissue—like bone, brain, and cardiovascular systems—is densely interconnected with estrogen signaling, which is to say a lot of cellular activity is taking place in which estrogen is essential. During perimenopause and menopause, when estrogen levels begin to fluctuate and eventually decline, this loss of hormonal input triggers a cascade of molecular changes that contribute to muscle loss, weakness, and delayed recovery. This isn't just aging; it's endocrine disruption at the cellular level.

Estrogen receptors (ERα and ERβ) are present throughout skeletal muscle, particularly in satellite cells, the stemlike cells responsible for muscle regeneration. Under normal hormonal conditions, estradiol promotes satellite cell activation and proliferation, supporting muscle repair and adaptation following exercise or injury. But during the menopause transition, as estradiol levels fall, satellite cell activity decreases, impairing the muscle's ability to regenerate and respond to anabolic stimuli like strength training.

In midlife women, the body not only loses muscle mass but also reduces the capacity to rebuild it. And with these losses, the downward slope toward sarcopenia is initiated.

Estrogen also plays a critical role in mitochondrial function within muscle cells. Mitochondria are responsible for generating adenosine triphosphate (ATP), the energy currency of muscle contraction and endurance. Estradiol enhances mitochondrial biogenesis and efficiency, reduces oxidative stress, and supports muscle endurance and recovery. When estrogen declines, mitochondrial dysfunction can occur, leading to decreased energy availability, increased fatigue, and slower post-exercise recovery—all of which make consistent movement and resistance training more difficult to maintain.

In addition, estradiol has anti-inflammatory effects within skeletal muscle. It suppresses the production of pro-inflammatory cytokines like IL-6 and TNF-α and promotes the expression of protective heat shock proteins and antioxidant enzymes. This hormonal buffering limits muscle damage and accelerates repair. Without it, systemic inflammation rises, muscle catabolism accelerates, and insulin sensitivity declines—all of which contribute to the metabolic derailment many women experience during perimenopause.

Many studies have reported 15 to 20 percent reductions in muscle mass and strength after the loss of ovarian function, with clear declines in satellite cell number, mitochondrial density, and protein synthesis. To wit, postmenopausal women consistently show reduced type II (fast-twitch) muscle fiber area, decreased peak force output, and lower lean mass compared with premenopausal women, even after adjusting for physical activity and age.

One longitudinal study, the Study of Women's Health Across the Nation (SWAN), found that women lost an average of 1 to 2 percent of lean body mass per year during the menopausal transition—most of it from the legs and trunk, areas that are critical for mobility, stability, and fracture prevention. These losses often go unnoticed until the emergence of functional deficits, such as difficulty rising from a chair, climbing stairs, or balancing on one foot.

And just as with bone, the timing of intervention matters. Hormone therapy initiated during the early postmenopausal window has been shown to preserve lean mass and improve muscle quality. Randomized controlled trials have shown that transdermal estradiol may help reduce muscle loss and improve strength, especially when combined with resistance training. Replacing estrogen alone isn't a miracle. It can buy you about a three-year window of opportunity, but after that, you go back to age-related decline. Hormonal signaling and mechanical loading, however, appear to have a synergistic effect. This is why it's imperative to focus on resistance training as a complementary tool in maintaining muscle tissue.

Despite all this, muscle is rarely discussed during perimenopause care. We measure weight but not composition. We encourage walking but rarely prescribe resistance training. And we tell women that fatigue, weakness, and overall physical decline are just natural parts of getting older, when they're often hormonal symptoms with modifiable roots.

Estrogen was never *just* about reproduction. It was the architect of muscular strength, regeneration, and endurance. When these recede, we need to recognize what's been lost and take strategic steps to preserve what we still have.

Sarcopenia and the Metabolic Domino Effect

Loss of muscle mass during the menopause transition sets off a domino effect that has an impact on nearly every aspect of a woman's health. From glucose regulation to fat distribution to inflammation, muscle is so much more than mechanical tissue. It's a metabolic organ, and its decline is central to the rise in cardiometabolic disease we see in women after menopause. In fact, as you'll see, it's tied to many of the metabolic disruptions outlined in chapter 7.

Skeletal muscle is the largest reservoir for glucose uptake in the body, which means it's responsible for pulling glucose from your bloodstream and putting it to use in tissues. So, it plays a critical role in maintaining insulin sensitivity and regulating blood sugar levels. As lean mass declines, it takes with it the capacity to clear glucose readily from the bloodstream. The result is fewer GLUT4 transporters—proteins that respond to insulin—in muscle cells and reduced mitochondrial efficiency, making room for insulin resistance to move in. In a lot of ways, this is what opens the metabolic door to unexpected weight gain, central adiposity (belly fat), and prediabetes during perimenopause even when your diet and exercise habits haven't changed.

This redistribution of body fat isn't just aesthetic. Loss of muscle mass is strongly associated with increased visceral fat, the metabolically active fat that I discussed in detail in chapter 7, which is stored around the abdominal organs and contributes to systemic inflammation, dyslipidemia (abnormal levels of lipids in the blood), and elevated cardiovascular risk. Several studies have shown that low muscle mass is an independent predictor of cardiovascular disease and mortality in postmenopausal women, regardless of BMI.

Adding to the shift in the metabolic milieu is the role of myokines, the signaling molecules secreted by skeletal muscle during contraction. These include anti-inflammatory cytokines like IL-15, irisin, and brain-derived neurotrophic factor (BDNF)—all of which support healthy metabolism, immune modulation, and even cognitive resilience. As muscle mass and activity decline, the production of these protective compounds diminishes. The result is a trend toward a more pro-inflammatory, insulin-resistant internal environment that accelerates aging across multiple systems.

The takeaway here is that these changes aren't isolated. They are hormonally mediated, deeply interconnected shifts in physiology that begin during perimenopause and—if left unaddressed—accumulate into chronic disease.

Muscle is medicine. It's glucose disposal, anti-inflammatory signaling, mitochondrial resilience, and physical autonomy wrapped into one tissue. Losing it isn't just a loss of strength—it's a loss of metabolic health and, with it, a loss of agency over how we age.

Dr. Gabrielle Lyon has called muscle "the organ of longevity," a phrase that couldn't be more accurate. In *Forever Strong*, she argued persuasively that skeletal muscle should be the starting point of preventive health in midlife, not an afterthought. I agree, and I would add that, for women, not only is muscle a longevity tool; it's also the key to strength, function, and self-trust during a time when so much feels out of our control.

Dr. Vonda Wright's book *Unbreakable* has also reshaped the conversation, reframing midlife not as the beginning of decline but as the ideal moment to invest in musculoskeletal resilience. Her concept of the musculoskeletal syndrome of menopause (see sidebar) is a call to action. In my own practice every day, women are asking not just how to look better but how to stay upright, independent, and powerful in the decades to come.

What makes sarcopenia especially challenging is that it often develops silently. It's not captured on a routine lab test. You don't see it on a scale. And unless a woman is undergoing serial body composition testing with DEXA or bioimpedance (the low-level electrical current used in InBody scans), her lean mass could be declining for years, even decades, before it leads to functional limitations or a serious fall.

The good news is that muscle loss is *reversible*. Unlike bone, where density is harder to rebuild, muscle responds rapidly to the right stimuli. With progressive resistance training, adequate protein intake, and—when appropriate—hormonal support, women can regain strength, improve body composition, and shift their metabolic trajectory.

But we have to act early. Waiting until muscle loss reaches clinical sarcopenia, when falls occur, when physical therapy is prescribed, when independence is already compromised, is far too late. The time to protect muscle isn't at seventy. It's in your thirties, forties, and fifties, when the first metabolic cracks begin to form.

The Musculoskeletal Syndrome of Menopause

The phrase *the musculoskeletal syndrome of menopause,* introduced by orthopedic surgeon and researcher Dr. Vonda Wright, reframes what many women experience in midlife: a progressive loss of bone, muscle, and functional strength—driven not just by aging but by hormonal decline.

This syndrome isn't formally recognized in most medical guidelines, but it's *very real* to the millions of women navigating it every day. What makes it so important is that it connects the dots between three systems that are often treated in isolation: the skeletal, muscular, and metabolic. Estrogen supports all three. As it declines during perimenopause, we see . . .

- accelerated bone resorption, leading to osteopenia and osteoporosis
- reduced satellite cell activity and protein synthesis, driving muscle atrophy
- changes in body composition, including increased visceral fat and decreased lean mass, which alter balance, mobility, and glucose control

Dr. Wright argued, in her 2024 research study published in the journal *Climacteric,* that these aren't just separate symptoms; they're part of a larger, interconnected syndrome that deserves proactive treatment. And she's right.

We don't screen for lean mass loss. We rarely measure functional strength. We wait until a fracture or fall occurs to intervene. But this approach is reactive, and by the time disability emerges, much of the damage has already been done. We need to be proactive instead.

Recognizing the musculoskeletal syndrome of menopause as a clinical entity allows us to shift from a treatment model to a prevention model. It means screening earlier. Prescribing resistance training like we prescribe medication. Supporting protein intake with the same urgency as calcium. And talking to women about muscle and bone health before they lose it.

Dr. Wright's work is part of a growing movement, alongside voices like Dr. Gabrielle Lyon and Dr. Abbie Smith-Ryan, that's redefining what women's health looks like in midlife. Dr. Smith-Ryan's research in exercise physiology and body composition has illuminated how resistance training and targeted nutrition strategies, particularly protein distribution and creatine supplementation, can help women preserve lean mass and metabolic function throughout the menopause transition.

This is the future of midlife medicine: not just preserving appearance, but protecting performance by securing muscle, movement, metabolism, and independence. See yourself in *this* future, not the present reality that plagues so many women living in later life today.

Strategies to Build and Preserve Muscle in Perimenopause and Beyond

You are not destined for a future defined by fraility simply because you were born with ovaries. Muscle is one of the most responsive tissues in the human body, and midlife isn't too late to intervene. With the right strategies, women can build and maintain lean mass, improve strength and mobility, and reduce their risk of disability, metabolic dysfunction, and loss of independence in later life.

The solution isn't singular. It's layered: movement, nutrition, and, when appropriate, hormonal support. The earlier we begin, the greater the impact. Let's explore the most effective muscle building and sustaining strategies.

Resistance and Functional Training

If estrogen withdrawal is the signal for muscle breakdown, mechanical loading is the antidote. Strength training is the most effective intervention we have to counteract sarcopenia. It stimulates satellite cell activation, upregulates muscle protein synthesis, and improves neuromuscular coordination, balance, and power.

The data is unequivocal. Studies show that twice-weekly progressive resistance training—using free weights, machines, or even body weight—can significantly increase lean mass, muscle strength, and functional performance in women over forty. In fact, postmenopausal women following resistance programs gain an average of two to four pounds of lean mass over twelve to twenty-four weeks, even in the presence of hormonal decline. (I know firsthand how counterintuitive it can feel to want to gain weight, but trust me—muscle building requires work, not magic, and you will feel so empowered as you witness your work transform into results. Not to mention, you will notice the strength, mobility, and energy benefits.)

Your focus with resistance training should be on consistency and progression; muscle adapts when it's challenged. When it isn't, it atrophies. Here are some points to consider in your workouts:

- High-load, low-repetition formats (lifting heavier weights for four to six reps) and moderate-load, higher-repetition formats (eight to twelve reps) have both been shown to be effective.

- Incorporating compound functional movements such as squats, lunges, rows, and loaded carries, translates directly to improved real-world strength and stability. These movements go beyond the goal of preserving muscle mass and specifically work to reduce fall risk, prevent fractures, and sustain the ability to live independently.

- Balance and power-based training (like kettlebell swings, box steps, or short plyometrics) may also be added, especially for women at risk of falls. Even simple interventions like walking with a weighted vest can increase lower-extremity strength and bone loading (see sidebar in chapter 8 for more on weighted vests).

The key isn't intensity at all costs. It's introducing an individually appropriate degree of challenge over time. This isn't always possible to accomplish on your own—that is, not everyone is built with the innate ability to push themselves through fitness progress or to even know what that looks like as it relates to muscle development. Group classes, workouts with friends, and/or an investment in personal training sessions may be necessary, and could introduce a bonus of fun to your pursuits.

Nutritional Interventions

Muscle is built in the gym, but in order to maintain it, we must align our nutrition intake with our physical efforts and implement strategic supplementation when appropriate. I encourage all women to pay attention to . . .

- **Protein intake.** This is a cornerstone of preserving muscle, yet most midlife women consume too little and distribute it poorly across meals. The current recommended dietary allowance of 0.8 g/kg/day is insufficient for preserving lean mass in women as they age. A growing body of evidence supports a target of 1.2 to 1.6 g/kg/day, divided across meals to optimize muscle protein synthesis. This means approximately twenty-five to thirty grams of protein *per meal* for most women—a threshold required to maximally stimulate the mTOR pathway (the regulator of cell growth) and muscle development.

- **Leucine.** Leucine is an essential amino acid that plays a particularly important role in initiating muscle protein synthesis. Including high-leucine sources—such as eggs, dairy, meat, soy, and whey protein—can help overcome age-related anabolic resistance.

- **Creatine monohydrate.** This is a compound made up of three amino acids that occurs naturally in the muscle tissues of the body. Long studied in athletes, creatine has emerged as one of the most promising evidence-based supplements for muscle health in women as they age. Dr. Abbie Smith-Ryan's research has been instrumental in shifting this conversation. Her work has shown that creatine supplementation in postmenopausal women, at doses of three to five grams per day, enhances lean mass gains and increases muscular power when paired with resistance training. Creatine may also support cognitive performance and bone density, offering a uniquely broad range of benefits during the menopause transition.

For women hesitant to start resistance training because of fatigue or slow recovery, creatine can make a meaningful difference. And unlike some supplements marketed to midlife women, its benefits are backed by high-quality, peer-reviewed trials.

- **Micronutrients.** Vitamin D (for muscle function and fall prevention) and magnesium (for muscle contractility and recovery) should also be optimized.

I must point out that some of these nutritional efforts will directly conflict with the message women still receive in midlife: that eating less is the answer to the metabolic dysregulation so many of us experience during this stage. Not only is this messaging inaccurate, but it can also be metabolically counterproductive: Inadequate nutritional intake may lead to the loss of vital muscle tissue. I prefer to promote eating smarter: Prioritize protein, making an intentional plan to eat an adequate serving of it with each meal, fill the rest of the plate with plants, and support your efforts on the plate with evidence-based supplementation when needed, not to replace effort, but to enhance response.

Menopause Hormone Therapy

Menopause hormone therapy isn't a substitute for training or nutrition, but it can be a valuable complement to your efforts in those areas.

Estrogen supports satellite cell function, mitochondrial efficiency, and post-exercise recovery. And some studies show that early initiation of estrogen therapy (within ten years after menopause) may modestly slow the loss of lean body mass in the short term, but this effect is small and not sustained over the long term. A review of forty-three studies on MHT (estrogen alone, estrogen and progestogen/progesterone, or tibolone) and sarcopenia published in June 2025 reported that while hormone therapy didn't have a negative effect on muscle, there was no consistent evidence to show that it improved muscle strength or mass in midlife women.

Transdermal estradiol, however, appears effective when paired with resistance training, as the combination seems to amplify anabolic responses and improve muscular adaptation in early menopause. What this makes very clear is that while MHT may be a tool in supporting muscle preservation, it should certainly not be the *only* tool.

Testosterone also deserves consideration. Women with low free testosterone may benefit from physiologic replacement, especially if they are experiencing fatigue, low libido, or persistent muscle loss despite intervention. Testosterone enhances muscle protein synthesis, increases neuromuscular efficiency, and improves body composition when dosed appropriately.

Testosterone and Muscle Health

Testosterone is often dismissed as a male hormone, but in women, it plays a crucial role in muscle maintenance. It's a key regulator of skeletal muscle mass, strength, and function. During midlife, women begin to experience a slow but steady decline in free testosterone, which accelerates in the years following menopause. This hormonal shift contributes to sarcopenia.

Clinical trials of physiologic testosterone therapy in postmenopausal women have demonstrated increases in lean body mass, reductions in fat mass, and improvements in muscle strength and physical function. One randomized controlled trial showed that women using transdermal testosterone for twenty-four weeks experienced a 2.1 percent increase in lean mass and improved leg-press strength, even at low doses designed to restore premenopausal androgen levels.

These findings suggest that testosterone therapy may be an important tool in addressing the musculoskeletal syndrome of menopause.

It isn't for everyone, and careful baseline and follow-up monitoring is essential. Testosterone should be prescribed only in doses that bring levels into the physiologic female range, and signs of androgen excess, such as acne, excess hair growth, or voice deepening, should prompt dose adjustment or discontinuation.

Still, for women with low testosterone symptoms, persistent sarcopenia, or bone loss unresponsive to estrogen therapy alone, this hormone deserves more attention. It isn't about replacing youth; it's about preserving strength, structure, and the freedom to age well.

While more data is needed on long-term outcomes, the current evidence supports a personalized, early, and physiology-informed approach to MHT for women concerned about strength and function.

The clinical take-home message on muscle is this: We screen for bone loss but not muscle loss. We track weight but not strength. And we tell women they're healthy as long as their BMI is within range—ignoring that two women with the same weight can have vastly different health outcomes depending on their lean mass and muscle quality. That needs to change.

In my clinic, we've started using a body composition scanner, which allows us to measure visceral and subcutaneous fat and make an essential assessment of each individual's muscle mass. Establishing this baseline is critical to staying on top of our efforts to increase patient awareness through meaningful markers and to highlighting any gaps in our strategic approach to lengthening health span. I hope this practice comes to be a part of standardized care for women in perimenopause.

Every woman deserves a strength plan as part of her approach to long-term health. Muscle isn't optional; it's protective, functional, and deeply modifiable. The earlier we intervene, the more we preserve—not just for aesthetics or metabolism, but for dignity and independence.

CHAPTER 10

Dreaming of Sleep in Perimenopause

I was in perimenopause by age thirty-eight, but I didn't know it. When I went to my OB-GYN teary-eyed and struggling both mentally and physically, I was referred to a psychiatrist and orthopedist. I was told I needed to work on my relationship with my husband as a response to my loss of sex drive. I was made to feel I had chemical imbalance and placed on psych meds when I began having what I now know are night sweats and insomnia. My mood swings would come out of nowhere and create so much drama. They revolved around my erratic periods that had always been so predictable. I developed pain in my hips and back, had a frozen shoulder, and was told this was all normal—I needed to exercise and stretch more (I have always been athletic). I was told I must be eating differently to have gained fifteen pounds—I was not. In a nutshell, I was gaslit through one of the most challenging transitions in my life by many doctors who should have known better, should have listened to me, and should have helped me put the pieces together.

—Caroline H.

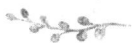

When patients tell me, "I've never had sleep problems in my life," I nod because I hadn't either. Indeed, before perimenopause, I never thought twice about sleep. I'd fall asleep easily, stay asleep, and wake up rested. But as my hormones began to shift, so did my nights. It started with occasional tossing and turning. Then came the full-body heat surges, the night sweats, the damp sheets—and always the 3 A.M. wake-up. Eyes open. Heart pounding. Mind racing. No clear trigger. Just wide awake in the middle of the night, night after night.

Once I started hormone therapy, the hot flashes subsided. The night sweats were gone. But that 3 A.M. wake-up? Still there. That was the part no one had warned me about.

And this is what I now tell my patients: Even with hormone therapy and even when it's working beautifully to address other symptoms, your sleep routine doesn't always snap back to how it used to be. Estrogen and progesterone play a major role in regulating the systems that support deep, continuous sleep, and shifting hormones during perimenopause and menopause can disrupt sleep's entire architecture. And once disturbed, that architecture often takes consistent, intentional effort to rebuild. Restoring hormones isn't the magic reset button we wish it could be, especially if other underlying causes are contributing to a pattern of chronically poor sleep.

As a woman in postmenopause, I know that I have to be religious about protecting my sleep. I guard my bedtime routine the way I used to do with my kids' nap schedules. I've learned that if I choose to drink alcohol, I'm also choosing not to sleep. That glass of wine might feel like a reward, but it almost guarantees I'll be staring at the ceiling at some point in the darkness of the night, well before sunrise. And I'm not alone; many of my patients and followers share this exact experience.

Research and data make it very clear: Perimenopause may be the moment when sleep starts to unravel. But it can also be the wake-up call we need to rebuild a relationship with rest and to create a non-negotiable plan for getting quality sleep.

In perimenopause, the brain becomes more sensitive to disruption. When we look at the changing hormonal environment, it's clear why sensitivity increases so profoundly. Less reliable ovulation reduces progesterone, which has a pronounced calming effect on the nervous system. Declines in estrogen lead to diminished melatonin production and cause cortisol spikes that are out of sync with your circadian clock. Without reliable hormonal buffering, anything that agitates the system—stress, sugar, alcohol, or screen time—can send sleep spiraling. Even when vasomotor symptoms (night sweats) are under control, your tendency toward early-morning waking can linger.

As women, we've learned to deprioritize our sleep needs and take pride in our ability to endure a subpar state of being; we clutch caffeine like it's a prized jewel and wander through our houses in a haze, gel under-eye patches stuck to our skin like NFL players ready to fight our way to the end zone of another day. As sleep medicine and women's health physician Dr. Andrea Matsumura shared with me in our discussion on sleep, "We have been socialized to suffer. Many women don't know that they should be sleeping well. They attribute a lack of sleep to life circumstances: 'I have kids; I have parents to care for; I have irregular periods; I am supposed to sweat and feel uncomfortable during perimenopause.'"

In this chapter, I want to help you understand the origins of sleep disturbances in perimenopause and provide you with the tools that can put you on a path to getting more restorative rest. I've learned to plan for sleep the way I plan for work or travel. It's not optional; it's fundamental to my ability to function and to access my intellect, compassion, and energy. When I prioritize sleep, I feel the difference in everything from my mood to my metabolism. And you will, too.

The Many Faces of Perimenopausal Sleep Disruption

If you're in your forties or early fifties and suddenly find yourself sleeping poorly, you're not alone (we could have a 3 A.M. We Can't Sleep Club Zoom call with millions of women). Epidemiological studies indicate that approximately 40 to 50 percent of women in perimenopause report significant sleep disturbances—with 40 percent reporting chronic insomnia, defined as trouble falling asleep or staying asleep at least three nights a week for three months or longer. This is compared with 16 to 42 percent of premenopausal women who report issues with sleep. I wish I could say postmenopausal women report a return to restorative rest, but the percentage of women in this group who experience poor sleep rises to roughly 47 to 60 percent.

These disturbances are disruptive to quality of life and carry long-term risks to physical and mental health. Daytime fatigue, anxiety, and cognitive complaints are common downstream effects of poor sleep during this transition.

The types of sleep disruption vary. For some, it begins with trouble falling asleep, referred to as increased sleep latency. For others, it's waking up multiple times through the night or, as was common in my experience, it's the dreaded middle-of-the-night wake-up that leaves you unable to fall back asleep. Even when total sleep time seems adequate, women often describe their sleep as light, fragmented, and unrefreshing.

Hot flashes and night sweats, also known as vasomotor symptoms, are often blamed—and for good reason. These sudden surges of heat and sweating can wake women from sleep and fragment the sleep cycle. For many of us, these symptoms persist for years, sometimes up to a decade.

But many contributors beyond vasomotor symptoms can disturb sleep in perimenopause. Other disruptive factors may include . . .

- **restless legs syndrome,** which becomes more common in midlife, with women reporting the urge to move their legs at night or frequent limb jerks that make it hard to stay asleep
- **obstructive sleep apnea (OSA),** the risk of which increases in menopause because of weight gain, fat redistribution, and the loss of hormonal protection (see sidebar for more on OSA and why doctors often miss it in women)
- **nocturia,** defined as frequent nighttime urination
- **feeling "tired but wired,"** the sensation of being physically exhausted but mentally alert and unable to quiet the mind

These symptoms are part of a broader physiological shift driven by our fluctuating and declining levels of estrogen and progesterone; these hormones support neurotransmitters and thermoregulation and stabilize circadian rhythm, and when they are in flux or fall away, sleep regulation suffers.

I see this every day in my practice. Women who once slept soundly now lie awake, wondering what changed. They've tried the sleep hygiene tips like adjusting their evening routines and even giving up their evening glass of wine, and still they wake unrefreshed. It's not a lack of effort. It's the hormonal reality of this life stage.

Understanding this reality can make a big difference or at least remove some of the mystery behind unexpected and sudden changes in sleep quality. When we consider the contribution of the hormonal zone of chaos, we can start rebuilding sleep from a place of biology.

The Overlooked Occurrence of Sleep Apnea in Women

Obstructive sleep apnea (OSA) is a sleep disorder that occurs when muscles in the throat relax and cause your airway to collapse. This structural failure leads to starts and stops in airflow and impedes breathing, creating fragmented sleep and sleep deficiency. OSA is associated with increased risk of heart disease, high blood pressure, and stroke.

OSA is often perceived as a condition predominantly affecting men. However, research indicates that menopausal women are at a comparable risk, though it's been estimated that nine out of ten women who have it don't know it! The decline in estrogen and progesterone during menopause contributes to changes in upper-airway anatomy and muscle tone, increasing the likelihood of airway collapse during sleep. Progesterone, in particular, acts as a respiratory stimulant; its reduction diminishes the drive to breathe during sleep, leading to sleep-disordered breathing.

Unlike men, women with OSA often present with atypical symptoms:

- persistent fatigue or feeling unrefreshed after sleep

- difficulty falling or staying asleep (insomnia)

- morning headaches

- increased anxiety or irritability

- depressive symptoms

- trouble concentrating or mental fog

- frequent nighttime urination (nocturia)

- episodes of waking with a racing heart or shortness of breath

These symptoms are frequently attributed to stress, aging, or hormonal changes, leading to overlooked diagnosis of sleep apnea and delayed treatment.

Untreated sleep apnea in women can exacerbate risks for cardiovascular disease, insulin resistance, depression, cognitive decline, and increased inflammatory markers. These risks are particularly concerning during the menopausal transition, a period already associated with heightened vulnerability to these conditions.

A 2016 systematic review highlighted the significant underdiagnosis of OSA in women, often due to clinical bias and differing symptom presentation compared with men. Women are more likely to experience REM-predominant OSA or upper-airway resistance syndrome, both of which require a higher level of clinical suspicion for accurate diagnosis. If a woman presents with unrelenting fatigue, mood changes, disrupted sleep, or cardiometabolic alterations during midlife, sleep apnea should be considered. A simple home sleep study can lead to a diagnosis that is both treatable and transformative.

Identifying and treating sleep apnea in perimenopausal and postmenopausal women is crucial not only for improving sleep quality but also for protecting brain, heart, and metabolic functions that support overall health.

Why Sex Hormones Matter for Sleep

As I've said above, the fluctuation and decline of our levels of estrogen and progesterone in perimenopause are very connected to our sleep. Let's take a closer look at how and why.

Estrogen plays a central role in regulating sleep. It helps modulate serotonin and melatonin, stabilizes body temperature, and supports the brain's natural circadian rhythms. When estrogen levels are stable and sufficient, these systems run smoothly. When estrogen levels follow a more chaotic pattern, it disrupts the finely tuned mechanisms that support falling asleep, staying asleep, and reaching the deep, restorative stages of sleep.

Research shows that lower or unstable levels of estradiol are directly linked to increased nighttime awakenings. (In part, this is due to estrogen's effect on cortisol, our primary stress hormone, which I'll discuss more a little later.) These disruptions persist even in women without hot flashes or mood disorders, confirming that the hormone shifts themselves—particularly lower estrogen and higher FSH—are driving the changes in sleep continuity.

Progesterone is no less important. Often referred to as the body's natural sedative, progesterone enhances the activity of GABA receptors in the brain, just like many prescription sleep aids. During regular ovulatory cycles, rising progesterone in the luteal phase promotes deeper sleep. But when ovulation becomes sporadic or stops altogether during perimenopause, that soothing influence disappears and the brain is left more exposed to stimulation. Sleep becomes lighter, and the nervous system becomes more reactive. Suddenly, a once-dependable night of sleep becomes as elusive as a pen in your purse.

The result is a phenomenon I hear about daily from my patients: "I'm so tired, but I can't sleep." Or "I fall asleep fine, but I'm wide awake in the middle of the night and can't turn my brain off." These anecdotal reports mirror textbook symptoms of hormone-driven sleep disruption. And they align with data from major studies like the Study of Women's Health Across the Nation (SWAN), which shows a sharp increase in chronic insomnia, sleep fragmentation, and non-restorative sleep in perimenopausal women compared with their premenopausal peers.

Sleep architecture, the structure and stages of sleep, also changes. Multiple studies confirm that perimenopause is associated with reduced slow-wave (deep) sleep and REM sleep, along with longer latency to reach those stages. Melatonin secretion patterns shift as well, suggesting that the entire hormonal ecosystem that supports circadian rhythm becomes less reliable.

What this means in practical terms is that women may go to bed at a reasonable hour and spend a full eight hours in bed yet still wake up exhausted. Their sleep is lighter and less restorative. They spend less time in the stages of sleep that support cognitive function, immune repair, and emotional regulation.

To make matters worse, mood disturbances and vasomotor symptoms can amplify the problem. If you have a history of depression, anxiety, or trauma, you are more likely to experience disrupted sleep in perimenopause.

When we put this all together, we see that the hormonal changes of perimenopause disrupt every layer of sleep, contributing to . . .

- more awakenings

- less deep and REM sleep

- a longer time to reach restorative stages

- a heightened vulnerability to stress

When I was experiencing these sleep disruptions, I blamed myself. I tried to do everything right: I wasn't drinking alcohol; I kept my bedroom cool and dark; I avoided screens before bed; I followed every sleep hygiene recommendation in the proverbial book. And still, night after night, I couldn't sleep. I would lie there, wide awake, growing increasingly anxious about how awful I'd feel the next day. Eventually, I developed what I can only describe as sleep anxiety. I would start panicking before the night even began, anticipating another battle with restlessness and exhaustion. It felt like my body was betraying me, and for a long time, I believed that somehow I was failing.

But I wasn't failing. I was experiencing a predictable change in physiology.

Cortisol and the Stress-Sleep Spiral

One of the most under-recognized disruptors of sleep in perimenopause is cortisol, the body's primary stress hormone. When we are premenopausal, we have robust and reliable estrogen levels that modulate the hypothalamic-pituitary-adrenal (HPA) axis, buffering the effects of stress and keeping cortisol responses in check. But as estrogen declines, that hormonal buffer disappears, leaving the stress response system more reactive, especially at night.

Cortisol is secreted in a pulsatile fashion from the adrenal glands in a natural circadian rhythm: It's highest in the early morning to help you wake up, and it tapers off throughout the day to allow for rest. But in perimenopause, that rhythm can become dysregulated, and you can be woken up in the middle of the night by a cortisol spike that triggers a racing heart, a spinning mind, or restless energy. Women tend to classify this sleep disruption as insomnia or a consequence of anxiety, but it would be more accurate to blame it on your biology. Even if you aren't experiencing or aware of acute stress, such spikes can occur.

Research published in the journal *Maturitas* in September 2024 confirmed this physiological pattern by reporting that women with higher nighttime cortisol levels experienced more awakenings and spent less time in deep, restorative stages of sleep—even when they didn't report feeling subjectively sleep deprived.

And it's not just about the sleep disruption itself. Chronic nighttime cortisol spikes have been linked to a host of downstream effects: insulin resistance, increased belly fat, poor memory consolidation, and heightened risk for anxiety and depression. In many cases, women are misdiagnosed or dismissed when they present with these symptoms, and the root issue of underlying hormonal chaos is never even discussed.

Understanding this connection is a critical piece of the perimenopause puzzle. If we focus only on the sleep hygiene checklist—no screens before bed; limited caffeine; cool, dark rooms—we're missing the bigger picture. Our physiology has changed. And unless we address the underlying hormonal instability and stress reactivity, women will continue to struggle.

That's why, in this chapter and throughout this book, we keep coming back to the same message: This is biology, not weakness. Disruptions to sleep during the menopausal transition aren't personal flaws or lifestyle missteps. They are the result of hormonal shifts, particularly the decline in estrogen and progesterone, that interfere with the brain's sleep architecture, thermoregulation, and stress response. The takeaway here is critical:

When we understand sleep disruption as a physiologic effect of perimenopause, we can stop blaming ourselves and start focusing on strategies that actually work.

Evidence-Based Treatment Strategies for Sleep in Perimenopause

Once we understand that sleep disruption in perimenopause is biologically driven, the next step is learning how to treat it effectively. This isn't about prescribing another generic sleep hygiene checklist—yes, these strategies do matter, but on their own, they may not make a meaningful difference. Instead, I'm going to provide you with some targeted, science-backed tools that can work alongside the more superficial strategies; the combination can support the body through hormonal transition and stabilize the systems that regulate rest.

Menopause Hormone Therapy

For many women, addressing the root hormonal fluctuations directly through menopause hormone therapy (MHT) can lead to a significant improvement in sleep quality. Estrogen therapy has been shown to reduce nighttime awakenings. Adding progesterone—particularly micronized progesterone, which has better absorption because of the reduced size of the particles—can make a marked difference in sleep, as it promotes deeper, more sustained rest through GABA receptor activation. Clinical trials have shown that micronized progesterone improves both sleep onset and sleep maintenance, especially in women reporting insomnia as a primary symptom of perimenopause.

MHT isn't a one-size-fits-all solution, and it's not appropriate for every woman. But for those without contraindications, it can be one of the most powerful tools we have for reclaiming restorative sleep. This is especially true if you are experiencing nighttime hot flashes, a.k.a. night sweats. Hormone therapy can be effective at managing these unpleasant disturbances (which make it virtually impossible to sleep) and can also address the deeper neurological and hormonal roots of fragmented sleep.

Cognitive Behavioral Therapy for Insomnia

Cognitive behavioral therapy for insomnia (CBT-I) is the gold standard non-pharmacological treatment for chronic insomnia. It's a structured, evidence-based approach that helps retrain the brain and body to restore healthy sleep patterns. It works by identifying and changing thoughts and behaviors that interfere with sleep. CBT-I addresses issues like racing thoughts, sleep anxiety, and poor sleep hygiene, using techniques such as stimulus control, sleep restriction, relaxation training, and cognitive restructuring. It's especially effective in perimenopause, where sleep disruptions are often reinforced by stress, worry, or conditioned wakefulness. CBT-I works by rewiring the brain's relationship with sleep, challenging unhelpful beliefs, improving sleep efficiency, and removing behaviors that unintentionally sabotage rest.

Several studies have shown that CBT-I is as effective as—and in some cases more effective than—pharmacological sleep aids, with longer-lasting results. Digital and telehealth-based CBT-I programs make this intervention more accessible than ever. Some of these programs are free, and others may be covered through insurance. They may reduce insomnia severity and are valuable options if you don't have access to a sleep specialist.

Evidence-Based Digital CBT-I Options (Available in the United States)

- **Sleepio:** Web-based CBT-I with a virtual therapist; improves sleep and mental health outcomes. Notable feature: Available direct-to-consumer.

- **Somryst (formerly SHUTi):** FDA-cleared prescription CBT-I app; more than 50 percent of users report significant improvement. Notable feature: Long-lasting effects.

- **CBT-i Coach:** Free app developed by Veterans Affairs (VA) for veterans and civilians with tools for tracking, relaxation, and sleep education. Notable feature: Designed to support therapy or for self-use.

- **Insomnia Coach:** Self-guided five-week CBT-I app, also from the VA; shown to reduce insomnia severity. Notable feature: Free and publicly accessible.

Lifestyle Interventions

The fundamentals of nutrition and exercise matter a great deal to sleep, but our approach to both needs to be highly nuanced in perimenopause if we want to see our efforts translate to results. I recommend a high-protein, anti-inflammatory diet to help stabilize blood sugar and cortisol levels. Regular strength training has also been shown to support more than muscle and metabolic health; it improves sleep quality as well.

You will want to pay closer attention to your evening routine, too, to see where you can make adjustments to support quality sleep. I suggest creating a wind-down period for yourself that includes dimming lights, reducing screen time, and keeping a consistent bedtime. These feel like small shifts, but they can play a big part in reinforcing circadian rhythms.

Perimenopause is when you may begin to notice the new intolerance to alcohol I mentioned earlier. What used to be a "relaxing" glass of wine may now lead to a rebound cortisol surge, shallow sleep, and 3 A.M. awakenings. Many of my patients are surprised to learn how dramatically sleep improves once they limit alcohol in the evening.

Targeted Supplements and Medications

For some women, temporary use of sleep aids like low-dose doxepin can help bridge the gap during periods of intense sleep disruption. Gabapentin and certain SSRIs/SNRIs can also support sleep, especially in women experiencing mood disturbances or severe night sweats.

Beyond prescription options, several nutritional supplements can help sleep:

- **Magnesium** acts as a natural NMDA (which "excites" the brain) antagonist and GABA agonist. It's been shown to reduce sleep latency and improve subjective sleep quality, though results vary and are more modest in older populations.

- **L-theanine** enhances calming neurotransmitters like GABA and serotonin and, when combined with magnesium as Mg-L-theanine, has been shown to increase slow-wave activity and improve overall sleep quality.

- **Melatonin,** the body's natural sleep hormone, can support circadian rhythm, reduce sleep latency, and improve subjective sleep quality, though individual responses vary widely.

Combination supplements, particularly those blending magnesium, L-theanine, and melatonin, have demonstrated reductions in time to sleep onset, increased sleep duration, and improved efficiency in both clinical trials and real-world settings. (The research on such combinations has been convincing enough for me to collaborate with board-certified sleep medicine specialist Dr. Andrea Matsumura on a version for my patients and others; you can find out more at thepauselife.com.) While results are mixed and often depend on formulation quality, these options may offer a helpful and generally safe adjunct for women seeking non-prescription support.

Managing Stress and Cortisol Reactivity

Daily stress management isn't optional in perimenopause; it's essential. Whether it's mindfulness meditation, breathing exercises, yoga, or simply carving out ten minutes of quiet, intentional downshifting of the nervous system is a non-negotiable for many women. Research shows that even short, consistent daily practices can lower cortisol, reduce nighttime wakefulness, and improve heart rate variability, all markers of a more resilient stress response.

Other Strategic Considerations for Stubborn Sleep Issues

If you find that your sleep challenges are nonresponsive to some or all of the strategies already noted, it's important to keep investigating, because good sleep is worth pursuing. In our discussion, Dr. Matsumura emphasized other considerations:

- Make sure to rule out sleep disorders like restless legs syndrome and sleep apnea, which, as mentioned, are often missed in women—especially during and after menopause.

- If you are a known snorer, regularly suffer from severe daytime fatigue, or experience frequent nighttime awakenings, a sleep study may be warranted.

- Low iron or vitamin D levels can also contribute to poor sleep and should be checked.

- For some women, a history of trauma or unresolved anxiety may be deeply intertwined with sleep issues, and therapy or trauma-informed care may be part of the healing process.

Believe It: Better Sleep in Perimenopause Is Possible

In my clinic, we pair sleep-restoring strategies with education. When women understand why their sleep is breaking down and what they can do to support it, everything shifts. The shame disappears and the helplessness lifts. And what's left is a clear, compassionate path to healing.

The bottom line is that sleep doesn't have to be another casualty of midlife. You don't have to suffer or accept a fate filled with sleepless nights and days spent dragging. With the right tools, we can rebuild sleep architecture—and, with it, restore the energy, clarity, and resilience that every woman deserves.

Part Three

SEX, PREGNANCY, AND PERIODS IN PERIMENOPAUSE

CHAPTER 11

When Desire Shifts: Perimenopause and Sexual Function

I didn't know perimenopause was a thing until I was about fifty-one years old and in the later stages of it (I'm fifty-three now). In hindsight, the first symptom I probably experienced was a very heavy period, starting in my mid-forties. When I googled the condition back then, some of the recommended treatments were ablation and hysterectomy, which scared me off and had me not seek treatment. When I finally sought HRT for other symptoms (vasomotor, sleep problems), my period returned to normal. While I regret that I didn't find hormonal treatment much earlier, I'm also glad I didn't get talked into a harsher treatment like some other women I've known.

The next symptom was a decline in sexual function, which started in my late forties. It snuck up on me initially—a bit less desire and less intense orgasms. It then accelerated rapidly in the last few years. This took me by surprise and has maybe been the most devastating.

—V.C.

We need to talk about something that too often goes unspoken: sex and perimenopause.

When I finished my OB-GYN residency and stepped into clinical practice, I thought I was well prepared to care for women. I had trained for years, memorized protocols, and logged countless hours on the wards. But when I began seeing patients in my clinic, real women in midlife, one pattern emerged almost immediately that I hadn't trained to help solve: They were struggling with sex. Not necessarily with pain, infection, or anything else that would light up a diagnostic chart. They were struggling with desire, with connection, with pleasure.

Repeatedly, I heard the same quiet confession: "I just don't want sex anymore, and I don't know why."

And I'll be honest. I didn't know either.

I felt embarrassed. Unprepared. *Powerless.*

Despite years of medical education, I had received almost *no* training on female sexual function, especially in the context of perimenopause. I went back to my textbooks. Nothing. I searched the journals, the guidelines, even my notes from residency. Still, very little. The silence in the medical literature mirrored the silence in our culture. Yet here it was, showing up in my clinic, day after day, woman after woman. I wanted to help, but I didn't know how. And that made me feel hopeless.

As I look back, there are things I told patients early in my career that now make me cringe. I was doing my best with what little information I had, but in hindsight, I know in some cases I probably caused more harm than good. I repeated the advice I had been given by mentors who also hadn't been properly trained. I told women to have a glass of wine and relax. I suggested they go on a vacation, get a babysitter, dress up, and make more time for date night. I thought I was being helpful, encouraging even, but I was completely missing the point. These women weren't lacking effort or romance. They were navigating a hormonal shift that none of us had been taught how to recognize, much less treat.

I now know that telling someone to "just try harder" when their body and brain are sending entirely different signals isn't just unhelpful; it can be shaming and deeply invalidating. I carry that with me. It's part of why I'm writing this chapter and why I'm so passionate about changing the way we talk about sex and perimenopause.

My Own Sex Education

I finally realized that if I wanted to become a better doctor, I needed to work harder to educate myself. I picked up *Mars and Venus in the Bedroom,* searching for anything that might help me understand the psychology of desire. It wasn't enough, so I kept reading, and I kept asking questions. And slowly, the right voices started to emerge—the ones that truly changed the way I understood female sexuality and helped me show up for my patients in the way they deserved.

What first cracked something open for me was the work of Dr. Kelly Casperson and her book *You Are Not Broken* (she has a podcast of the same name). Her ability to blend science, story, and radical compassion reframed everything I thought I knew about female sexual function. She dared to say out loud what so many of us had been taught to tiptoe around: that women deserve pleasure, that sexual dysfunction is treatable, and that shame has no place in the exam room. I had been a board-certified OB-GYN for decades, but what she offered—clear, evidence-based information delivered with empathy and confidence—felt revolutionary.

Then I read Dr. Emily Nagoski's *Come as You Are*, a master class in understanding arousal, desire, and sexual well-being through the lens of neuroscience, psychology, and real-life complexity. She validated what I had seen over and over in clinic: that women's sexual responses aren't linear and that the brain is just as important as the body. Her work helped me understand the role of context, safety, and emotional connection in unlocking desire and gave me a new framework to explain it to my patients.

And then there's Dr. Lauren Streicher, whose clinical wisdom, research, and plainspoken approach to women's health have made her a true beacon in this field. She speaks the language of both the academic and the everyday woman, bridging the gap between rigorous science and relatable care. Her guidance around menopause, hormone therapy, and vulvovaginal health gave me clinical strategies I could implement immediately and the confidence to talk about topics I was never trained to navigate.

Finally, let's talk about Dr. Rachel Rubin, the urologist and sexual medicine specialist whose appearance on Peter Attia's *The Drive* podcast should be required listening for every clinician practicing in the area of women's health. This podcast was a master class. Dr. Rubin brought the data, the heat, and the full, unapologetic truth about testosterone, clitoral anatomy, and the wildly underdiagnosed sexual dysfunctions that too many women suffer through in silence. She didn't just educate; she electrified. She made it very clear that if you're not talking about the clitoris, you're not practicing medicine. Period.

The plain truth is that these women—and many others like them—have changed the way I practice medicine. They gave me the language I never learned in school, the tools I wasn't handed in training, and the courage to go beyond the status quo. Together, they've helped create a new foundation for women's sexual health, one built on science, inclusivity, and the belief that every woman deserves to feel seen, heard, and whole.

What they collectively helped me understand is that sexual health *is* health. It's not a luxury or an afterthought. It's a core part of physical, emotional, and relational well-being. And during perimenopause, a time when hormones shift, energy wanes, tissues change, and emotional landscapes evolve, it becomes even more critical. Sexual dysfunction isn't rare. It's pervasive and incredibly under-discussed.

When estrogen, testosterone, and progesterone fluctuate and fall, it affects everything from vaginal tissue and lubrication to blood flow, brain chemistry, and sleep. The result? Many women feel disconnected from their bodies, from their desire, and from their partners. But instead of naming it, we're taught to internalize it. To assume that it's just "aging." Or that it's our fault. This must change.

In this chapter, I will offer you—and the clinicians who care for you—the information we should have had access to all along. My goal is to deliver an understanding of what's really happening to our bodies and to introduce—or reintroduce—you to the right you have to feel connected, alive, and empowered in your sexual self. Because midlife isn't the end of our sexual stories. It's just a new chapter. And you deserve a voice, a vocabulary, and a care plan that honors the whole you.

What Changes During Perimenopause?

The hormonal shifts of perimenopause can be deeply destabilizing not just physically but emotionally, sexually, and relationally. For many women, the changes in sexual desire and function are among the earliest and most confusing signs that something is shifting. These aren't simply mood changes or lifestyle issues; they're biological consequences of complex hormonal transitions.

Let's look at the hormones with the biggest impact on sexual function.

Estrogen. Estradiol is the most potent form of estrogen during reproductive years. It supports the health of vaginal and vulvar tissues, promoting blood flow, maintaining lubrication, and sustaining elasticity. When estrogen levels begin to drop as they do during perimenopause, those protective effects diminish. Vaginal tissues become thinner and less resilient. Lubrication declines, and sexual activity can become uncomfortable or even painful. For many, this leads to a natural avoidance of sex, not from lack of desire, but to avoid discomfort or embarrassment.

These changes are now understood as part of the genitourinary syndrome of menopause (GSM), a term that reflects not just vaginal symptoms but also urinary tract symptoms and changes in sexual function. What makes GSM especially challenging during perimenopause is that symptoms can begin well before periods stop, when most women (and many providers) aren't yet looking for them.

But estrogen's influence on sexual health isn't just local. It also affects blood flow and tissue responsiveness throughout the pelvic region. Declining estrogen leads to reduced genital engorgement and lower sensitivity, which can make arousal feel muted and orgasm harder to reach. In short, even when the mind is willing, the body may not respond the way it used to and that disconnect can be distressing, especially in relationships where sex was once a source of joy and connection.

Testosterone. Alongside estrogen, testosterone plays a critical role in sexual function—particularly libido and sexual satisfaction. While it's often overlooked in conversations about female health, testosterone is essential for women's sexual well-being.

Unlike estrogen, testosterone doesn't fluctuate dramatically during perimenopause. Instead, it declines gradually and steadily with age, beginning as early as a woman's mid-twenties. By the time a woman reaches her late forties or early fifties, her testosterone levels may be less than half of what they were in her younger years. While perimenopause doesn't drive testosterone levels lower, the effects of its slow, quiet decline are often amplified by the more erratic and dramatic drop in estrogen.

Research has shown, clearly and repeatedly, that low testosterone levels in women are associated with reduced spontaneous desire, fewer sexual thoughts, diminished responsiveness, and lower overall sexual satisfaction. We have decades of data. We have clinical consensus. And we have thousands of women walking into our clinics every year saying the same thing: *I don't feel like myself anymore.*

Yet despite all this, there is still no FDA-approved testosterone therapy for women in the United States. Not one. While men have multiple formulations, delivery systems, and commercial products for testosterone replacement, women are left to patch together treatment with off-label solutions or compounded hormones, or they are left with nothing at all.

I want to be clear: It's not because the science isn't there. It's not because the need isn't real. It's because the regulatory system has failed women. Again.

Even worse, testosterone is not only left out of treatment; it's often left out of the conversation entirely. Most clinicians aren't taught to ask about sexual function. Most patients don't know they're *allowed* to bring it up. And for women in midlife, whose libido shifts are routinely blamed on aging, stress, or relationship issues, the suggestion that there could be a physiological solution is too often met with a shrug or dismissal.

The irony? The Endocrine Society and the International Society for the Study of Women's Sexual Health have already issued guidance supporting the use of testosterone therapy for postmenopausal women with hypoactive sexual desire disorder (HSDD). The experts are on board and the data is there. But the system has been too slow, too silent, and, frankly, too steeped in paternalism to act. Both medical societies have made it clear, too, that perimenopausal women shouldn't be left out of the conversation despite lags in population-specific research—if you are in perimenopause and are experiencing HSDD with low testosterone, your clinician should consider you for a trial of testosterone therapy. Many of us in menopause care are using it in women with HSDD in perimenopause and having excellent results. (As a reminder, testosterone levels change because of age-related decline, which means that testosterone therapy may be beneficial regardless of your menopausal status.)

What Is Hypoactive Sexual Desire Disorder (HSDD)?

Hypoactive sexual desire disorder (HSDD) is one of the most common sexual concerns reported by women during perimenopause and menopause. It's characterized by a persistent or recurrent lack of sexual desire that causes personal distress or difficulty in relationships. This is different from a temporary dip in libido that can happen with stress or fatigue. In HSDD, the loss of interest in sexual activity persists for months or longer and negatively affects quality of life.

During perimenopause, fluctuating and declining levels of estrogen and testosterone can contribute to changes in sexual desire. These hormonal shifts can alter brain chemistry involved in sexual motivation and pleasure, reduce genital blood flow and sensation, and worsen vaginal dryness or discomfort during intimacy. Mood changes, sleep disruption, chronic stress, and relationship factors can also play a role, making HSDD a complex, multifactorial condition.

The diagnosis of HSDD is clinical and requires both a persistent low desire and personal distress about that loss of desire. Importantly, not every woman with low desire is distressed by it. Treatment approaches may include counseling, addressing contributing medical or psychological factors, optimizing hormone therapy, and, in some cases, considering FDA-approved options such as flibanserin or bremelanotide. Testosterone therapy may also be considered off-label in some cases after careful evaluation.

Women deserve more than silence. They deserve options. They deserve access to therapies backed by evidence, whereas too many are buried by bureaucracy or bias. The absence of FDA-approved testosterone for women isn't just an oversight; it's a failure of the system to take female sexual health seriously.

In my own practice, I've had countless patients express shame or confusion about their declining interest in sex. And I've felt their frustration because I lived it myself. The truth is, these changes aren't imagined, nor are they failures of personality or effort. They're the direct result of neuroendocrine shifts, and they deserve to be acknowledged, studied, and treated with the same seriousness we apply to any other hormone-driven disorder.

Sexual changes in perimenopause aren't just about "getting older." They're about *the loss of hormones* that once supported healthy desire, arousal, and satisfaction. When estrogen crashes and testosterone fades, the result is a body that may feel foreign and unresponsive. But this doesn't have to mean the end of sexual pleasure. It means we need new tools, new conversations, and far better education, for women and for clinicians alike.

The Overlooked Impact of Pain and Lubrication: Understanding GSM

One of the most common yet least discussed drivers of sexual pain in midlife is the genitourinary syndrome of menopause (GSM). This condition results from the loss of estrogen in the tissues of the vulva, vagina, and lower urinary tract, including the bladder. And this is not just about dryness but about structural change. The vaginal epithelium thins, collagen and elasticity decline, and the vaginal opening can narrow. Over time, these changes lead to burning, irritation, tearing, urinary discomfort, and pain with penetration—what we refer to clinically as dyspareunia.

GSM is incredibly common and highly treatable, yet it remains largely invisible in routine care. The result is that too many women suffer in silence, believing pain during sex is something they just have to accept. That is simply not true. Symptoms of GSM are a clear signal that your body needs support.

The problem is that when pain becomes the expectation, even the possibility of pleasure starts to fade. Many women begin to anticipate discomfort before touch even begins, and the nervous system learns to associate intimacy with pain, not connection. Once this pattern sets in, even when desire is still present, the body withdraws. Arousal becomes harder to reach, and sexual activity shifts from something enjoyable to something stressful or something to avoid.

This is why we must normalize conversations about vaginal moisturizers and lubricants and local estrogen therapy. These aren't luxury products. They are essential tools that help restore tissue integrity, improve comfort, reduce infection risk, and bring ease back into touch. In some cases, DHEA or vaginal testosterone may be appropriate (see more in chapter 14). For others, pelvic floor physical therapy can be transformative, especially if muscular tension or prior trauma is involved.

But none of this happens if we don't name it. If women aren't asked, if clinicians aren't trained, if discomfort is waved off as inevitable, then treatable problems become chronic burdens. The troubling nature of sexual discomfort is that it's a burden that doesn't stay in the body alone—it affects identity and relationships and begins to erode the belief that pleasure is still possible.

Clinical Considerations: New AUA Guidelines on GSM Care

In 2025, the American Urological Association (AUA) released new clinical guidelines to improve the identification and treatment of the genitourinary syndrome of menopause (GSM). These recommendations support a proactive, evidence-based, and patient-centered approach to care. I will cover this topic in greater detail in chapter 14, where I focus on the hormonal treatment options in perimenopause.

One of the notable highlights was the emphasis on shared decision-making—that is, clinicians should center treatment decisions on each patient's values, goals, and preferences, using the best available evidence (the opposite of this would be a one-size-fits-all treatment protocol).

The AUA also made some important updates to guidelines in a range of categories:

SCREENING AND DIAGNOSIS:

- Screen all at-risk patients with a focused medical, sexual, and psychosocial history.
- Conduct a genitourinary exam in all symptomatic patients.
- Educate patients on the hormonal origins of GSM symptoms.
- Evaluate for other genitourinary conditions and refer when necessary.
- Consider referrals to licensed therapists for sexual or psychosocial concerns.
- Refer to pelvic floor physical therapists when dysfunction is present.

HORMONAL THERAPIES:

- Offer local low-dose vaginal estrogen to improve dryness, discomfort, and dyspareunia.
- Offer vaginal DHEA for similar symptoms.
- Consider ospemifene as an oral option for vulvovaginal discomfort.
- Offer local estrogen or DHEA even to patients already on systemic estrogen.
- Use local estrogen to treat GSM in patients with co-morbid conditions like overactive bladder or recurrent urinary tract infections.

NON-HORMONAL THERAPIES:

- Recommend vaginal moisturizers and lubricants alone or alongside other treatments.
- Counsel patients that supplements have no proven benefit for GSM.
- Advise avoiding irritants and harsh cleansers that may worsen symptoms.

ENERGY-BASED THERAPIES:

- Inform patients that CO_2 laser, ER:YAG laser, or radiofrequency devices for treating GSM are not supported by current evidence.

- If used, they should be offered only with full disclosure and to patients who cannot use or prefer to avoid FDA-approved treatments.

CANCER CONSIDERATIONS:

- Local vaginal estrogen does not increase the risk of breast or endometrial cancer.

- Vaginal DHEA and ospemifene also show no increased cancer risk.

- Local vaginal estrogen may be used in breast cancer survivors after shared decision-making with their care team.

- Routine endometrial surveillance is not required for patients using local therapies or ospemifene.

FOLLOW-UP:

- Reassess treatment response regularly.

- Prepare patients for the potential need for long-term therapy and monitoring.

How Physical Symptoms Influence Emotional Intimacy and Identity

One of the most heartbreaking dynamics I've witnessed in practice is the way sexual disconnection, usually brought about by physical discomfort, can quietly erode emotional closeness and how emotional disconnection, in turn, can suppress sexual desire. It becomes a loop, a feedback cycle that intensifies over time. The less intimacy a couple shares, the more they drift apart emotionally. The more they drift, the harder it becomes to initiate or respond sexually.

I've had patients sit on my exam table and, in the quietest voice, say things like "I love my partner, but I just can't bring myself to initiate. It doesn't feel good anymore, and I don't want to fake it." Many of them feel anxious, embarrassed, or avoidant—not because they've lost interest in intimacy or no longer love their partners, but because they're trying to protect themselves from discomfort, disappointment, or shame. And over time, that avoidance is often misread as rejection or a lack of interest, breeding emotional distance, hurt feelings, and relationship strain. What starts as a hormone shift becomes a communication breakdown. What begins in the tissues of the vulva and vagina begins to echo in the silence between two people in bed.

Many women carry the weight of this shift as a personal failure. *We blame ourselves for not wanting sex, for pulling away, for not being "fun" or "spontaneous" anymore.* We internalize self-criticism, and it ripples out and begins to erode our broader sense of self, our identity as sexual beings, and our connection with our partners. I've sat with countless women who whisper through tears, "I miss the way we used to be, but I don't know how to get back there."

The reality is that the blame is entirely misdirected. What has happened is a result of the accumulation of years of unspoken needs, invisible labor, and physical changes that were never acknowledged, much less treated. It's the complicated manifestation of how we as women were taught to respond to pain, to frustration, to grieving what once came easily.

Let me be abundantly clear: The physical changes that can come with perimenopause—vaginal dryness, decreased arousal, slower orgasmic response, and even discomfort with penetration—are not your fault.

The tragedy is that so many of these issues are treatable, with the right education, the right tools, and the right clinical support. But instead of being offered evidence-based solutions, women are often left to internalize the problem. They're told to relax or try harder, or they're offered nothing more than a dismissive "This is just what happens when you get older." (To any of my past patients to whom I offered little more guidance than to suggest a glass of wine, I'm sorry.)

We need to start acknowledging this for what it really is: hormone depletion, not just aging, not personal failure or absence of desire. This is structural change. The lack of understanding that has harmed so many women is the result of decades of silence, medical oversight, and a culture that has failed to teach women how their bodies work and how to care for them through every stage of life. Sexual well-being is a fundamental part of health and quality of life. And every woman deserves to feel safe, informed, and empowered in her own body.

Libido Isn't a Light Switch: Responsive Desire Versus Spontaneous Desire

In the early years of my clinical practice, I thought of female libido as something simple, like a light switch—it was either on or off. You wanted sex or you didn't, and if you didn't, it must be hormonal or psychological. Flip the right switch, and everything should come back on.

But the more I listened to my patients and the more I studied the work of modern sexual health experts like Dr. Emily Nagoski, Dr. Lauren Streicher, Dr. Kelly Casperson, and Dr. Rachel Rubin, the more I realized how wrong that assumption was. Female desire isn't a switch. It's more like the cockpit of a 747: complex, dynamic, and highly sensitive to internal and external cues. Everything from hormones to history, stress to safety, self-image to partnership—it all matters. During perimenopause, when hormones are shifting and life responsibilities are peaking, that flight deck gets even harder to navigate.

Another major shift in how we understand female libido comes from the concept of responsive versus spontaneous desire. Many of us were raised to believe that desire should hit us out of the blue, that we should feel a sudden wave of arousal like we're in a movie scene. That's spontaneous desire, and while it's more common in men and in the early stages of a relationship, it's not the norm for most women, especially in long-term relationships or during midlife.

Instead, what's far more common is responsive desire: desire that follows physical or emotional intimacy, not precedes it. It's the kind of desire that emerges once you feel safe, touched, and connected. If women don't know this, they often think something is broken when spontaneous desire fades, but this is *normal*. And when we reframe expectations around desire, we create space for a new kind of intimacy, one that's just as real but often slower and more deliberate.

The Role of Stress, Fatigue, and Caregiving

Perimenopause doesn't exist in a vacuum. It often arrives as an uninvited guest during one of the most demanding chapters of our lives. It collides head-on with the pressures of raising children, managing demanding careers, caring for aging parents, supporting partners, maintaining homes, and staying connected to friends and community. For many women, this decade of *all the things, all at once* requires a relentless juggling act that leaves very little space for rest, let alone desire.

The result? Chronic stress, poor sleep, and a state of near-constant nervous system activation. And all these factors, independent of hormones, are well-established suppressors of sexual desire.

Our nervous system is wired for survival, not seduction. When the brain is busy triaging stress hormones and coping with fatigue, libido takes a back seat or disappears altogether. Research shows that elevated cortisol, our primary stress hormone, interferes with the brain's arousal pathways, dulling the physiological and psychological responses needed for sexual engagement. In other words, it's incredibly hard to feel turned on when your body is stuck in fight-or-flight.

But it's not just stress; it's *burnout*. It's the kind of fatigue that sleep doesn't fix, the kind of emotional depletion that comes from carrying the invisible weight of everyone else's needs. Women in midlife are often the emotional center of their families, workplaces, and communities. And when that mental load collides with hormonal shifts that affect mood, energy, and sleep, the result is a perfect storm for low desire.

In truth, many cases of low libido in perimenopause aren't just about hormones. They're about context. They're about a life that has crowded out autonomy and rest. They're about a nervous system that hasn't had a moment to downshift in weeks, months, or even years. Before we rush to pathologize low desire, we need to ask better questions: *Does this woman have help? Does she have time? Does she have space to reconnect with herself?* Because desire is something we have to *make room for.*

Desire Is Non-Binary

Desire is a relational experience. It thrives in environments of safety, curiosity, tenderness, and mutual care. And when those conditions begin to erode through stress, fatigue, resentment, or physical discomfort, desire doesn't necessarily disappear. It just gets quieter. It hides. It waits.

Yet our culture treats desire as something binary: It's either there or it's not. But midlife teaches us that desire is more nuanced than that. It's responsive and contextual. It adapts, withdraws, and returns depending on how we're living, how we're treated, how we feel in our bodies, and how emotionally connected we are to our partners.

When the body no longer responds the way it once did, when arousal takes longer, when orgasm becomes elusive, when pleasure feels replaced by pressure, it's not a sign of brokenness. It's a sign that the signals have changed. And we need to change how we listen.

For many couples, the first step back toward intimacy isn't more sex. It's more safety and more truth telling. More curiosity without pressure. I often remind my patients, *You're not the problem. You're responding to a problem.* And when you begin to understand the patterns and the physiology behind the shift, you can stop blaming yourself and start building something new.

Because desire may go quiet, but that doesn't mean it's gone. It just needs a different kind of invitation.

The Role of Communication and Connection

In my experience, open communication is one of the most powerful tools for reigniting intimacy during perimenopause. That includes conversations about how your body is changing, what feels good (or doesn't), and what kind of emotional support you need. For many couples, these conversations have never happened before, and they can be awkward at first. But when they do happen, something shifts. Shame turns into understanding, and frustration becomes collaboration.

Research consistently shows that emotional closeness, communication, and feeling valued by one's partner are more predictive of sexual satisfaction in women than hormone levels alone. That doesn't mean we ignore biology. It means we treat the whole picture.

There is no single path back to intimacy in perimenopause, but there are many tools. Some are medical, some relational, and some emotional. But the first step is understanding that what you're experiencing is valid, common, and treatable. Female sexuality in midlife isn't broken. It's changing. And with the right support, it can change into something just as meaningful, sometimes even more so.

Diagnosing the Problem: What's Really Going On?

Sexual difficulties in midlife are incredibly common—but they are rarely diagnosed and even more rarely addressed. Why? Because women often don't bring them up. And when they do, providers frequently don't know what to do with them. This silence—on both sides of the exam table—is one of the great failings of modern medicine.

As I've mentioned, in my early years as a physician, I was one of those providers. I wasn't trained to assess sexual function. I didn't have a reliable script or tool to start the conversation, and I certainly wasn't given a road map to guide treatment. I was never taught that sexual dysfunction should be evaluated like any other medical issue—systematically, thoughtfully, and without shame.

But over time, I learned to ask the questions. I learned to create a space where women felt safe sharing the truth about their changing bodies, their shifting relationships, and their private frustrations. What I also learned is that sexual function in women is multidimensional and no one symptom tells the whole story.

That's why it's important to use evidence-based screening tools to identify the full scope of what's going on.

A Tool to Open the Conversation: The Female Sexual Function Index (FSFI)

One of the most widely used and validated tools in clinical and research settings is the Female Sexual Function Index (FSFI)—a nineteen-item questionnaire that assesses six key domains of sexual health: desire, arousal, lubrication, orgasm, satisfaction, and pain. I often use the FSFI in practice, not just to gather data, but to normalize the experience and to open the door to deeper, more nuanced conversations. Women are often relieved to see their symptoms reflected in a structured tool; it validates what they've been feeling and gives them the language to talk about it.

Below I've printed what is known as the FSFI-6, a brief, evidence-based screening tool adapted from the FSFI questionnaire and designed to assess sexual function in women.* It isn't a diagnostic test but can help identify areas where you may benefit from medical, psychological, or sexual health support.

You can note your scores below or just keep a mental tally. If you find that many of your responses indicate low satisfaction or function, consider taking this questionnaire to a practitioner who is trained in female sexual medicine.

---

* Adapted for self-awareness and clinician-guided discussion.

OVER THE PAST FOUR WEEKS...

1. How often did you feel sexual desire or interest?

    0—Almost never or never

    1—A few times

    2—Sometimes

    3—Most times

    4—Almost always or always

2. When you felt sexual desire or interest, how strong was it?

    0—Very low or none at all

    1—Low

    2—Moderate

    3—High

    4—Very high

3. How often were you able to become sexually aroused during sexual activity or intercourse?

    0—Almost never or never

    1—A few times

    2—Sometimes

    3—Most times

    4—Almost always or always

4. How satisfied were you with your level of sexual arousal during sexual activity or intercourse?

    0—Very dissatisfied

    1—Dissatisfied

2—Moderately satisfied

3—Satisfied

4—Very satisfied

5. How often did you achieve orgasm during sexual activity or intercourse?

    0—Almost never or never

    1—A few times

    2—Sometimes

    3—Most times

    4—Almost always or always

6. Overall, how satisfied have you been with your sexual relationship with your partner?

    0—Very dissatisfied

    1—Dissatisfied

    2—Moderately satisfied

    3—Satisfied

    4—Very satisfied

SCORING GUIDANCE: Each response is scored 0–4. A total score of 19 or less (out of a possible 24) may indicate concerns worth exploring further with your clinician.

How Practitioners Can Better Support Their Patients

Despite the prevalence of sexual dysfunction in perimenopausal and postmenopausal women, the medical system continues to treat it as peripheral. It's not. Sexual health is foundational to quality of life, emotional well-being, and overall health. Yet most women navigating midlife will never be asked about sexual dysfunction during a routine visit. Most will never be screened for it. And most clinicians, even in women's health, will have received little to no formal training in how to diagnose or manage it.

I know because I was one of those clinicians.

For years, I treated hot flashes and irregular bleeding with ease. But when a patient quietly confessed that she no longer wanted sex, that sex had become painful, or that she felt numb and disconnected, I used to freeze. I didn't know what to do with that information, let alone how to help. I wasn't taught how to assess libido. I wasn't given language for responsive desire. I certainly wasn't trained to offer treatment.

Yet these conversations were happening daily in my clinic.

This disconnect between women's lived experience and the clinical framework used to evaluate them isn't just frustrating; it's damaging. When women are told "Everything looks normal," "It's just aging," or "Maybe it's in your head," they internalize that shame. They stop asking questions. They stop believing there are answers. This isn't just medical oversight; it's medical gaslighting, and it's one of the quiet epidemics in women's midlife care.

We urgently need change at every level of the system:

- Medical education on female sexual function must be comprehensive and include evidence-based training that addresses hormonal, psychological, relational, and physical contributors.

- Routine screening for sexual dysfunction should be normalized in midlife care—right alongside blood pressure checks, mammograms, and cholesterol labs.

- Clinical guidelines must reflect the multidimensional nature of sexual health and acknowledge the legitimacy of both hormonal and non-hormonal treatments.

- Research funding must support more studies on women's sexual function in midlife—focusing not just on pharmaceutical interventions but on integrative and lifestyle-based approaches as well.

This isn't just about better sex. It's about restoring dignity to women's health. It's about giving clinicians the tools they need to listen, validate, and offer help. And it's about empowering women with knowledge so they no longer have to suffer in silence.

Even without formal tools, clinicians can begin to make sexual function a part of every routine visit with midlife women. It can be as simple as asking...

- "Are you experiencing any changes in your sexual desire or satisfaction?"
- "Is sex comfortable for you?"
- "Have you noticed any changes in how your body responds during intimacy?"
- "Would you like to talk about ways to improve your sexual well-being?"

These questions aren't intrusive. They're essential. They tell a woman that her sexual health matters, that it's not an afterthought but a core part of her overall well-being.

What's more, we need to dig deeper than just the presence or absence of libido. We need to ask about vaginal dryness, discomfort or pain, difficulty with orgasm, relationship stress, body image concerns, and past trauma, all of which can influence sexual function. And we need to listen without judgment.

Here's what I know after years of listening, practicing, reading, and learning: When women are believed and supported, they thrive. When we stop ignoring sexual function as a vital sign, we help women reclaim joy, confidence, and connection. That's what they deserve. That's what we all deserve.

Let's Explore: The Many Tools and Therapies That Can Help with Sexual Pain and Pleasure

When I started hearing about low libido, painful sex, and a sense of sexual disconnection from my midlife patients, I felt unprepared. I knew something hormonal was happening. I could see the pattern clearly, but I didn't have the tools. I wasn't trained to manage sexual dysfunction. And the standard advice—"try lube" or "reduce stress"—felt woefully inadequate.

But the truth is, there are solutions. Effective, evidence-based therapies exist. And just as importantly, they need to be tailored to the unique biology, relationship context, and lived experience of each woman.

This section is about what helps. Not one silver bullet, but a tool kit—one that includes hormones, lifestyle interventions, and medications.

Menopause Hormone Therapy

Menopause hormone therapy (MHT) can be profoundly helpful for many women experiencing sexual dysfunction in perimenopause and postmenopause. Estrogen therapy, specifically, helps restore vaginal moisture, elasticity, and blood flow, addressing the core physical symptoms of the genitourinary syndrome of menopause (GSM) and improving comfort during sex.

When used locally (as a cream, tablet, or vaginal ring), estrogen is low dose, safe for most women, and incredibly effective in treating vaginal dryness, irritation, and pain with penetration.

In addition to local therapy, systemic MHT (oral, transdermal, or injectable estrogen, often combined with progesterone) can support overall mood, sleep, and energy, creating the hormonal and emotional conditions that support sexual well-being.

Some women may also benefit from DHEA vaginal suppositories or testosterone therapy, particularly those with persistent low libido not relieved by estrogen alone. In international guidelines, testosterone is supported for the treatment of hypoactive sexual desire disorder (HSDD) in postmenopausal women. While there's no FDA-approved formulation for women in the United States, off-label prescribing can be done responsibly with proper monitoring.

Non-Hormonal Therapies: More Than Just Lube

Hormones are helpful, but they're not the whole story. Many women benefit from non-hormonal strategies, particularly when hormonal therapy is contraindicated or not preferred.

- **Vaginal moisturizers and lubricants:** Moisturizers are used regularly, like with skincare, and lubricants, used during sexual activity, are first-line, over-the-counter solutions. Look for water- or silicone-based products free from irritants like glycerin or parabens. (We created our own at The 'Pause Life that you can try out, but there are many good options on the market now.)

- **Pelvic floor physical therapy:** Many women in perimenopause have pelvic floor dysfunction due to tight muscles, scar tissue, or altered tone that can contribute to pain and reduce sensation. Working with a pelvic health specialist can be transformative.

- **Neuromodulators:** Medications like flibanserin and bremelanotide are FDA-approved treatments for low sexual desire in premenopausal women. These may be considered when desire issues are persistent and distressing.

Lifestyle: The Underrated Power of Movement, Sleep, and Nourishment

Midlife women are often told to "just relax" when they mention sexual difficulties. But instead of relaxation, what they really need is restoration of energy, hormone balance, strength, and mental clarity.

- **Resistance training** improves blood flow, body image, and energy—all of which feed into sexual health.

- **Quality sleep** supports hormonal rhythm, desire, and emotional resilience. Prioritizing sleep isn't optional; it's therapeutic.

- **Anti-inflammatory, whole-food nutrition** supports vascular and neurological health, essential to arousal and orgasm. Omega-3s, antioxidants, fiber, and plant-based estrogens (like flax and soy) can help create a nourishing foundation.

Emerging Therapy: GLP-1s

New classes of medications like GLP-1 receptor agonists (such as semaglutide and tirzepatide) have shown promise not just for weight loss but for improving insulin resistance and reducing systemic inflammation. A recent study found that when paired with lifestyle changes, GLP-1 therapy led to up to 30 percent total body weight loss and improved energy, mobility, and confidence, factors that indirectly support libido and emotional intimacy.

And while direct studies on GLP-1 therapy and sexual function in women are still lacking, what I'm seeing in clinical practice is impossible to ignore. Many of my patients, particularly those in loving, long-term relationships where desire was once strong but had gone quiet, are noticing that as their visceral fat decreases, inflammation lowers, and sleep improves, something else is waking back up: their libido. They aren't just feeling better in their bodies; they're feeling more alive, more connected, and more open to intimacy. One patient put it this way: "I didn't expect to feel this much like myself again. It's not just about sex. It's about wanting to be close."

We need more research. But as a clinician, I want to report what I'm seeing in practice: For some women, GLP-1 therapy is doing more than reshaping bodies; it's helping restore connection, confidence, and a part of their identity they feared was gone for good.

The Next Chapter: You Get to Write the Future of Your Sexual Health

There is nothing wrong with you.

Your body is going through a profound and complex transition. Your hormones are shifting. Your libido might feel unfamiliar. Intimacy may be different, distant, or confusing. But none of this means that you're defective or that something essential has gone missing. You're still whole. You're still you.

For far too long, we've allowed outdated narratives and clinical blind spots to shape how we talk about female sexuality in midlife. We've medicalized desire without contextualizing it. We've ignored pain and blamed fatigue. We've left women alone to figure it out with little support and even less education.

When I began practicing, I felt those gaps. My patients were asking for help I hadn't been trained to give. I had the clinical tools to manage bleeding and hot flashes but not the knowledge and confidence to talk about pleasure, arousal, or libido. I went searching for answers, and when I didn't find them in medical textbooks, I turned to experts outside the system. I started listening differently. And what I discovered changed everything.

Because here's the truth: Your sexual health is worthy of care. It's not superficial. It's not shameful. And it doesn't end when your periods do.

Whatever you're feeling—grief, frustration, curiosity, confusion—it's all valid. And more importantly, there are tools and treatments, and there are people who can help. A new and updated version of intimacy is waiting for you—it might look different from the past but can still be rich, connected, and deeply satisfying.

This chapter isn't a prescription; it's an invitation. To shift the narrative. To ask better questions. And to advocate for yourself. You're entitled to explore what intimacy means for *you*, in this phase of life, in this body, right now.

Midlife isn't the end of your sexual story. It's the beginning of a new chapter. And you get to write it.

CHAPTER 12

Fertility Changes and Challenges: The Clock Is Real, but So Is Your Power

> I had no knowledge about menopause or that perimenopause even existed. What little I thought I knew was inaccurate, which resulted in years of suffering that culminated in me being fairly certain that I had developed early-onset dementia. Two of the biggest falsehoods I believed that put me years away from any menopause-related symptoms were that I had started my periods very late (a few months shy of sixteen), and I'd had a baby at age forty-three, which I thought meant I was still very much in prime fertility. Having a baby at that age put me at a severe disadvantage to recognize that the symptoms I developed (brain fog, sleep disturbances, memory lapses, and so on) were something else and not just postnatal hormone shifts. My doctors never mentioned anything either. It took me four years post-pregnancy to realize that there was no way these symptoms were related to his birth, and I found Dr. Haver's videos on YouTube. I'm so grateful for the knowledge and that my daughters won't suffer.
>
> —Julie S.

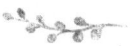

For women who have postponed having children, the late reproductive years can represent an urgent, confusing, and often emotionally fraught time of their lives. What can make this time even more distressing is the lack of clarity and absence of conversation around the intersection of fertility and perimenopause. I've witnessed the impact of this stressful overlap, and I'm here to offer some insightful information that's anchored to biological reality. While this may not fully put your mind at ease, it will hopefully grant you some peace of mind that comes with understanding.

Fertility Changes and Challenges: The Clock Is Real, but So Is Your Power

In my clinical practice and in conversations with friends, I've seen women blindsided and caught between their desire to become a mother and a body quietly entering a hormonal transition. These women are often experiencing subtle shifts in their state of being; they may be having heavier or lighter periods or mid-cycle spotting, or they may be being hit with worsening fatigue and mood instability. Yet they are often reassured—by their own thinking and even by clinical validation—that everything is normal because their cycles are still coming . . . until they aren't.

To demystify this critical life stage, I reached out to my friend and colleague, Dr. Natalie Crawford, a fertility specialist and board-certified reproductive endocrinologist. Dr. Crawford has dedicated her career to helping women understand their fertility with honesty, compassion, and scientific rigor. Her insights, combined with the latest research and my own professional background, provide a road map for navigating the complex overlap between diminishing fertility and midlife transition.

What Happens to Fertility After Thirty-Five?

Fertility decline is often described as a cliff: One day you are fertile, and the next you are not. But in truth, it's more like a slow erosion, a gradual wearing down that becomes dramatically more pronounced after the age of thirty-five.

The biology is clear: In a woman's twenties, the chance of conceiving per menstrual cycle is approximately 20 to 25 percent. By the age of forty, that probability plummets to less than 5 percent. By forty-five, natural conception is rare, with only a small fraction of women able to achieve pregnancy without assistance.

This steady decline is driven by two intertwined biological processes: a reduction in the number of remaining eggs and a decline in their quality. Both processes unfold silently, often without noticeable signs—until the disruption in hormonal balance begins to affect the menstrual cycle. Between the ages of thirty-five and forty-five, there is a steep drop in ovarian reserve. As the ovaries become less responsive, the brain compensates by increasing its output of follicle-stimulating hormone (FSH) in an attempt to prompt ovulation. This results in observable shifts: Cycles may shorten at first, then begin to lengthen unpredictably, and ultimately become more and more irregular (that is, irregular may become your new regular). These aren't random changes; they are signals from a hormonal system straining to maintain equilibrium with fewer and less functional eggs.

Let's take a more detailed look at changes to both egg quantity and quality.

Egg Quantity

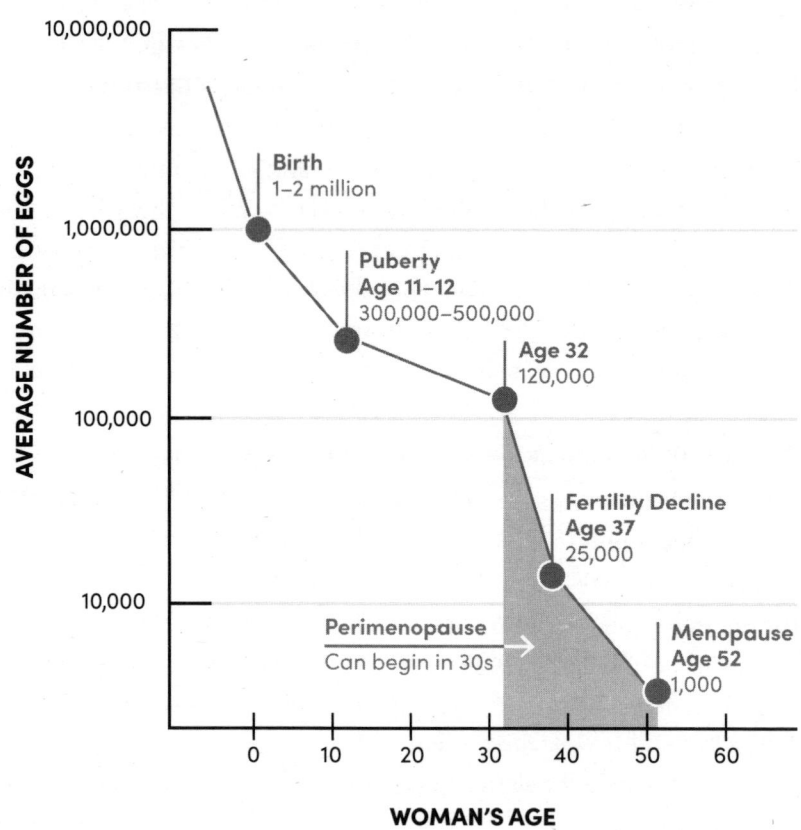

Adapted from "How many eggs does a woman have?" published by *Medical News Today*

Fertility Changes and Challenges: The Clock Is Real, but So Is Your Power

At birth, your two ovaries contain between them all the eggs, or oocytes, you'll have throughout your life. The exact number varies by individual, but it's estimated that we all begin with a primordial pool of between one and two million eggs. This pool will be reduced as you age and pass through various stages of life, and of the total number of eggs you are born with, only about four hundred of them will be ovulated.

At puberty, the egg count has already dropped to about three hundred thousand to five hundred thousand because of a naturally occurring process called atresia. Once you start your period, each menstrual cycle will sacrifice up to one thousand eggs to ovulate one premium oocyte. (During our peak reproductive years, we can afford to lose this many eggs during each recruitment stage of our cycle because the selection pool is still so large. By the age of thirty-five, we see the rate of loss drop to between twenty and two hundred follicles per menstrual cycle.)

For some, looking at the chart on the left can be distressing. But I share this level of detail to provide context for the numbers and to emotionally drive home why timing matters. My intention is not to provoke fear but to inspire proactive, informed decision-making (and to encourage you to act sooner rather than later if you feel it's necessary based on the information you've just read). The biological clock isn't a scare tactic; it's biology, which means it's clear, trackable, and navigable when we acknowledge it as truth. Facing this reality head-on allows women to pursue fertility options and life planning with power rather than panic.

The shortening of cycles, where periods come closer together, is one of the first signs that your ovarian reserve is diminishing. Yet most women—and even many providers—don't recognize it for what it is. Only later, when cycles become erratic, do they realize they are transitioning toward menopause.

This physiological chaos mirrors what I described in earlier chapters as "the zone of chaos," the stage of perimenopause where hormonal signaling becomes disordered, unpredictable, and volatile. Fertility decline is woven into the fabric of this very same chaos.

Even women with outwardly normal periods often experience hidden internal changes:

- a lengthened follicular phase (the time between menstruation and ovulation)
- weaker mid-cycle estrogen surges
- more frequent low-estrogen days

These internal changes affect more than fertility. Low-estrogen days can independently bring about increased fatigue, worsening insomnia, heightened brain fog, declining sexual desire, and subtle but centralized weight gain (in the abdominal region).

Egg Quality

Egg quality is a measure of an egg's ability to undergo normal cell division and form a healthy embryo; it's a reproductive element that diminishes even faster than egg quantity. Aging is the primary factor that can lessen egg quality, and it's been suggested that smoking, excessive alcohol intake, chronic stress, and a consistent dietary pattern of poor nutrition may also downgrade follicle quality. Unfortunately, it's difficult to isolate factors that influence egg quality in humans, so the evidence is either based on animal studies or inconclusive. We clearly need more research in this area.

Changes in egg quality increase the chances of chromosomal abnormalities, which make it less likely for an embryo to implant and develop successfully. This is one of the reasons that rates of miscarriage increase as you advance in age; more than half of all pregnancies in women in their early forties are reported to end in miscarriage. At this time of our lives, we also see the risk of conditions like Down syndrome, trisomy 18, and other genetic disorders rise exponentially.

According to Dr. Crawford, "For the vast majority of women, our eggs lose chromosome integrity before we actually run out of eggs or enter ovarian failure." In other words, fertility after thirty-five isn't just about how many eggs you have—it's the *health* of those eggs that matters most.

The Moving Target of Optimum Fertility in Perimenopause

As if the narrowing window of fertility weren't enough, perimenopause introduces a hormonal "wild card" phase that makes understanding one's fertility even harder.

During perimenopause, the regular feedback loop between the brain and ovaries begins to falter. As ovarian reserve declines and the ovaries become less responsive, the brain responds by pulsing out stronger and more erratic signals, particularly of follicle-stimulating hormone (FSH) and luteinizing hormone (LH). This chaotic hormone signaling disrupts the normal rhythm of ovulation. As a result, cycles that once ran like clockwork—ovulation on day 14, a predictable luteal phase, and a regular menstrual flow—become increasingly irregular.

Women may notice changes like . . .

- shorter cycles (periods coming every twenty-one to twenty-four days)
- longer cycles (skipping a month or bleeding every thirty-five to forty-five days)
- mid-cycle spotting or unpredictable bleeding
- heavier or lighter periods without warning
- occasional anovulatory cycles (no ovulation despite a bleed)

Because of this instability, traditional fertility-tracking methods, such as ovulation predictor kits and basal body temperature (BBT) charting, become less and less reliable. Rising baseline LH levels can produce false-positive ovulation tests, making it seem like ovulation is imminent when it's not. These fluctuations can make it more difficult to detect ovulation and time intercourse.

Similarly, shifts in sleep patterns, metabolism, and nighttime hot flashes can distort basal temperature readings, undermining fertility-tracking tools that rely on BBT.

Research supports this reality: Studies show that estrogen and progesterone levels during perimenopause vary wildly, leading to unpredictable fertile windows that are difficult, if not impossible, to map using traditional cycle-tracking methods.

This confusion has real emotional and clinical consequences. Many women misinterpret these chaotic signs as indications of pregnancy, leading to repeated cycles of hope and disappointment. Others, reassured that irregular bleeding is simply normal perimenopause, may miss early opportunities for fertility evaluation and intervention and as a result lose precious months they can never regain.

Adding to the complexity, something called hormonal withdrawal bleeding can become more common in late perimenopause. Hormonal withdrawal bleeding happens when the body experiences a bleed not because of a successful ovulation but because of a sudden drop in estrogen. Because the bleeding mimics a real menstrual cycle, women assume they are still ovulating regularly when they may not be.

Here's the truth that needs to be broadcast beyond the pages of this book: As the term *zone of chaos* suggests, during perimenopause biology becomes unpredictable, feedback loops destabilize, and even the most carefully laid plans for conception can feel like they're shifting underfoot. This doesn't mean pregnancy is impossible or even unlikely, but it does make it more complicated to achieve. This fact is a product of biology, not personal failure. If navigating fertility during perimenopause feels challenging, it's not because you're not smart enough or dedicated enough or you don't want it enough to figure it out; it's because your body is no longer following the pattern you've known for decades. Period. This isn't a gray area, and we need so much more education focused on this topic to help dispel confusion and self-blame (this is why I'm such a big fan of people like Dr. Crawford who are working so hard to make evidence-based fertility knowledge more accessible).

When you truly allow yourself to understand that fertility unpredictability in perimenopause is biological and not personal failure, you accept an empowering reality. You allow yourself to say,

"I'm going to seek help sooner."

"I'm going to advocate for a thorough evaluation."

"I'm going to make informed decisions about how to move forward."

Testing, Timing, and Treatment

For women in their late thirties and early forties, early and comprehensive fertility evaluation is essential. The traditional definition of infertility, which tells you to wait to see a doctor until you've spent six to twelve months trying unsuccessfully to get pregnant, simply isn't a viable strategy when ovarian reserve is declining rapidly. The time to get an exam is now.

According to Dr. Crawford, a comprehensive evaluation will include . . .

- ovarian reserve testing (includes serum measurements of AMH, FSH, and estradiol)
- antral follicle count via ultrasound
- anatomic evaluation (uterus and fallopian tubes)
- semen analysis for the partner

If you hope to have more than one child, she also emphasizes a strong consideration of embryo banking with in vitro fertilization (IVF) to save embryos for the future. This is a topic of conversation that you can address with the reproductive endocrinologist who does your exam.

You will also likely discuss whether you want to pursue IVF or intrauterine insemination (IUI). IVF involves fertilizing a mature egg with sperm in a lab to form an embryo and implanting this embryo in the uterus. IUI involves placing sperm directly into the uterus, increasing the chances of fertilization (versus penetrative sex). IUI is often an attractive option because it's less complicated and not as costly; however, data shows that older patients may want to consider moving directly to IVF rather than wasting time and money on multiple IUI attempts. IVF can ultimately lead to faster, more cost-effective outcomes.

It should be noted that IVF success rates do decline significantly after age thirty-eight, and perimenopausal patients often face additional challenges such as poor ovarian response, elevated baseline FSH, and premature ovulation.

> ### When Postpartum Meets Perimenopause: The Overlooked Collision
>
> If you are able to get pregnant and have a child in your late thirties or early to mid-forties, it's important to be aware of an overlooked intersection between postpartum and perimenopause. Low estrogen, brain fog, mood swings, sexual health challenges, and persistent amenorrhea (lack of your period) that occur after birth may be blamed on normal postpartum recovery, but it's also possible that ovarian failure is progressing underneath. "Some women never fully resume menstruation after childbirth and are actually in early menopause," notes Dr. Crawford. "We must do better at monitoring postpartum hormones in women thirty-eight and older."
>
> Screening for ovarian reserve after late-maternal-age births, especially if periods don't resume within six months post-weaning, should be part of routine care.

Hormone Therapy and Reproductive Planning

The question many women face is, Can you treat perimenopausal symptoms without jeopardizing fertility goals? The answer is yes, with careful management. I consulted Dr. Crawford for her insight on this topic because it's highly nuanced. "There are very few risks from starting MHT if done carefully," she said. "Low-dose estrogen and strategic progesterone can relieve symptoms without blocking ovulation." This strategy involves using low-dose estrogen to stabilize symptoms, while allowing spontaneous ovulation to occur, and adding progesterone after confirmed ovulation or administering it cyclically if periods are absent.

Achieving both symptom management and fertility preservation will require careful monitoring, but it's absolutely possible.

The Emotional Toll of Midlife Infertility

Struggling with fertility in midlife is layered with unique grief. It's not just the potential loss of motherhood; it's the confrontation with aging, shifting identity, and societal expectations. It can also require an all-consuming level of attention to detail and be extremely isolating; holding space simultaneously for uncertainty, deep longing, *and* lab work, ovulation timing, and so much more. The combination can be distinctly draining and feel like it has literally extracted you from the rest of your life.

Because fertility struggles have this pronounced capacity to isolate, I highly encourage seeking psychological support or connecting with peer groups with whom you can have honest communication about your fertility. Give yourself permission to speak candidly, and make room for waves of grief and hope.

Now Is the Time for Advocacy and Empowerment

One of the greatest myths told to women is that waiting to have children won't cost them anything. In reality, fertility loss happens silently until it becomes irreversible. Don't wait for this to happen to you. Knowledge isn't fearmongering. Knowledge is freedom. Take time now to learn more about ovarian reserve, egg quality, the effects of inflammation and environment, and how lifestyle factors including diet, gut health, and toxin exposure can influence your fertility potential. An excellent resource on this topic is Dr. Crawford's book, *The Fertility Formula*.

Fertility isn't just a matter of fate or luck; it's a combination of biology, environment, and an informed choice. Whatever your future path holds, it's critical to remember that your worth isn't determined by your reproductive timeline. We are such complex beings—our lives branch out and our dreams change shape—which is why I want to make sure you give yourself grace for doing your best to meet your hope for pregnancy with clear-eyed information, strong medical partnerships, and fierce self-compassion in tow. That way, you can move through this transition empowered, not defeated.

CHAPTER 13

When the Bleeding Becomes a Mystery: Uterine Changes in Perimenopause

My menstrual cycle was a problem. I had horrible cramps, super heavy bleeding, and it was unpredictable. In 2017, I had the worst year ever. I was under a lot of stress, having marital issues, and had no time. My period got so bad that I would leak through a super tampon with a heavy pad. Between periods I still bled. I would maybe get four to five days with no bleeding. Finally, one day at my desk at work, I felt so tired that I was ready to pass out. My family doctor got me in early the next morning. She immediately said that we needed to run some blood tests. It turned out that my hemoglobin was so low I needed to get a blood transfusion. I saw an OB-GYN that same day who prescribed birth control, but it did not help. I then had an ultrasound and they found a bunch of fibroids. It was recommended that I have an ablation or hysterectomy, and I opted for a hysterectomy. Six years later, I started having weight gain, brain fog, IBS, and hot flashes every forty-five minutes or so. I wish I had understood better what menopause was like before choosing a hysterectomy.

—Kathryn J.

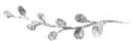

According to the Menopause Society, perimenopause is "the period around the onset of menopause that is often marked by various physical signs such as hot flashes and menstrual irregularities." Let me stop right there. Menstrual irregularities deserve their own entire chapter. So here we are.

If there's one thing that catches almost every woman off guard during perimenopause, it's how these menstrual irregularities present themselves. You may have a period that involves excessive bleeding or that lasts for too long . . . or shows up too early . . . or shows up too late . . . or vanishes for months, only to return with a vengeance. This stage of life can feel like one long guessing game, especially when it comes to what your uterus is doing.

In many ways, this time of our lives can feel a lot like puberty. In fact, I often hear people describe perimenopause as the mirror image of adolescence because just as our bodies transitioned *into* reproductive life during our teen years, perimenopause represents the winding path *out*. And like adolescence, perimenopause can be messy, hormonal, and unpredictable.

One of the ways we can lessen at least some of the unpredictability of this stage is to enhance our understanding of what's going on—knowledge really is the most effective way to weaken the power of mystery. In this chapter, you will learn that perimenopausal menstrual irregularities, while mystifying, aren't so mysterious after all and are most often a direct reflection of the underlying zone of hormonal chaos. I will also walk you through how a clinician might evaluate menstrual irregularities. You shouldn't have to guess what's going on with your body or suffer through it silently.

Defining Irregular Bleeding

The average age of menopause in North America is around fifty-two, but perimenopause can start much earlier and last several years. One of the reasons women seek care during this time is abnormal uterine bleeding (AUB), which is just a clinical way of saying, *"My periods are no longer following the rules."*

Here's the nuance: To most women, any bleeding is "a period." But medically speaking, a true period means that ovulation occurred and was followed by a rise and fall in progesterone. In perimenopause, ovulation becomes sporadic or stops altogether. When that happens, your bleeding may still come, but it won't be predictable.

Abnormal uterine bleeding is defined as flow that falls outside the boundaries of what's considered normal for volume, duration, frequency, or regularity. And it's *incredibly common*. One-third of all visits to a gynecologist are because of AUB, and among women in perimenopause and postmenopause, it accounts for more than 70 percent of consultations. AUB may present itself in a variety of ways:

- **Changes in menstrual symptoms** such as intensity of cramps and PMS symptoms happen as a result of hormonal changes, structural changes, endometriosis, or adenomyosis.

- **Irregular spotting,** light bleeding that occurs between periods, is common in perimenopause and can happen as a result of hormonal or structural fluctuations.

- **Lighter periods** may be caused by decreasing hormone levels.

- **Heavier periods** may be caused by fluctuations in estrogen and progesterone, and are more likely in the late transition and are more common in obese women and in women with fibroids.

- **Shorter cycles** are more common in early perimenopause, as hormone fluctuations can lead to less time between periods.

- **Longer cycles** are more likely to occur in late perimenopause, as shifting hormones can disrupt the regularity of ovulation and lead to more time between periods.

- **Missed periods** happen when your ovaries stop releasing eggs regularly.

If you are postmenopausal, that is, it's been more than twelve months since your last period, and you experience bleeding, it's critical that you get evaluated by a gynecologist. Your physician will be able to rule out endometrial and cervical cancer and atrophic vaginitis/GSM. Atrophic vaginitis is a common cause of postmenopausal bleeding and, if diagnosed, will be treated with topical estrogen therapy or lubricants/moisturizers.

The clinical approach to AUB is to first rule out serious causes like precancer or cancer. In most cases, what we find is something benign and treatable. The treatment in some cases is simply reassurance that there is nothing wrong; in others, we will introduce strategies to lessen the severity of bleeding abnormalities.

Let's get into the why and the what-you-can-do-about-it of bleeding in perimenopause.

Why Periods Get So Unpredictable

When it comes to abnormal bleeding during perimenopause, the causes can be surprisingly complex and can include hormone fluctuations, the body's response to certain medications, and/or physical changes inside the uterus that we can see on an ultrasound or during a procedure.

To guide diagnosis and establish a treatment plan, doctors use a system called PALM-COEIN to sort the possible causes into two buckets:

- structural (something we can see)
- non-structural (related to how your body is functioning)

Let's break it down into plain language.

Structural Causes (PALM)

These are physical changes in or around the uterus:

- **P—Polyps:** Small growths that can form inside the uterus or cervix. Polyps are typically non-cancerous but can sometimes cause bleeding, especially between periods or after sex.
- **A—Adenomyosis:** When the lining of the uterus grows into the muscle wall of the uterus. This usually leads to cramping and heavier periods—but not always.
- **L—Leiomyoma (also known as fibroids):** Benign (non-cancerous) muscle tumors that grow in the wall of the uterus. Some women

never know they have them, while others experience very heavy or prolonged bleeding because of them.

- **M—Malignancy (cancer) or hyperplasia:** Abnormal or precancerous thickening of the uterine lining, or uterine cancer. It's especially important to rule this out in anyone with bleeding after menopause or irregular, heavy bleeding in midlife.

Non-Structural Causes (COEIN)

These are causes related to how your body works, rather than something we can see on a scan:

- **C—Coagulopathy:** A fancy word for a bleeding disorder, where your blood doesn't clot as well as it should. Some women have always had heavy periods and didn't know a clotting issue was part of it.

- **O—Ovulatory dysfunction:** When your body doesn't ovulate regularly (*which happens a lot in perimenopause*), your periods become irregular, unpredictable, or unusually heavy. This can also be related to conditions like PCOS, thyroid issues, high stress, weight changes, or extreme exercise.

- **E—Endometrial (uterine lining) problems:** Sometimes the problem is how the lining of your uterus breaks down and sheds—even if you're still ovulating. The bleeding might be heavy or prolonged, without any clear structural cause.

- **I—Iatrogenic (caused by medications or devices):** This includes bleeding caused by hormonal treatments (like birth control or hormone therapy), IUDs, or other medications that can affect the uterus or hormone levels.

- **N—Not yet classified:** Some causes are still being studied or don't fit neatly into any of the above categories.

You don't need to memorize these lists—but it's important to understand that irregular or heavy bleeding in midlife can have multiple causes.

It's a hormonal shift *plus* a fibroid. It's an anovulatory cycle *plus* an endometrial lining that's grown unchecked. Sometimes it's thyroid dysfunction. Sometimes it's something else entirely.

But here's what I want you to hear loud and clear.

It's not your fault.

It's not just your age.

And it's *definitely* not just stress.

One of the hardest parts of this phase is how quickly women blame themselves. "Maybe it's because I haven't taken care of myself." "Maybe I'm just overreacting." No, you are not overreacting. You are responding to real, physiological changes. As a clinician, I've seen what happens when we validate those symptoms and investigate what's actually going on. When we take women seriously, we get answers. And with the right care, we can stop the chaos, preserve your health, and give you back a sense of control.

So please, don't carry shame for what your body is doing. This is biology and not a personal failing. And you deserve support that reflects that truth.

Once your practitioner can identify the root cause of menstrual irregularities, they can then determine options for the best next step, whether that's watchful waiting, medication, hormone therapy, or something more.

You deserve answers and options, and as a patient, you are going to have to do your part in pursuing both. I wish I could say reading this book will be enough, but it won't; it's going to take a trip to the gynecologist.

When It's "Just Perimenopause"—What Are Your Options?

After a thorough evaluation, your gynecologist may determine that your irregular or heavy bleeding is due to perimenopause—and not from other causes such as fibroids, endometrial hyperplasia, or cancer. While this can be reassuring, many women still feel frustrated by the unpredictability of their cycles and the disruption it brings to daily life.

It's important to understand that just because it's common doesn't mean you have to live with it. Once serious conditions have been ruled out, several well-established strategies can help manage abnormal uterine bleeding (AUB) caused by perimenopause. These options range from conservative approaches to more definitive procedures, and the right choice depends on your symptoms, health goals, and personal preferences.

Expectant Management

Sometimes the best approach is simply watching and waiting. Known as expectant management, this strategy involves keeping track of your bleeding pattern over time, monitoring your hemoglobin or iron levels if necessary, and checking in regularly with your provider. This may be a good option if your bleeding isn't heavy, painful, or affecting your quality of life.

Hormonal Therapies

When we talk about treatment options for irregular or heavy bleeding in perimenopause, it's important to be clear: Traditional menopause hormone therapy (MHT) isn't designed to do this job.

The doses used in MHT, whether it's transdermal or oral estradiol with a progestogen, are effective for managing vasomotor symptoms, sleep, mood, and bone health. But they aren't high enough to inhibit ovulation or fully suppress the menstrual cycle. So, if your primary concern is cycle regulation or bleeding control, MHT alone isn't the right tool.

Instead, we need to look at hormonal therapies that are specifically tailored for menstrual regulation:

- **Oral contraceptives (the Pill):** These contain higher doses of estrogen and progestin and are often used to stabilize the endometrium, reduce menstrual flow, and offer predictable bleeding patterns. They're especially helpful in early to mid-perimenopause when ovulation is still occurring sporadically.

- **Progestogens:** For women who can't take estrogen—or prefer not to—cyclic or continuous progestogen therapy can be used to thin the endometrial lining and reduce bleeding. This can be delivered orally or via intramuscular injections, depending on the clinical situation.

- **Hormone-releasing IUDs (like Mirena):** These are one of my go-to tools in practice. The levonorgestrel IUD delivers progestin directly to the uterus, minimizing systemic exposure while significantly reducing or even eliminating bleeding. It can also help manage cramping and is often effective for up to eight years.

These therapies can also offer broader symptom relief. Some formulations may improve hot flashes and PMS-like symptoms, especially in women whose hormonal cycling is still active but erratic.

Every woman's needs are different, and treatment should always be individualized. But we need to stop pretending that "just waiting it out" is a valid strategy. When heavy or unpredictable bleeding is interfering with your life, there are safe, effective options to get it under control—and help you reclaim your quality of life.

Nonsteroidal Anti-Inflammatory Drugs (NSAIDs)

Drugs like ibuprofen or naproxen, taken during menstruation, can not only relieve cramps but also reduce blood loss by decreasing prostaglandin production. Often underutilized as a first-line option, NSAIDs can be helpful especially for women with mild to moderate bleeding.

Antifibrinolytics

Some women bleed heavily because their bodies break down blood clots too quickly—a process known as fibrinolysis. In these cases, medications like tranexamic acid can reduce menstrual blood loss without affecting hormones. These are taken (orally) only on the days you're bleeding and are a good option for women who want a non-hormonal solution.

Dilation and Curettage (D&C)

This is a short outpatient procedure in which the lining of the uterus is gently scraped or suctioned to remove tissue. A D&C can be both diagnostic (to rule out abnormalities) and therapeutic (to temporarily reduce heavy bleeding). It's not a long-term solution but may offer short-term relief or help confirm a diagnosis.

Endometrial Ablation

For women who no longer wish to have children, endometrial ablation may be considered. This procedure permanently destroys the uterine lining using heat, cold, or other techniques. In many cases, this results in lighter periods—or no periods at all. While effective for some, it's not suitable for everyone and should be discussed carefully with your doctor.

Hysterectomy

In the most severe cases—or when other treatments have failed—a hysterectomy may be considered. This surgery removes the uterus and sometimes the cervix. While a hysterectomy provides definitive relief from bleeding, it's rarely the first step and comes with important considerations. Even when the ovaries are left intact, a hysterectomy reduces blood flow to them and leads to earlier menopause, on average about 4.4 years sooner than if the uterus were left in place.

A Note on Hysterectomy

It still shocks me how often I ask a patient why she had a hysterectomy and she doesn't really know. Sometimes the answer is clear: fibroids, adenomyosis, endometriosis, or unmanageable bleeding that didn't respond to other treatments. These are legitimate medical indications, and for some women, a hysterectomy can be truly life changing. But almost half the time, what I hear is this: "My doctor said I didn't need my ovaries and uterus anymore." Or even worse: "They told me it would cure my menopause."

Let me be clear: Hysterectomy isn't a treatment for perimenopause. It won't stop the hormonal chaos of fluctuating estrogen and progesterone, and it won't cure hot flashes, mood swings, or sleep disruption. If the ovaries are left intact, you'll still go through the hormonal transition. If they're removed, you'll be thrust into sudden menopause, which is often more severe than the natural transition.

A hysterectomy is major surgery. It carries risks: surgical complications, infection, long recovery time, changes in pelvic floor function, and even long-term impacts on sexual health and bladder function. That doesn't mean it's never appropriate, but it does mean we should treat the decision with the seriousness it deserves.

The essential takeaway is this: The uterus isn't disposable. It's not something you remove just because "you're done having kids" or "you don't need it anymore." It's a complex organ that plays a role beyond reproduction—including structural support in the pelvis and emotional significance for many women.

So, if you're being told you need a hysterectomy and you're feeling rushed, uncertain, or confused, pause. Ask questions. Get a second opinion. Make sure your concerns are heard and your diagnosis is clearly explained. This is your body, your future, and your decision. We owe it to ourselves—and to one another—to demand care that honors that.

What to Consider When Choosing a Treatment

Choosing a treatment isn't one-size-fits-all. Factors including your age, bleeding severity, risk factors, medical history, desire for contraception, and proximity to menopause should all be considered. A shared decision-making approach—with you and your doctor working together—is essential.

Remember, your symptoms are real, your comfort matters, and help is available. Whether you're hoping for lighter periods, fewer surprises, or simply a sense of control over your body again, there are solutions. You don't have to white-knuckle your way through perimenopause. Let's get you the support and relief you deserve.

Part Four

A WINDOW OF OPPORTUNITY (FOR PREVENTION)

CHAPTER 14

Treating Hormonal Fluctuation with Hormones: A Deep Dive into MHT to Treat Perimenopause

At thirty-nine, I began experiencing night sweats, joint pain, dry skin, hair loss, and sudden intolerance to red wine. The worst was four years of insomnia, which deeply affected my nervous system. I was also diagnosed with functional depression. In summer 2024, I gained ten pounds in two months. My cholesterol and triglycerides skyrocketed, and my blood work showed I was close to prediabetes. I knew something was wrong. My gynecologist dismissed me, saying I was forty-three and that Latina women don't enter perimenopause until forty-nine. After I insisted, she tested my hormones and said everything was normal. I felt unheard.

A menopause specialist reviewed my labs and confirmed low hormones and vitamin D deficiency, warning me about osteoporosis. She prescribed hormone therapy, and within six months, I felt like myself again. As a Hispanic woman, I know menopause is rarely discussed. But we deserve to be heard. No doctor should dismiss our reality.

—Lilly R.

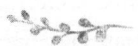

As I hope is clear by this point, perimenopause isn't just a transition. It's a window. A critical and often-overlooked opportunity to pause, assess, and take control of our long-term health. This phase of life isn't the beginning of the end. It's the beginning of a new conversation with our bodies. It's when we are most likely to be told that everything is fine while feeling anything but. It's when our risk for disease starts to quietly increase, when our resilience can either erode or be rebuilt, and when the cracks in the system—medical, cultural, and personal—begin to show. But this is also the moment when we can intervene. We can challenge outdated assumptions. We can stop tolerating suffering as the price of admission to midlife. We can choose strength, clarity, and prevention.

Perimenopause is the turning point. If we recognize it, respect it, and respond with action, it can become one of the most powerful inflection points in our lives. This is our chance to shift the status quo and demand more for ourselves, for our daughters, and for every woman still waiting to be seen.

Despite the significant impact of perimenopause on women's health and quality of life, there remains a striking lack of large, prospective studies focused on its treatment. As I pointed out in chapter 1, a search of the top scientific database in the world reveals around 7,000 studies have been conducted on the topic of perimenopause (this is compared with nearly 1.2 million on pregnancy). Add to this the fact that a lot of the research we do have comes from studies done on animals that *don't go through perimenopause,* and you can see why we don't have a lot of rock-solid evidence on which to base our clinical practice.

This glaring gap in research leaves healthcare providers relying on data extrapolated from studies on postmenopausal women, which often fail to address the unique hormonal fluctuations and symptoms of perimenopause. These factors make the treatment of perimenopause . . . in a word, complicated.

As a physician, I was never taught to *treat* perimenopause. It wasn't framed as a condition that could warrant intervention. Instead, it was framed as a normal, albeit sometimes-uncomfortable, transition. Even now, many doctors cling to outdated criteria, insisting you must go one year without a period before being considered eligible for even a discussion on treatment options. This leaves countless women in limbo, struggling with life-altering symptoms while being told to wait it out.

What I realize *now* is that I was taught to silo *each* symptom of perimenopause and address them separately and was never taught that they could *all* be related to hormone changes. I knew that bleeding problems were common in perimenopause, but I wasn't taught that abnormal uterine bleeding could be a direct result of underlying hormonal chaos. I also saw an increase in mental health changes, but I wasn't educated on the fact that declining/fluctuating estrogen could be to blame. This fragmented approach ignores what is most often the root cause of perimenopausal symptoms and leads to a patchwork form of care that results in little more than incremental improvements of overall quality of life.

The question is this: Now that I know so much more about perimenopause after years spent poring over research, hundreds of hours invested in conversations with brilliant specialists, and a new focus on a patient profile made up almost entirely of perimenopausal and postmenopausal women, have I landed on the guaranteed formula for the treatment and management of symptoms in perimenopause? Do we treat the symptoms one by one, with sleeping pills for insomnia, antidepressants for mood changes, and NSAIDs for heavy periods? Or do we address the hormonal instability itself, potentially with low-dose hormone therapy to smooth out the peaks and valleys of estrogen?

There's no one-size-fits-all solution. Every woman's experience of perimenopause is unique, and treatment needs to be tailored to her specific symptoms, health history, and goals. But the lack of clear guidelines and comprehensive research means that many women and their clinicians are left navigating this complex phase with little guidance and even less validation.

In my experience and in the experience of my colleagues sitting face-to-face with patients doing perimenopause care, what we have found is that if we do decide to treat, it tends to require much trial and error. What works well during one era of perimenopause often needs adjustments as hormonal fluctuations continue and symptoms evolve until full menopause is reached. This dynamic and individualized approach reflects the reality of treating a condition that is as variable as the women experiencing it. It also underscores the importance of regular monitoring, open communication, and a willingness to adapt the approach to meet a woman's changing needs.

In this chapter, we'll explore the hormonal options for managing perimenopause, from symptom-specific treatments to systemic approaches. These treatment options are the result of consultations with colleagues in perimenopause care and direct learning from the experiences of my patients. Given the scant guidelines currently available for treatment during perimenopause, these strategies represent a collective effort to provide effective care in the absence of robust research. Ultimately, the goal is to empower you to advocate for yourself and make informed choices about your care in a time when the medical establishment often fails to provide the answers you need.

Hormones 101: What's Actually Changing in Perimenopause

Throughout this book, you have learned so much about the hormones that are most influential during the menopause transition and the many ways fluctuations in their long-stable presence can disrupt your body and overall well-being. Before I get into the details on the use of menopause hormone therapy (MHT) in perimenopause, I want to step back and offer you a recap of these key hormones and how they work. I know there is a lot of confusion on MHT use in perimenopause and whether it should be considered in the first place and, if it is used, whether it will be helpful, safe, or affordable. I think this brief overview will provide proper context for you to grasp fully why MHT can be so effective during this hormonal stage.

So, first things first: Hormones are chemical messengers. They travel through the bloodstream to communicate with cells, telling them what to do—whether that is building tissue, metabolizing fuel, regulating mood, or supporting reproduction. Hormones interact with receptors located on the surface of or inside cells. In chapter 4, I described this interaction as being similar to a track athlete (the hormone) in a relay passing off the baton to the next runner (the receptor). We can also think of the hormone as the key, and the receptor as the lock. When the right key finds the right lock, the system activates. No matter which way you look at it, the relationship between hormones and their receptors is one of great biological significance; in fact, it's responsible for nearly every action that takes place within the body.

When hormone levels drop or become erratic, as they do in perimenopause, the communication between hormones and cells begins to break down. Cells are left waiting for the signal to act, or they receive conflicting messages. Over time, this dysregulation can lead to physical and emotional symptoms and open the door to disease risk.

> ### A Name Change in the Future for MHT?
>
> Menopause hormone therapy (MHT) is a phrase many in the menopause healthcare space have worked hard to reclaim and clarify. It is a step up and away from the term *hormone replacement therapy,* which proved to be too limiting and misleading. Yet many of my colleagues and I have begun to realize that MHT may itself again need revising because it implies that hormone therapy is *only* for those who are menopausal. And that its use begins with the cessation of menstruation.
>
> When we describe it as menopause hormone therapy, we risk the very label leaving out the perimenopausal woman whose ovaries are still firing erratically and leaving a trail of symptoms in their wake; the postpartum woman with genitourinary syndrome of lactation, who is experiencing dryness, UTIs, and painful intimacy. We dismiss the woman on ovulation-suppressing medication whose testosterone has plummeted, and the people, of all genders and ages, who experience clinically significant hormonal deficiencies and need support.
>
> We need language that reflects the full scope of physiological reality, and a new nomenclature is in the works. The proposed term is PET hormones, which stands for Progesterone, Estrogen, Testosterone.
>
> We are not abandoning the word *menopause,* but we are recognizing that hormone therapy should not be limited by it. PET hormones can support health far beyond the menopause label, across midlife, postpartum, post-surgical, and medically induced hormone loss.

Estrogens

Most people think of estrogen as a single hormone, but there are actually three primary estrogens in the body.

Estradiol is the most potent and the one produced primarily by the ovaries during the reproductive years. It's the dominant estrogen before menopause and plays a central role in regulating the menstrual cycle, brain function, metabolic activity, and bone health. During perimenopause, estradiol levels don't simply drop—they swing wildly. You may experience surges followed by crashes. This instability contributes to many of the hallmark symptoms including night sweats, mood swings, brain fog, and cycle irregularity.

Estrone becomes the dominant estrogen after menopause. It's mainly produced in adipose and other tissues, but its effects are weaker and less reliable than estradiol.

Estriol is mostly produced during pregnancy by the placenta. While it can have some benefit in very low doses for local tissue support such as vaginal atrophy, it isn't a major player in systemic hormone regulation for perimenopausal or menopausal women.

Progesterone

Progesterone is produced after ovulation and plays an essential role in preparing the uterine lining for potential pregnancy. It also has important effects on the brain, supporting sleep, mood stability, and a sense of calm.

In perimenopause, ovulation becomes irregular, so even when estrogen is still present, progesterone often isn't. This leads to an imbalance that can drive anxiety, poor sleep, breast tenderness, heavy periods, and more. Supplementing with oral micronized progesterone during this phase can have a calming effect on the brain and body, even in the absence of full menopause.

Androgens

Androgens such as testosterone, DHEA, and androstenedione are typically thought of as male hormones, but they play an essential role in female health, too. They support sexual function, energy levels, muscle tone, and mood. Androgens are produced by the ovaries and adrenal glands, and while levels decline more gradually than estrogens or progesterone, some women may experience noticeable symptoms as they taper, particularly in the years after ovulation begins to slow.

In chapter 11, I mentioned that some women in perimenopause may develop hypoactive sexual desire disorder (HSDD), defined as a lack or loss of sexual desire, including the absence of sexual thoughts or fantasies, that creates personal distress and difficulty in relationships. If HSDD is suspected, your practitioner should consider you for a trial of low-dose testosterone therapy. This approach to HSDD in perimenopause has thus far proved to be very effective in my patients.

Should We Treat High Estrogen with Estrogen?

If estrogen levels are already fluctuating wildly and sometimes even soaring to levels we don't see outside pregnancy, why would we give a woman more estradiol? It's a fair question and one I hear often. But here's the key: Perimenopause doesn't begin in the ovaries. It begins in the brain. The hypothalamus in the brain is constantly scanning for a stable, sufficient level of estradiol to maintain homeostasis. When estradiol levels begin to destabilize in perimenopause, even briefly, the pituitary receives a signal from the hypothalamus to send increasingly intense bursts of LH and FSH to the ovaries in an attempt to get more estrogen through ovulation. The ovaries, now nearing the end of their reproductive capacity, respond unpredictably: Sometimes they ignore the signals entirely; other times they send out a massive surge of estrogen that overshoots the mark and then crashes. This is the roller coaster of perimenopause: not just low estrogen, but unstable estrogen.

I was never taught about this in medical school, and I know many practitioners out there have similarly not been educated on the nature of extreme fluctuations in perimenopause. What I've come to understand is that if we run a woman's labs during one of these peaks, we see an estradiol level that looks surprisingly high. *But this is a transient moment,* not a steady state. And almost always, it's paired with low or absent progesterone because ovulation is becoming sporadic. This hormonal mismatch—high estrogen with no progesterone to balance it—can lead to a range of symptoms like mood swings, sleep disruption, breast tenderness, and heavy periods.

What we are aiming to do with low-dose estradiol in perimenopause is not to add to the chaos but to calm it. These physiologic doses bind to estrogen receptors in the hypothalamus and help stabilize the feedback loop between the brain and the ovaries. In doing so, they can reduce the frequency and intensity of those dramatic hormonal swings. The brain, sensing that estradiol is finally present, may stop pushing the pituitary to stimulate the ovaries so aggressively. And with that, the system settles.

My patients do very well with this approach in perimenopause. It doesn't block ovulation outright, as these aren't high enough doses to fully suppress the system, but it takes some of the volatility out of the equation. This can be especially helpful in supporting sleep and mood when paired with progesterone in the luteal phase or given continuously. Progesterone is always given alongside estrogen in patients with a uterus because of its role in protecting the endometrium.

The Nuance of Hormone Therapy in Perimenopause

Hormone therapy during perimenopause isn't just about replacing what is lost; it's about stabilizing what is dysregulated. You aren't in menopause yet, which means your system is still active but often out of rhythm. Restoring that rhythm with carefully dosed estradiol, progesterone, or sometimes testosterone can calm the chaos, reduce symptoms, and protect long-term health. This isn't about giving back what you no longer have. It's about supporting the hormonal systems you still do.

When we consider treatment of perimenopause from a root cause perspective, there are two schools of thought: suppress and replace hormones or support the fluctuations (remember the zone of chaos). These approaches vary mostly based on the type and dose of hormones used, and they each serve a purpose depending on the individual's symptoms and menstrual cycle status.

Suppress and Replace

When we suppress and replace, we are using higher hormone doses such as those found in contraceptive hormones. This can be the best option if the patient has symptoms that may be related to perimenopause and is also seeking contraception. High-doses hormone options can be used, too, if a patient is experiencing heavy periods. Either contraceptive hormones or a progestin-containing IUD effectively controls heavy periods by stabilizing and regularly shedding the endometrial lining. (Note: The progestins contained in IUDs are locally acting and not systemic; some women may benefit from the use of such IUDs for control of abnormal uterine bleeding whether or not there is a need for contraception.)

Support

If you don't need contraception or treatment for heavy cycles, a supportive approach may be a better option. This approach is usually in the form of low-dose hormone therapy, designed to stabilize the fluctuating ovarian hormone levels seen in perimenopause. By providing steady hormone levels, the therapy feeds back to the hypothalamus and calms the surges of FSH that drive many of the symptoms during this transition, without fully suppressing ovulation.

To give you a couple of examples of how supportive hormones work, if you are perimenopausal with regular periods and you are experiencing sleep disruptions in the luteal phase (the twelve- to fourteen-day phase that occurs after ovulation), progesterone alone may produce noticeable improvements. Or if you have perimenopausal depression, transdermal estradiol has been found to be an effective treatment, even more so than a traditional SSRI.

Both approaches have their merits and challenges, and there's no objective best way—it's incumbent on a clinician to evaluate a patient thoroughly to determine the appropriate starting strategy for them (and on both the clinician and the patient to be ready and willing to wade through some trial and error). Every woman's hormone landscape, symptom burden, and personal goals should be used to guide the treatment choice—and when all of this is taken into consideration, either approach can be safe, evidence based, and transformative.

Another critical point of consideration will be to determine with your doctor if for you the benefits of MHT outweigh the risks; hormone therapy isn't right for everyone, and there are absolute contraindications when it comes to its use. There are also many misconceptions about who can and can't take it. A contraindication is a specific condition or reason that a drug or procedure shouldn't be used because it may be harmful to the person. You shouldn't use MHT if any of the following safety concerns are present:

1. **Known or suspected breast cancer or other estrogen- or progestogen-sensitive cancer:** MHT can stimulate the growth of hormone-sensitive cancers, so it's not recommended for individuals with a history of these types of cancers.
2. **Undiagnosed abnormal genital bleeding:** Any unexplained unusual vaginal bleeding needs proper diagnosis before considering MHT, as it could be a sign of an underlying condition.
3. **Active or recent arterial thromboembolic disease:** Conditions like recent heart attack or stroke pose risks when combined with MHT, as it may increase the risk of blood clots.
4. **Active or recent venous thromboembolic disease:** Conditions like deep vein thrombosis or pulmonary embolism can be aggravated by oral estrogen therapy, leading to further clotting risks.
5. **Known or suspected pregnancy:** Hormone therapy isn't appropriate during pregnancy because of potential effects on fetal development.
6. **Active severe liver disease or dysfunction:** Individuals with *significant* liver impairment might not metabolize hormones properly, making MHT unsafe.

7. **Hypersensitivity to any components of hormone therapy:** Prior allergic reactions to components of MHT can prohibit you from using them again.

MHT shouldn't be used if any of these specific conditions are met, because the risks for the patient are known to be greater than the benefits. The same exclusion does not extend to related conditions even though some clinicians have misconstrued contraindications in ways that have excluded patients from MHT. Here are some of the most common misconceptions:

1. *A history of endometriosis or adenomyosis excludes you from MHT.* **False.** The data to suggest that MHT will reactivate endometriosis and cause pain is theoretical. If endometriosis led to the need for a hysterectomy, I would always add progesterone to decrease the reactivation of any lesions, especially in perimenopause.
2. *A family history of heart disease, liver disease, or breast cancer **automatically** excludes you from MHT.* **False.** The latest research and expert consensus challenge the notion that family history alone should disqualify a woman from MHT candidacy.
3. *Concern over an increased risk of clotting excludes you from MHT.* **False.** While it's true that oral estrogen formulations have been associated with an increased risk of clotting, the same isn't true of estrogen formulations in other delivery systems. Non-oral forms of estrogen, such as patches or creams, don't elevate clotting risk over baseline levels.

The decision to embark on MHT in perimenopause should always be based on your unique medical history, risk factors, and symptoms. And your healthcare provider will ideally be referencing current research and clinical guidelines to provide for you the most up-to-date recommendations. Perimenopausal women have been denied access to a discussion on hormone therapy for far too long—it's time for this to change.

Contraceptive Hormone Therapy Versus Menopausal Hormone Therapy: What's the Difference?

In everyday conversation, many people refer to any hormonal treatment as birth control, but this can be misleading, especially in midlife care. What we often call birth control is more accurately described as contraceptive hormone therapy (CHT). These therapies, while sometimes used to prevent pregnancy, are also frequently used in perimenopause to manage symptoms like heavy or irregular bleeding.

CHT isn't just about pills—it includes rings, patches, implants, and IUDs. The key point is this: CHT and menopause hormone therapy (MHT) both involve giving hormones to women, but the intention, hormone type, and dosage vary significantly.

Whether we are prescribing hormones for contraception, for symptom relief, or for both, the goal is always to meet the patient where she is in her reproductive and hormonal journey—with the safest and most effective options available.

1. **Hormone dosages:** CHT contains higher hormone doses than MHT. This is because CHT is designed to suppress ovulation and prevent pregnancy, which requires a strong hormonal signal to override the body's natural cycle. In contrast, MHT aims to supplement or stabilize hormone levels to alleviate menopausal symptoms and support overall health. The lower doses in MHT are sufficient to manage symptoms like hot flashes and vaginal dryness without suppressing ovulation or significantly altering the menstrual cycle (if it's still occurring).

2. **Hormone formulations:** The types of hormones used in CHT and MHT also differ. CHT typically contains a synthetic version of estrogen (ethinyl estradiol) and a progestin, which are chemically different from the hormones naturally produced by the body. These synthetic hormones are potent and designed for contraceptive effectiveness. MHT, on the other hand, often uses bioidentical hormones, which are chemically identical to the body's natural

hormones. Common examples include estradiol for estrogen and micronized progesterone for progestogen. These formulations are chosen to mimic the body's natural hormone activity and are generally considered safer and better suited for long-term use.

Types of Menopause Hormone Therapy

When we are discussing hormone therapy for perimenopause, we are usually talking about estradiol, progesterone, and, in some cases, testosterone. Hormone therapy for perimenopause can be confusing, in part because of the many overlapping and sometimes-misleading terms used to describe treatment options. You may hear *conventional, natural, traditional, bioidentical, synthetic,* and *compounded.* The easiest and most useful way to think about hormone therapy is to consider how your body sees it: Is the hormone chemically identical to what your body used to make or is now making less of? Or is it a copy of a copy, therefore having less molecular resemblance? Let me explain further.

Bioidentical hormones have the same molecular structure as the hormones naturally produced by your body. These are usually derived from plant sources and are made in a lab to be structurally identical to human estrogen, progesterone, or testosterone.

Synthetic hormones are also made in a lab but aren't molecularly identical to your body's hormones. Your body may need to convert them into usable forms, and they may interact differently with hormone receptors.

Both bioidentical and synthetic hormones are manufactured. The key distinction is not where they come from but whether their structure matches what your body is designed to use.

In my practice, I prefer bioidentical hormones whenever possible. It makes intuitive and clinical sense to give the body a form it already knows how to use.

As a menopause specialist, I'm deeply grateful to have access to bioidentical forms of MHT like estradiol and micronized progesterone for my postmenopausal patients and for perimenopausal patients when it's the right fit. But when I need higher doses—for contraception or reliable cycle control in perimenopausal women—I hit a wall. There is no FDA-approved, even partially bioidentical combination available in the United States for these purposes, and I have to resort to using synthetic forms of contraceptive hormone therapy. (While these aren't bad, I would love to see a biologically equivalent option on the market.)

I'll tell you why this is incredibly frustrating—there is a product that contains bioidentical estradiol plus a synthetic progestin, and it's offered in doses high enough to inhibit ovulation *and* provide contraception. It's called Zoely. Amazing. Except it hasn't been approved for use in the United States. It has been used in Europe since 2011 and in dozens of other countries. Here in the United States, we seem destined to go on without a combined option even though it's clearly possible to create one. The issue to me seems purely a matter of economics—no pharmaceutical company has stepped up to combine estradiol and progesterone in a dose that can reliably suppress ovulation, because the profit margins aren't high enough to justify the cost of development, testing, and FDA approval. Synthetic formulations continue to dominate the U.S. market. This remains true even though we don't have testing of synthetic versus bioidentical options that compares safety and efficacy. We need more research.

The Sudden End of Perimenopause: Surgical Menopause Changes Your MHT Needs

If your path leads to the need for surgical intervention and your ovaries are removed, your perimenopause stage will be over immediately and you will be in surgical menopause. In this case, it's highly important to discuss with your clinician an MHT protocol that addresses sudden symptoms and rising risks that come with the abrupt loss of estrogen. The risks are even more amplified the younger you are when you lose the function of your ovaries. This is not to scare you but to make sure you know taking action is essential.

FDA-Approved Versus Compounded Hormone Therapy

Within the bioidentical category, there are two major types: FDA-approved bioidentical hormone therapy and compounded bioidentical hormone therapy.

FDA-approved bioidentical hormone therapy is made by pharmaceutical companies, standardized for dose and purity, and regulated under strict guidelines. These products are prescribed in known amounts, come in specific delivery forms, and are typically covered by insurance.

Compounded bioidentical hormone therapy is prepared in compounding pharmacies, often customized by a provider to a specific dose or delivery method (such as troches, creams, pellets, or capsules). While customization can be helpful for women who have allergies or unique dosing needs, compounded hormone therapy isn't regulated to the same degree as FDA-approved versions. This means variability in quality and dosing, and compounded products are usually not covered by insurance.

There is also a lot of misinformation in the marketplace. I have found that a lot of women leave their practitioner's office convinced that the only way to access estradiol and progesterone is through a compounding pharmacy—this isn't true. You can get non-compounded, bioidentical transdermal estradiol and micronized progesterone through a traditional pharmacy, and they will likely cost less out of pocket.

Some compounding pharmacies and their promoters claim their customized blends are safer or more effective than FDA-approved hormones, especially those containing estriol. These claims aren't supported by clinical trials.

Another area of concern within the space of perimenopausal care is the push toward saliva or urine hormone tests, such as the DUTCH test, to guide diagnosis or dosing. These tests are expensive, not covered by insurance, and not validated for use in determining precise hormone therapy prescriptions—especially not in the constantly shifting landscape of perimenopause. I don't use them, and I don't recommend them, and to be completely frank, I find their use to be borderline predatory on women in perimenopause. Hormone levels during this phase fluctuate too widely to be captured reliably with one-time lab tests.

Hormone Therapy Delivery Systems

Hormones are delivered two primary ways: systemically and locally.

Systemic therapy delivers hormones into the bloodstream and throughout the body. These therapies are most commonly used to treat whole-body symptoms like hot flashes, mood shifts, and sleep disturbances.

Systemic estrogen can be delivered in several forms:

- **Pill (oral):** easy to take but increases liver activation and comes with a slightly higher risk of clotting, hypertension, and changes in lipids
- **Patch:** applied to the skin, bypasses the liver, preferred in women with clot risk
- **Gel or spray:** applied daily to the skin, also bypasses the liver
- **Ring:** inserted vaginally
- **Injection:** long-acting, typically used in specialized settings
- **Creams or pellets:** typically compounded and not FDA approved

Local estrogen therapy is used to treat vaginal and urinary symptoms. These medications come in creams, tablets, rings, and suppositories. They are low dose and have minimal systemic absorption. *You can safely combine local and systemic therapy if needed.*

One of the primary reasons for the prescription of localized estrogen therapy is to treat the genitourinary syndrome of menopause (GSM), which can cause symptoms such as vaginal dryness, irritation, pain during intercourse, increased urinary frequency and urgency, and UTIs.

The table below reflects the updated guidelines from the American Urological Association (released in 2025) on hormonal interventions for

GSM. I'm including it here so that you can share this page with your practitioner if your symptoms match those I just described.

FDA-Approved Treatments for GSM				
CATEGORY	COMPOSITION	COMMONLY USED STARTING DOSE	COMMONLY USED MAINTENANCE DOSE	TYPICAL SERUM ESTRADIOL LEVEL (PG/ML)
VAGINAL CREAMS	17β-estradiol 0.01% (0.1 mg active ingredient/g)	0.5–1 gram daily for 2 weeks	0.5–1 gram 1–3 times/week	Variable, 3–5a
	Conjugated estrogen (0.625 mg active ingredient/g)	0.5–1 gram daily for 2 weeks	0.5 grams 1–3 times/week	Variable
VAGINAL INSERTS	17β-estradiol inserts	4 or 10 µg/d for 2 weeks	1 insert twice/week	3.6 (4 µg) 4.6 (10 µg)
	Estradiol hemihydrate tablets	4 or 10 µg/d for 2 weeks	1 insert twice/week	5.5
	Prasterone (DHEA) inserts	6.5 mg/day	1 insert/day	5
VAGINAL RINGS	Silicone polymer with a core containing 2 mg estradiol	7.5 mcg/day for 3 months	1 ring/3 months	8
ORAL TABLETS	Ospemifene	60 mg/day	1 tablet by mouth/day	N/A

The American Urological Association 2025 Guideline on the Genitourinary Syndrome of Menopause

SERMs (Selective Estrogen Receptor Modulators)

SERMs are medications that act like estrogen in some tissues and block estrogen in others. They may be used in women who aren't candidates for traditional estrogen therapy, such as those at higher risk for breast cancer. Common SERMs include tamoxifen, raloxifene, ospemifene, and Duavee (a combination of estrogen and a SERM that protects the uterus).

Progestogens

If you still have a uterus and are using systemic estrogen, you also need a progestogen to protect the uterine lining. Options include . . .

- micronized progesterone (bioidentical, oral)
- synthetic progestins (often combined with estrogen in pills or patches)
- progestin IUDs (local protection only)
- vaginal gels, suppositories, or injections (less commonly used)

I generally prefer continuous daily progesterone over cyclic regimens because it simplifies treatment and supports consistent symptom control. Oral micronized progesterone is also beneficial for sleep, and if sleep disruption is a major complaint of perimenopause, daily dosing tends to benefit the patient.

Important note: Transdermal progesterone creams are popular in wellness circles but don't provide adequate endometrial protection. They aren't absorbed consistently and shouldn't be used as the sole progestogen when taking systemic estrogen for endometrial protection.

Androgens: Testosterone

There is currently no FDA-approved testosterone product formulated specifically for women. However, the off-label use of testosterone is increasingly common in menopause care. I typically prescribe testosterone using FDA-approved male formulations, such as AndroGel or Testim, in carefully adjusted doses appropriate for female physiology.

These formulations are applied as a gel and absorbed through the skin. The goal is to use the smallest effective dose to alleviate symptoms such as low libido, fatigue, or poor muscle tone—without pushing testosterone levels into the male range. Monitoring is essential, and I strongly caution against overuse. Compounded testosterone creams are also an option, but again, proper dosing and lab follow-up are key.

The Truth About Testosterone Pellets

One of the most aggressively marketed—and controversial—forms of testosterone therapy for women today is pellet-based hormone therapy, often under brand names like Biote. These pellets are inserted through a small incision, typically in the gluteal area, and release hormones over time. For many women, the appeal is clear: no daily creams, no weekly patches—just one procedure every few months.

But convenience can come at a cost. And in this case, the cost is high both medically and ethically. *Nearly 100 percent* of my patients who've had testosterone pellets inserted test in the supratherapeutic range within three months—and most stay elevated for months afterward. I routinely see total testosterone levels above 300 ng/dL, well into the male physiologic range (typically 260–1000 ng/dL), while the normal range for women is closer to 15–70 ng/dL. These levels aren't just excessive; they're experimental. *There is no solid clinical evidence that testosterone at these doses is safe for women,* and we have no long-term data supporting their use.

Yet this therapy is booming. Testosterone pellet therapy is now a billion-dollar industry. And not a cent of that revenue, as far as I can tell, is being reinvested in high-quality research to better understand female hormone needs in midlife. Instead, we see a business model that preys on vulnerable women, promising revitalization and often offering only one option: pellets. No education, no alternatives, no discussion of risks.

Women deserve better.

Testosterone therapy can be beneficial—but should be prescribed in female physiologic doses, monitored with regular blood work, and used in the context of shared decision-making. That's how we avoid side effects like...

- deepening of the voice and clitoral enlargement (both often irreversible)
- increased body hair, oily skin, and acne
- aggression, mood swings, and anxiety
- elevated LDL and decreased HDL cholesterol
- liver stress and abnormal liver enzymes
- menstrual suppression or irregular bleeding
- increased visceral fat and higher risk of cardiovascular events

The reality is this: *Your hormones aren't a business model.* Any clinician who promotes only pellet therapy without discussing other FDA-approved, evidence-backed options isn't practicing responsible medicine; they're selling a product.

If you're considering testosterone therapy, ask questions. Demand monitoring and insist on transparency. Because while testosterone can be part of a thoughtful, science-informed menopause plan, no single method should ever be treated as the only path forward.

DHEA

DHEA is a hormone precursor that converts into other hormones like testosterone and estradiol. Vaginal DHEA (Intrarosa) is FDA approved and effective for GSM. Oral DHEA, which offers systemic hormone therapy, is unregulated and not FDA approved, and I generally don't recommend it. The reason is that I think it's offered based on a faulty sort of logic—why would I want to give a systemic precursor to a hormone that is barely being eked out by a failing system when I could just give the actual hormone the body needs? My experience is that women who are recommended systemic DHEA are often not offered a full explanation of how it works.

A Word About Supplements and Natural Remedies

There is no shortage of products claiming to balance your hormones or cure perimenopause by targeting so-called root causes like vitamin deficiencies, high cortisol, or adrenal fatigue. I've seen it all. But the truth is, the root cause of perimenopause isn't mysterious. It's the natural decline and dysfunction of ovarian hormone production. That is it. Your ovaries are running out of eggs. No supplement will resuscitate their function. It's just not going to happen, and any product that claims otherwise is selling unrealistic hope, not science.

That said, many women are drawn to the idea of natural remedies. It's a common question I receive in practice: *Are there supplements or natural treatments that can replace the hormones my body no longer produces?* While no supplement can restore estrogen or progesterone to pre-perimenopausal levels, certain nutrients and botanicals may support the body through this transition.

For example, black cohosh, red clover, and soy isoflavones may reduce mild hot flashes or mood symptoms in some women. Magnesium and melatonin may improve sleep. Omega-3 fatty acids and vitamin D are often recommended for general health and may support mood regulation and bone health and help lower inflammation. But results vary. The scientific evidence behind many of these options is mixed, and individual response is highly variable.

It's also important to remember that supplements aren't regulated as rigorously as prescription medications. Quality and potency can vary widely between brands. You should be cautious, seek guidance from a trusted healthcare provider, and choose products from reputable manufacturers. At The 'Pause Life, we are committed to offering the highest quality supplements, with third-party testing to ensure accuracy and safety. But even then, we are clear with our messaging—we don't promise to reverse menopause or cure hormone loss. Our goal is to support women through this transition with honesty and integrity.

Natural remedies can play a role, but they should never be seen as a replacement for evidence-based therapies. For women with moderate to severe symptoms or those at increased risk of conditions like osteoporosis or cardiovascular disease, menopause hormone therapy or other medical treatments are the gold standard. The key is a thoughtful, informed discussion with a clinician who understands the complexity of this life stage. Supplements can support you, but they are most effective when integrated into a holistic plan that includes lifestyle shifts, appropriate medical care, and a commitment to long-term well-being.

You Asked—Can MHT Be Considered If I Have . . .

Endometriosis?

For women with a history of endometriosis, menopause brings both relief and new challenges. The sharp decline in estrogen after menopause can finally halt the cycle of inflammation and pain that has plagued so many for years. But for those seeking MHT to manage menopausal symptoms, the decision isn't always straightforward.

Endometriosis is an estrogen-driven condition, meaning that reintroducing estrogen through MHT can, in some cases, trigger recurrence of endometriotic lesions—even after a hysterectomy. In rare cases, there is also concern about malignant transformation, making it critical to carefully tailor MHT choices for women with a history of endometriosis.

UNDERSTANDING THE RISKS

Studies have shown that estrogen-only MHT, often prescribed after a hysterectomy, carries a higher risk of endometriosis recurrence. This is especially true for women who had severe disease with deep peritoneal involvement. Without progesterone to counteract estrogen's stimulating effects, any residual endometrial-like tissue may reactivate, leading to symptoms that were thought to be left in the past.

However, this doesn't mean that hormone therapy is off-limits for women with a history of endometriosis; it simply means the approach matters.

MHT OPTIONS: FINDING THE RIGHT BALANCE

- **Combined MHT (estrogen + progesterone):** Using both estrogen and progesterone is generally recommended, as studies suggest that combined MHT may reduce the risk of recurrence compared with estrogen alone.

- **Tibolone:** This synthetic steroid is often considered a safer alternative for women with a history of endometriosis. Unlike traditional MHT, tibolone hasn't been shown to significantly increase recurrence risks, and it offers benefits for menopausal symptoms, bone health, and cardiovascular protection.

THE IMPORTANCE OF MONITORING AND INDIVIDUALIZED CARE

For women with endometriosis, MHT must be carefully individualized. This means . . .

- **Close monitoring:** You should have regular follow-ups with a physician to assess for symptoms of recurrence.

- **A personalized treatment plan:** Your hormone therapy protocol should be tailored based on severity of prior disease, surgical history, and risk factors.

- **Weighing benefits versus risks:** While recurrence risk is a concern, MHT remains the most effective option for managing menopause symptoms, preventing bone loss, and supporting long-term health.

Menopause doesn't erase the impact of endometriosis, and for many women, the decision to use MHT feels overwhelming. But the reality is that there are options, and with the right approach, it's possible to manage menopausal symptoms without unnecessarily increasing the risk of recurrence.

This is where individualized, evidence-based care is essential. If you have endometriosis and are considering hormone therapy, know that your experience matters and your concerns deserve to be heard. With the right hormonal strategy and thoughtful monitoring, you can feel your best in menopause, without fear of reigniting the past.

Fibroids?

When we talk about hormone therapy in menopause, we often focus on its benefits, relief from hot flashes, protection for bones, improved sleep, and even cognitive support. But what about women who also have uterine fibroids? Can MHT affect these benign but sometimes troublesome growths?

This is a question I hear often in my practice, and the answer, like so much in medicine, isn't one-size-fits-all. Yes, MHT can influence fibroid growth, but the effects vary significantly depending on the type of hormones used and how long they are taken.

WHAT THE SCIENCE TELLS US

We know that fibroids are estrogen-sensitive, which means that, in the presence of estrogen, they may continue to grow—even after menopause. Some studies show that MHT, particularly transdermal estrogen combined with progestins like medroxyprogesterone acetate, can cause fibroids to increase in size, especially in the first two years of use. But this isn't the full story.

- Different hormone therapy formulations lead to different outcomes. Some regimens, such as those containing tibolone, don't appear to significantly affect fibroid size, while others may contribute to growth.

- Fibroid growth from MHT may stabilize over time. Research suggests that although fibroids may enlarge early on, their growth often levels off after three years of therapy.

- Size doesn't always equal symptoms. Just because a fibroid grows doesn't mean it will cause discomfort, heavy bleeding, or other complications. Many postmenopausal women on hormone therapy with fibroids remain asymptomatic.

If you have fibroids, it doesn't automatically mean that MHT is off the table for you. The key is careful monitoring and individualization of treatment. If you are considering hormone therapy and have a history of fibroids, here's what you should keep in mind:

- **Close monitoring:** If you have fibroids and are on MHT, an ultrasound may be useful to track any changes in size.

- **A personalized treatment plan:** The type and dose of estrogen and progestogen can make a difference in how fibroids respond.

- **Considering lifestyle factors:** Obesity and MHT together have been linked to a higher likelihood of fibroid growth, so nutrition, exercise, and metabolic health can be important factors in management.

In postmenopause, fibroids aren't a strict contraindication for MHT, but you will continue to need thoughtful decision-making and potentially require intermittent monitoring to notate any significant changes in fibroid size. If fibroids begin to enlarge and cause symptoms, adjustments to the regimen, such as changing the type of progestogen, altering the delivery method, or discontinuing therapy, may be necessary.

Every woman's perimenopausal journey is unique, and you deserve options that support your overall health without unnecessary fear or restriction. If fibroids have been part of your story, know that, with the right guidance, you can still find your way to the approach that's right for you.

It's Time for More Discussion, Less Dismissal

Hormone therapy during perimenopause continues to be a complex, evolving field. In the midst of this clinical fluidity, you deserve access to providers who are up to date, who are willing to listen and discuss openly your options, and who understand that symptoms—not just lab results—should guide care. The goal is to stabilize, support, and protect, not to chase perfect numbers or follow outdated rules.

CHAPTER 15

The Foundation for Resilience: The Lifestyle Factors That Matter Most

I'm a fifty-two-year-old breast cancer oncology nurse. I went through perimenopause in my late forties with the classic symptoms and by fifty was postmenopausal. Throughout my journey I was caring for breast cancer patients with symptoms similar to mine, and often worse. I counseled them on the usual clinical recommendations, but it was not effective. At fifty, I experienced a fifteen-pound weight gain, poor sleep, hot flashes, and anxiety. I knew I needed to do something different to help my breast patients. I started moderate weight lifting two or three times a week and cardio workouts two or three times a week and yoga once a week, I consumed thirty grams of protein with each meal. I started sleep hygiene. I saw changes! I became stronger, more confident, slept better, and my hot flashes went away. I was happy. I certified as a personal trainer. I now combine the nursing and counsel patients on resistance training and lead health workshops on fitness and movement. I'm reaching our cancer population to get them stronger and improve health outcomes.

—Allison G.

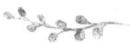

The gender health gap is real and wide. On average, women live longer than men, but we also live sicker. Statistically, women spend on average 25 percent more of their lives in poor health compared with their male counterparts. That translates to years, sometimes decades, spent dealing with chronic illness, frailty, pain, cognitive decline, and reduced quality of life. And this gap doesn't begin in old age. It starts in midlife, often right at the threshold of perimenopause, when the first signs of hormonal decline start to quietly influence every system in the body.

This isn't about blaming individual clinicians. Most are doing their best within a medical system that was never designed with women's midlife health in mind. I practiced within that system, too, and I know how many good, well-intentioned providers are doing heroic work every day. But the system itself—the way we fund research, write guidelines, structure training, and prioritize care—is failing women. It's not one giant failure but death by a thousand tiny cuts. A missed screening here. A dismissed symptom there. A treatment delayed. A referral never made. And over the course of a lifetime, those missed opportunities add up.

The gap in health is stark. But I believe it's also preventable. When women are informed, supported, and empowered to make proactive decisions, we can begin to close that gap. We can change this trajectory. We can grab ahold of the opportunity presented to us within perimenopause to avoid negative and evadable health outcomes by committing to strategic intervention.

And that is what this chapter is about. This is where we shift the trajectory.

Because here's what the science and my clinical experience make clear: Perimenopause is one of the most important leverage points for preventing disease and preserving health across the lifespan. This is the moment to act.

It doesn't require perfection. It doesn't require rigid rules or punishing routines. What it does require is clarity, consistency, and compassion for our bodies, for our future selves, and for the generations of women coming up behind us who deserve better than the silence we inherited.

From research, from my practice, and from my own experience, I've learned that small, strategic changes made consistently can have an outsize impact. The way we eat, the way we move, the way we rest—these things compound. They create a foundation not only for symptom relief now but also for strength, stability, and independence in the decades to come.

It starts with reframing our goals. We aren't chasing skinny or counting calories. We are building strength and prioritizing nutrient density and blood sugar stability. We are no longer dieting for summer; we are fueling for longevity. We aren't shrinking; we are fortifying.

And this isn't just motivational fluff. It's evidence based. A 2023 study published in *Menopause* found that cardiorespiratory fitness, a measure of how efficiently your heart, lungs, and muscles work together, is a significantly stronger predictor of long-term health outcomes in midlife women than BMI. In other words, how well you move matters far more than the number on the scale. Fitness protects against cardiovascular disease, type 2 diabetes, osteoporosis, depression, and even cognitive decline. And contrary to what we were told in our twenties, it's absolutely possible to gain strength and improve body composition in your forties, fifties, and beyond.

Similarly, research on resistance training in menopausal women shows improvements in bone mineral density, insulin sensitivity, visceral fat reduction, and mental well-being, often rivaling or exceeding pharmacologic interventions. Adequate dietary protein, omega-3 fatty acids, fiber, and vitamin D all contribute to muscle health, cognitive function, and inflammation control. These are not abstract wellness trends but are instead foundational strategies grounded in physiology and supported by decades of data.

Perhaps most importantly, we are working toward preserving autonomy alongside disease prevention. Again and again, my patients tell me what they're really afraid of: not just heart disease or dementia or osteoporosis—but the possibility of losing themselves. Losing the ability to drive, live alone, or climb stairs . . . to travel and dance at their grandchildren's weddings. In other words, to choose for themselves how they want to live and age.

That is what this work is about. How to build a lifestyle that supports not just your body but your brain, your energy, your metabolism, your confidence, and your joy. Because the perimenopausal body is a foundation to be fortified, not a problem to be fixed. In this chapter, we'll break down the *how*:

How to eat.
How to move.
How to recover.

Let's begin.

The Four Fundamentals of Perimenopausal Health (Besides Hormones)

There are four fundamentals of health that are most important to focus on in perimenopause: nutrition, movement, sleep, and stress reduction. Let's go through each of these areas and how you can optimize them to your advantage.

Nutrition

Good nutrition is the cornerstone of maintaining health, strength, and vitality during perimenopause. This phase of life is an opportunity to embrace a philosophy of "strong over skinny" and "nutrition over calories," shifting the focus to building a resilient, well-nourished body rather than chasing restrictive dieting or unrealistic body standards. The hormonal changes of this transitional phase can influence your metabolism, weight, and overall energy levels, making it essential to adopt a diet rich in nutrients to support your body.

In my practice, I've seen how a well-rounded nutrition plan can transform the health and confidence of my patients. Women often come to me feeling overwhelmed by the changes happening in their bodies, but with guidance, they begin to see how prioritizing nourishment can empower them during this transition. By focusing on the quality of your food, you can address key concerns like bone health, inflammation, and muscle maintenance while supporting long-term wellness.

ANTI-INFLAMMATORY NUTRITION IN PERIMENOPAUSE: A CRITICAL LIFESTYLE SHIFT

One of the most profound and underappreciated shifts that occur during perimenopause is the slow, systemic rise in chronic inflammation. As estrogen levels decline, a cascade of changes affects nearly every tissue in the body: The gut becomes more permeable, visceral fat accumulates, the brain becomes more vulnerable to oxidative stress, joints become inflamed, and bone remodeling slows in favor of resorption. These aren't isolated phenomena; they are interconnected, and at the root of much of this dysfunction is inflammation.

But here's what matters most: We have control over this. While we can't stop the natural transition of perimenopause, we can dramatically influence how our bodies respond to it through food. In my clinical experience caring for patients in midlife and in my training as a certified culinary medicine specialist, I've seen how applying the deeply established science of anti-inflammatory eating can benefit the unique hormonal landscape of the perimenopausal body. We can improve quality of life and lower long-term risk for serious chronic diseases simply through the power of strategic nutrition choices.

Why Inflammation Increases in Perimenopause

Estrogen is a powerful anti-inflammatory hormone. It downregulates the expression of pro-inflammatory cytokines like IL-6 and TNF-α and helps maintain gut barrier integrity and vascular health. When estrogen begins its unpredictable decline in perimenopause, this regulatory function falters.

The gut, in particular, becomes more vulnerable. Estrogen supports the tight junctions that keep the gut lining sealed; its loss can lead to increased intestinal permeability, or "leaky gut," allowing bacterial endotoxins to enter circulation and trigger an inflammatory immune response. This process has been linked to the development of insulin resistance, mood disorders, and even osteoporosis.

Simultaneously, hormonal shifts promote the accumulation of visceral fat, a metabolically active tissue that secretes pro-inflammatory cytokines. These cytokines elevate systemic inflammation and disrupt insulin signaling, lipid metabolism, and endothelial function.

With anti-inflammatory nutrition, we help break the unwelcome inflammatory cycle by providing the body with the nutrients it needs to modulate immune activity, support metabolic function, and protect against oxidative damage. My online program the Galveston Diet (and book of the same name) was built on this way of eating, and countless women have reported on the profound positive effects they've noticed when they've reduced systemic inflammation with food.

The goal isn't to eliminate inflammation completely, because, when acute, it's a vital defense mechanism that we rely on. But we must prevent the chronic, unresolved inflammation that contributes to disease progression and accelerates aging.

A diet built around anti-inflammatory principles can . . .

- reduce markers of systemic inflammation, such as CRP and IL-6
- preserve cognitive function by lowering brain oxidative stress and supporting neuronal plasticity
- improve insulin sensitivity and help stabilize blood glucose
- reduce muscle loss and support mitochondrial health
- protect against cardiovascular disease and atherosclerosis
- support the gut microbiome and gut barrier integrity
- slow bone turnover and reduce osteoclastic activity

KEY COMPONENTS OF AN ANTI-INFLAMMATORY DIET

Based on the literature and clinical outcomes, these are the core nutritional strategies I recommend to women navigating perimenopause:

- **Omega-3 fatty acids:** Long-chain omega-3s (EPA and DHA) from fatty fish such as salmon, sardines, and mackerel reduce inflammation through multiple mechanisms, including suppression of NF-κB signaling and downregulation of COX-2 enzymes. For those who don't consume fish regularly, algae- or fish oil–based supplements can be effective alternatives.

- **Antioxidant-rich plant foods:** Beets, cruciferous vegetables, berries, and other deeply pigmented fruits provide a dense source of carotenoids, flavonoids, and other polyphenols. These compounds reduce oxidative stress and regulate immune signaling.

- **Gut-supportive fiber:** Soluble and insoluble fibers found in legumes, vegetables, nuts, and seeds feed beneficial gut bacteria and help maintain mucosal integrity. Prebiotic fibers also enhance the production of short-chain fatty acids (SCFAs) such as butyrate, which have potent anti-inflammatory effects.

- **Polyphenols and other phytonutrients:** Found in foods like green tea, turmeric (curcumin), olive oil, beets, cruciferous vegetables, and deeply pigmented fruits, these plant compounds inhibit inflammatory signaling pathways, reduce oxidative stress, and modulate immune responses at the cellular level.

- **Healthy fats:** Monounsaturated fats such as olive oil and avocado oil reduce oxidative LDL formation and support endothelial health.

- **Spices with therapeutic potential:** Turmeric, ginger, garlic, and cinnamon contain bioactive compounds that directly inhibit inflammatory enzymes and cytokines.

This approach isn't about rigid rules or restrictions. It's about creating a sustainable and nourishing way of eating that supports the distinct physiological needs of the perimenopausal woman. The foods you choose can either fuel inflammation or help resolve it.

The sooner you begin supporting your body with anti-inflammatory nutrition, the more resilience you'll build for the years ahead and the better you can feel today.

A Simple Gut Health Strategy for Midlife Inflammation

One of the easiest and most effective nutrition strategies I recommend to my patients in perimenopause is to aim for *thirty different plant foods per week*. I learned this from the researchers behind ZOE, a large-scale nutrition science initiative that helped illuminate the links between gut health, metabolic function, and inflammation. Greater microbial diversity in the gut is associated with lower inflammation, better blood sugar control, and improved overall metabolic health. These are critical factors as hormone levels begin to shift during the menopause transition.

This plant diversity target includes not just fruits and vegetables but also nuts, seeds, herbs, legumes, and whole grains. Each plant contains unique types of fiber and phytonutrients that feed different strains of beneficial gut bacteria. These microbes help regulate everything from mood to immune function to body weight. If the balance of these microbes is disrupted—a condition known as gut dysbiosis—you can become more vulnerable to symptoms like joint pain, brain fog, and hot flashes.

Fiber also plays an important role in estrogen metabolism. The gut helps break down and eliminate estrogen through a specific collection of microbes. A diverse, fiber-rich diet supports this system and may keep hormone levels more stable and symptoms better controlled.

If the idea of tracking thirty plants feels overwhelming, think of it as a weekly goal rather than a strict requirement. A handful of mixed nuts, a few types of leafy greens, some different berries, and a spoonful of hummus all count. This is a more strategic way of following the advice to *eat the rainbow*. The more colors, textures, and types of plants you include, the more resilience you build against the inflammation and metabolic shifts of midlife.

FIBER: THE HUMBLE HERO OF HORMONE AND METABOLIC HEALTH

Fiber plays an essential role in hormone regulation, gut health, and the prevention of chronic diseases such as diabetes and cardiovascular conditions. But its benefits go much deeper, especially for women navigating midlife.

High-fiber foods like oats, beans, flaxseeds, and berries are nutritional powerhouses. Not only do they improve satiety and support weight management, but they also help regulate insulin, reduce systemic inflammation, support estrogen metabolism, and improve gut microbiota diversity. Increasing your fiber intake is simple: Swap refined grains for whole grains, add beans or lentils to soups and salads, and keep your plate filled with colorful fruits and vegetables.

Most women in the United States aren't getting nearly enough fiber. On average, women consume only about fifteen grams of fiber per day. That's far short of the recommended twenty-five to thirty grams per day for adult women. This deficiency has real implications, from increased weight gain and insulin resistance to higher risks of cardiovascular disease and colon cancer.

Closing the fiber gap in midlife can be a preventive health measure and offer therapeutic benefits. In fact, for women navigating perimenopause, optimizing fiber intake becomes an essential tool in managing hormonal shifts, metabolic changes, and long-term disease risk.

- **Body composition:** Research has shown that consuming fiber may preserve muscle mass and reduce body fat—two wins as we focus on healthy body composition in perimenopause. Even modest increases in daily fiber intake help prevent the slow creep of weight gain over time, independent of physical activity or calorie intake.

- **Metabolic and hormonal benefits:** Fiber helps stabilize blood sugar and improve insulin sensitivity. Diets rich in whole grains, legumes, and vegetables reduce fasting glucose and insulin levels, lowering the risk of developing type 2 diabetes. These benefits extend to pregnancy as well. High fiber intake in pregnant women improves glycemic control, reduces the need for insulin therapy, and lowers triglycerides.

    While more research is needed in postmenopausal women, fiber's ability to support liver and gut function makes it a foundational strategy for hormone balance at every life stage.

- **Increased satiety:** Fiber-rich foods enhance satiety, which is the feeling of fullness. Soluble fibers, in particular, slow gastric emptying and modulate hunger hormones, leading to longer-lasting fullness and more stable energy levels throughout the day.

A high-fiber diet is one of the simplest, most powerful interventions for women in midlife. It supports weight stability, insulin regulation, hormonal balance, and long-term metabolic health. For women navigating perimenopause, fiber isn't just a digestive aid; it's a hormonal ally.

ADEQUATE PROTEIN INTAKE

Currently, the FDA recommends a protein intake of 0.8 grams per kilogram of body weight (0.36 grams per pound) per day for adults. However, this guideline is designed to prevent deficiency rather than to optimize health, and it may fall short for midlife adults, particularly women who are transitioning into menopause and will eventually be postmenopausal.

Ensuring adequate protein intake is a critical component of maintaining musculoskeletal health in women. Reviews of the Women's Health Initiative (WHI) and other studies have gleaned the critical importance of protein consumption in mitigating the risks of osteoporosis and sarcopenia, both of which become increasingly prevalent with age. The WHI findings underscore that a higher protein intake, about 1.2 grams per kilogram of body weight (0.54 grams per pound), particularly from animal sources, is associated with better muscle mass retention and bone health outcomes.

Dr. Gabrielle Lyon, author of *Forever Strong*, has been a vocal advocate for increasing protein intake even further, emphasizing the profound need for women—especially those with established risk factors for sarcopenia and osteoporosis—to consume more than the standard dietary guidelines suggest. She argues that higher protein consumption is essential to support bone health and muscle protein synthesis, aligning with evidence that suggests intakes of 1 gram of protein per pound may maximize gains in muscle mass in individuals who are resistance training. Her recommendations are grounded in the belief that a proactive approach to nutrition can help prevent the debilitating consequences of muscle and bone deterioration, ultimately promoting longevity and independence.

The contrast between the FDA's general recommendation and the insights provided by the WHI and experts like Dr. Lyon is clear. The latter advocate for a higher daily intake of protein to effectively prevent osteoporosis and sarcopenia. The consensus emerging from the science is that an increased protein intake, when combined with regular physical activity, is essential for maintaining muscle and bone health as we age.

I have done an intellectual download of all of the available information on protein and adapted it into clinical practice in a way that is customized to my patients' individual needs. I accomplish this by measuring a patient's body composition with an InBody scan, then recommending protein intake based on the results. In patients who have normal to above average muscle mass, the goal is maintenance, and I suggest consuming about 1.2 to 1.6 grams of protein for every kilogram of ideal body weight (that is, the healthy weight they want to maintain), or 0.54 to 0.73 grams per pound. And for patients who have low muscle mass or are even sarcopenic, I recommend a higher intake of 1.6 to 1.8 grams of protein for every kilogram of ideal body weight, or 0.73 to 0.82 grams per pound.

Women navigating perimenopause and beyond deserve evidence-based nutritional guidance that prioritizes their long-term well-being. With a growing body of research supporting the role of protein in musculoskeletal health, it's crucial that healthcare providers encourage higher protein intake as part of a comprehensive strategy to promote healthy aging. By doing so, we can empower women to take proactive steps in safeguarding their mobility, independence, and overall quality of life.

MAXIMIZE NUTRIENTS FROM FOOD

Along with anti-inflammatory foods, I recommend a focus on eating a variety of whole foods to ensure your body receives the full spectrum of nutrients it needs. When you minimize ultra-processed foods, which are inherently low in nutrients and high in added sugars and unhealthy fats, this becomes easier because you make room to prioritize the abundance of fresh whole foods available. I often counsel patients to start with small steps—like swapping sugary snacks for nutrient-rich alternatives—and they are amazed at how these changes improve their mood, energy, and overall well-being. This is often motivation enough to keep overhauling pre-existing nutrition habits that were misaligned with their health goals.

In perimenopause, it's important to look to foods to increase your intake of key supportive nutrients:

- **Calcium and vitamin D:** Both are critical for bone health. Incorporate sources such as dairy products, fortified plant-based milks, leafy greens, and fatty fish into your meals.

- **Omega-3 fatty acids:** Omega-3s reduce inflammation and support heart health and can be found in salmon, walnuts, and flaxseeds.

- **Iron:** One of the most common deficiencies in women is in iron. Dietary efforts to support healthy iron levels can include eating red meat, seafood, poultry, eggs, beans, lentils, and dark green leafy vegetables. (Note: Even though iron deficiency is common in women, it's not a certainty that you are in fact deficient. While dietary sources of iron are safe and recommended, you will want to have your iron and ferritin checked before considering supplementation.)

SOME PRACTICAL TIPS TO ENCOURAGE HEALTHY EATING

Almost everything in life these days seems to be overwhelmingly complicated—but creating balanced meals doesn't have to be one of those things. In my own life, I apply a few strategies to increase my chances of staying on target with my nutrition goals—and you might be successful with these strategies as well.

Use the plate method as a guide: Fill half your plate with fruit and vegetables, a quarter with protein, and the remaining quarter with whole grains. Remember, too, to see your plate as a palette that you can fill with colorful fruits and vegetables, and aim to eat the rainbow.

Meal prepping can be a game changer: I live by meal prepping when I'm busy. My advice is to dedicate time each week to preparing ingredients that you can later build into meals. One of my favorite things to make this way is what I call the Kelley Salad (named for my friend Kelley Sullivan Georgiades, who gave me the recipe), which has broccoli, brussels sprouts, kale, romaine, and fresh mint. To this, I'll add different proteins, seeds, healthy fats, and more depending on my goals each day.

Engage in mindful eating practices: Try to eat meals away from distractions such as your phone or TV and focus on savoring each bite. I know it sounds a little silly, but give it a try—this habit can connect you a bit more to hunger and fullness cues.

To support your nutrition goals, I've included five days of meal plans in the appendix.

THE BIG PICTURE OF EATING FOR HEALTH IN PERIMENOPAUSE

By adopting the mindset of "strong over skinny" and "nutrition over calories," you prioritize the long-term health and functionality of your body over temporary aesthetic goals. With fiber, nutrient-dense foods, and practical meal strategies, you can fuel your body effectively during perimenopause. These changes not only support your immediate health but also lay the foundation for resilience and vitality in the years to come.

Small, consistent steps can make a significant difference, empowering you to navigate this phase with confidence and strength. If you're looking for additional support, you can check out The 'Pause Life (we've partnered with HelloFresh to offer some meal options) for resources.

SUPPLEMENTS: BRIDGING NUTRITIONAL GAPS WITH PURPOSE AND PRECISION

In a perfect world, every woman would meet her nutritional needs through colorful vegetables, high-quality proteins, fiber-rich grains, and healthy fats. But in clinical practice and in my own experience, that's rarely the reality. For perimenopausal women in particular, achieving optimal nutrient intake through diet alone can be an uphill battle.

Before I recommend any supplement to a patient, I almost always suggest one foundational step: Track your nutrition for two to three weeks. The best way to do this is to use an app that will automatically calculate your nutrient consumption for you. With this information, you can gain an understanding of any gaps in your dietary intake. Once you have a clearer picture of your baseline intake, you can identify what gaps can realistically be filled through whole foods and what may require supplementation.

I also like to get lab values for iron and vitamin D before supplementing these two. When considering a supplement, I ask the patient why they're thinking about taking it:

- Are you correcting a nutritional deficiency?
- Supporting a specific health goal?
- Aiming to increase your health span?
- All of the above?

This level of intentionality is essential. The supplement industry is saturated with products promising energy, weight loss, better skin, and youth in a bottle, but most are untested, underdosed, or poorly absorbed. That's why evidence-based, targeted supplementation can be a powerful adjunct to lifestyle but only when used with purpose.

Take vitamin D, for example. It's a fat-soluble hormone-like vitamin that plays a central role in calcium absorption, immune regulation, and muscle and bone function. As women age, levels tend to decline because of lower sun exposure, changes in skin synthesis, and dietary insufficiency. Despite its importance, a large proportion of women in midlife are vitamin D insufficient or deficient, increasing their risk for osteoporosis, falls, and possibly cardiovascular disease.

Another common gap is fiber. As we've seen, the average American woman consumes much less than the recommended daily amount of fiber, important for cardiovascular risk reduction, glycemic control, and gut health. Meeting that goal requires a highly intentional diet, one that's rich in legumes, whole grains, nuts, seeds, fruits, and vegetables. For many women, this is easier said than done.

These two examples, vitamin D and fiber, are why I often recommend supplements in my clinical practice. I often suggest other supplements to patients in perimenopause, because they can support overall goals of building muscle, improving sleep, and more. Some of the key supplements I recommend include the following:

- **Vitamin D:** supports bone, immune, and cardiovascular health
- **Fiber:** assists with digestive regularity and weight management
- **Collagen:** can support dermal integrity and bone matrix strength
- **Turmeric:** a potent anti-inflammatory to help manage joint pain, metabolic inflammation, and oxidative stress
- **Creatine:** clinically shown to support muscle mass, cognitive function, and energy metabolism in aging women
- **Magnesium:** has a significant impact on sleep, helps maintain normal blood glucose levels, and supports bone development
- **B vitamins:** play an important role in maintaining functions of the nervous system

Supplements aren't intended to be a replacement for nutrient-dense food, movement, stress management, or sleep. But when used strategically, they can be an essential tool to help women navigate this transition with more energy, strength, and resilience.

My philosophy is simple: Test, track, personalize. Support your body with what it needs and nothing it doesn't.

Movement

Exercise is one of the most effective tools for preserving physical health. In perimenopause, it can be an unparalleled asset against muscle loss, decreased bone density, and metabolic dysfunction, all of which can be initiated by persistent hormone fluctuations. By incorporating regular physical activity into your daily life, you can counteract these negative effects while maintaining strength and stability and supporting your overall health.

Physical activity can also be highly beneficial for your mental health. It increases the production of beta-endorphins, your body's natural mood boosters, and helps lower stress hormones and reduce anxiety. Exercise also promotes better sleep, having been shown in research to improve sleep quality and reduce sleep latency (the time it takes to fall asleep), and in insomnia, it may be an effective non-pharmacological approach to getting less-disrupted sleep.

If you're starting from a sedentary lifestyle, take small steps to ease into regular activity. Walking just thirty minutes a day has been shown to decrease the risk of diabetes by 50 percent, offering a tangible and accessible way to begin. Meet yourself where you are and focus on gradual progress. Building confidence in your abilities is just as important as the activity itself.

Your goal should ultimately be to include both aerobic activities and resistance training.

Aerobic activities, such as brisk walking, swimming, and cycling, done at moderate intensity are recommended. The key is that you must push yourself into a moderate-intensity zone to maximize the benefits. Studies have shown that engaging in at least 150 minutes of moderate-intensity aerobic exercise per week reduces the risk of cardiovascular disease and helps maintain healthy metabolic function.

Resistance training includes strength-based exercises, such as weight lifting, body-weight movements, and/or resistance-band workouts. This type of training is critical to incorporate as your estrogen levels decline and you begin to lose bone and muscle tissue in response. Research indicates that a minimum of two resistance training sessions per week can increase bone density and muscle mass, reducing the likelihood of fractures and enhancing your overall strength. These activities also make daily tasks easier and promote long-term functional independence.

Don't overlook flexibility and balance exercises, which are essential components of a well-rounded approach to fitness. Practices like yoga, tai chi, and Pilates improve flexibility, joint mobility, and core strength, helping you stay agile and reducing stiffness. Balance-focused exercises, such as standing on one leg and heel-to-toe walking, mitigate the risk of falls and related injuries. A study published by researchers at the Institute for Musculoskeletal Health at the University of Sydney found that balance-focused activities reduced fall risk among older adults. Adding these to your routine ensures greater stability as you age.

Starting an exercise routine doesn't have to be overwhelming. Begin with small, manageable changes, like incorporating ten-minute movement breaks throughout your day. If you want to enhance bone health further, consider using a weighted vest during certain activities. Research has demonstrated that walking with a weighted vest can improve bone mineral density over time, offering an accessible and effective strategy for strengthening skeletal health.

To maintain consistency, focus on finding activities that you enjoy. Whether it's dancing, hiking, or joining a group class, make exercise something you look forward to. Adding a social element, such as exercising with a friend, can also enhance motivation and commitment. The goal is to establish a routine that fits seamlessly into your life, ensuring long-term benefits.

By integrating aerobic, resistance, flexibility, and balance exercises into your lifestyle, you can address the unique challenges of perimenopause head-on. This holistic approach not only strengthens your body but also enhances your overall well-being in such a profound way.

Sleep Optimization: Restoring and Rejuvenating the Body

Sleep is foundational to nearly every aspect of health, especially during perimenopause, when hormonal shifts begin to interfere with rest. Deep, consistent sleep supports physical recovery, cognitive clarity, immune regulation, and emotional balance. But for many women in midlife, restful nights become elusive.

The most common sleep disruptors I hear about in clinical practice include night sweats and middle-of-the-night waking—all of which become more common as estrogen and progesterone decline. What's often missed in these conversations is the critical role of progesterone in sleep quality.

Progesterone interacts with the GABA-A receptors in the brain, the same receptors targeted by anti-anxiety medications like benzodiazepines. Through this mechanism, progesterone has a natural calming, sedative effect, which promotes sleep onset and deeper, more restorative stages of rest. As progesterone levels decline in the late reproductive years and perimenopause, women often experience more difficulty falling and staying asleep.

I've seen this in my patients time and time again, and I've experienced it myself. One of the key changes some women report after starting hormone therapy is finally being able to sleep through the night. Estrogen can reduce nighttime hot flashes (a.k.a. night sweats), and progesterone promotes calm in the brain, both beneficial to better rest.

STRATEGIES FOR BETTER SLEEP

While hormonal therapy may play an important role, lifestyle changes also make a significant difference:

- **Stick to a consistent sleep schedule:** Going to bed and waking up at the same time every day supports your circadian rhythm.

- **Keep your bedroom cool, dark, and quiet:** Body temperature regulation is essential during perimenopause.

- **Limit caffeine and alcohol:** Both can worsen sleep quality and increase nighttime waking.

- **Use relaxation techniques:** Progressive muscle relaxation, breath work, and guided imagery can lower stress and improve sleep onset.

- **Try physical sleep aids:** Weighted blankets and white noise machines can improve sleep depth and reduce anxiety.

Sleep is a biological necessity, not a luxury. And during perimenopause, it often requires a proactive, multipronged strategy. With the right combination of hormonal support, environment, and lifestyle practices, restful sleep becomes possible again.

Stress Reduction: Managing the Invisible Load

We can't talk about health during perimenopause without talking about stress. Chronic stress is more than an emotional burden; it's a biological disruptor. It contributes to systemic inflammation, weight gain, poor sleep, and hormonal imbalance, all of which are already shifting during this life stage.

This season of life can feel like a perfect storm: caring for aging parents, raising children, navigating career pressures, and managing relationships, all within a cultural and economic climate that feels more overwhelming than ever. I don't know a single woman right now who isn't stressed out about something.

In my clinical experience, patients don't need a lab to tell them they're stressed. That's why I rarely check cortisol levels anymore; most women already intuitively know. They feel it in their minds and bodies: the tension, the fatigue, the sense of always being "on." Chasing numbers isn't nearly as useful as helping them build practical tools to self-regulate.

What has worked for me and for many of my patients is learning to tune into stress and gently unwind it. Techniques like cognitive behavioral therapy (CBT), meditation, and journaling have made a tangible difference in my own life and in the lives of the women I care for.

STRATEGIES FOR STRESS MANAGEMENT

- **Mindfulness practices:** Meditation, deep breathing, or body scans help regulate the nervous system.

- **Restorative activities:** Journaling, creative hobbies, and spending time in nature promote mental clarity and calm.

- **Digital tools:** Meditation apps like Insight Timer, Headspace, or Calm can help you build a consistent practice.

- **Identifying and prioritizing stressors:** Even small acts of delegation or setting boundaries can make space for self-care.

Stress may be inevitable, but chronic overwhelm isn't. With intention, support, and practice, we can create micro-moments of calm that ripple outward—and help our bodies feel safe enough to heal.

Bringing It All Together: A Holistic Approach

Perimenopause isn't just a phase—it's a powerful window of opportunity to redesign your health strategy. The interconnected nature of nutrition, movement, sleep, and stress regulation means that progress in one area often amplifies the others. This systems-based thinking reflects the latest science in lifestyle medicine, which demonstrates that even modest, consistent interventions can dramatically reduce disease risk and improve quality of life.

In both my clinical and my personal experience, the key isn't perfection; it's sustainability. We aren't chasing short-term fixes. We are laying a strong foundation for decades of strength, independence, and cognitive clarity. I've seen countless women reclaim their energy, reframe their mindset, and rebuild trust in their bodies—simply by starting with small, repeatable steps.

This entire chapter has focused on creating and reinforcing habits that will not only support you now but also *prepare your body for a smoother transition into menopause*. The decisions you make in perimenopause—how you eat, how you move, how you sleep, how you manage stress—form the scaffolding for your future health. And while hormone therapy is an incredibly powerful and effective tool that many women benefit from (particularly when started near the menopause transition), it works best in the context of a resilient body and healthy habits.

What motivates so many of my patients at this stage in life isn't the way their bodies look; it's the way they perform. They want to avoid the chronic conditions that plagued our mothers and grandmothers: cardiovascular disease, type 2 diabetes, frailty, dementia. And perhaps most critically, they want to avoid the loss of independence that marked the last decade of life for too many of the women who came before us.

They want to be the women in their seventies and eighties whose brains

The Foundation for Resilience: The Lifestyle Factors That Matter Most

are sharp, whose muscles are strong, and who move confidently through the world. They want to thrive, not merely survive. They want to travel, hike, lift their grandbabies, live alone if they choose, and remain present and vibrant in their relationships.

This will become our new status quo.

The beauty of this approach is that every strategy we've discussed in this chapter—nutrient-dense food, physical activity, sleep, and stress reduction—has been shown in research to reduce the risks of each of these conditions.

This isn't about perfection or punishment. *It's about building the body that will carry you forward into the next decades of life with strength and vitality.* The work we do now shapes that outcome.

CHAPTER 16

Talking Points and Lab Tests: Everything You Need for Your Next Appointment

> Where do I even begin?! I'll be forty-three in October, and I started experiencing symptoms, at random, about five years ago, but it came on strong last year. It started with my period. I went from having a four-day cycle to a twelve- to fourteen-day cycle. Then came everything else! Hot flashes, night sweats, mood swings, brain fog, itchy scalp and ears, hair loss, insomnia, overstimulation . . . I have a huge list! This is like puberty with a vengeance! And no one gave me a guidebook to navigate this!
>
> —Michelle M.

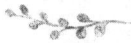

If you are feeling frustrated trying to find relief from your perimenopausal or menopausal symptoms, you aren't alone. In fact, it's all too common for women who are experiencing disruptive, even debilitating, symptoms during this stage of life to be dismissed or ignored. Few women are offered a discussion of treatment options despite the fact that we have safe, effective therapies that not only can improve quality of life but may also reduce the risk of long-term diseases.

I know this to be true based on what I hear from patients and from women who reach out to me via social media. This reality has also been confirmed in research. When Yale researchers analyzed insurance claims from more than five hundred thousand women, they determined that 60 percent of them sought medical care for significant menopausal symptoms and, of this group, more than 75 percent left their visits without receiving any treatment at all.

We can do better. You deserve better.

How to Prepare for Your Appointment

I want to help you make the most of your time with your healthcare provider and be ready to advocate for the care you need and deserve. Ideally, you are working with someone who listens, respects your input, and is committed to helping you feel well. But even with a supportive provider, time is limited and preparation matters.

Here are some suggestions for getting the most out of your time in your practitioner's office.

Ask for an early appointment with extra time. Try to schedule your visit as the first appointment of the day if possible, when your provider is likely to be less rushed.

If you are using the traditional insurance model, it's important to know that a perimenopause consultation will likely not be covered under a routine wellness exam. Insurance companies often require this to be billed as a separate problem-focused visit. Be clear when scheduling and ask specifically for a problem visit related to menopausal symptoms. Request as much time as the office is able to offer so you aren't squeezed into a standard ten- or fifteen-minute slot.

Arrive in a fasted state. I also suggest arriving in a fasted state if you anticipate needing blood work, since certain labs require fasting and having come prepared for this can avoid unnecessary delays.

Write down your family history of major health conditions. Note which relative had the condition and at what age they were diagnosed. This can influence not only what labs are ordered but also whether insurance will cover them. For example, fatigue combined with a family history of hypothyroidism may justify a full thyroid panel. Your family history may also help determine whether you are a good candidate for certain hormone therapies.

Keep a symptom journal. Track any changes in your sleep, mood, cognition, weight, digestion, menstrual cycle, energy level, and sexual health. These seemingly disconnected symptoms can form a pattern when viewed together and will help guide a more comprehensive evaluation.

Reflect on your preferences. It's helpful to have done a little homework as it relates to your preferences. For example, would you like to explore hormone therapy? Would you prefer to try lifestyle changes or nonhormonal treatments first? This is your body and your decision, and your provider is there to help you make informed choices, not to make them for you. Have your preferences or any questions written down or typed into your Notes app so you don't rely on memory when you're put on the spot.

Bring credible information. One of the biggest barriers I see is that many clinicians simply haven't been trained in perimenopause care. A survey of OB-GYN residents in the United States found that only one in five had received formal education in perimenopause medicine. The majority wanted more training. Sharing information from trusted sources can start a meaningful conversation and show your provider that you have done your homework.

For example, The Menopause Society has published a clear position statement on hormone therapy: For healthy women younger than sixty and within ten years of menopause onset, the benefits of hormone therapy far outweigh the potential risks. Unfortunately, we are still waiting for formal guidelines that address perimenopause specifically. Hormone therapy isn't one-size-fits-all. There are many options to consider, including different FDA-approved formulations and routes of administration, all of which should be matched to your symptoms, goals, and medical history.

Research also shows that hormone therapy, when combined with nutrition and other supportive lifestyle strategies, is associated with better cardiovascular outcomes and lower long-term disease risk. This isn't fringe science. This is endorsed by organizations such as the American Heart Association and supported by a growing body of high-quality evidence.

What to Say and How to Say It

It isn't always easy to speak up, especially if you have been dismissed in the past. But your health matters and your symptoms are valid. Consider starting your visit by setting the tone. You might say, "In the past, I have felt dismissed when I brought up my symptoms. I want to make sure I'm heard today."

If your provider tells you your labs are normal but you still feel unwell, don't doubt yourself. You can say, "I'm relieved that everything looks normal, but I still feel off. I would like to explore what else might be going on."

If the appointment feels rushed or incomplete, ask for a follow-up or request a referral to a specialist. And if your efforts to get the care you need still fall short, please don't give up. There are perimenopause-trained providers and online options like telemedicine clinics who can help. On our website, thepauselife.com, we have a clinicians list, which is a database of testimonials from our followers who have referred their own clinicians. I don't endorse any one group, but I encourage women to keep looking until they feel truly supported.

What You Should Not Accept

Perimenopause is a natural stage of life, but that doesn't mean you are required to suffer through it. You shouldn't be told that this is just your new normal and that nothing can be done. You also shouldn't be told that hormone therapy is never an option. If your provider doesn't offer it, they should explain why based on your individual medical history. If they dismiss the topic entirely, it's time to seek another opinion. You can find certified menopause specialists through The Menopause Society's practitioner database.

Be cautious of unnecessary limitations, like providers who say they will prescribe hormone therapy only for one year or who refuse to continue it based on outdated guidelines. Hormone therapy is a conversation that evolves over time, and if your symptoms persist, you deserve continued support.

The Lab Tests I Run for My Perimenopausal Patients

The basic metabolic panel that is typically run with an annual wellness exam can provide a lot of intel on your health, but I think this panel could be significantly improved—especially for perimenopausal and postmenopausal women. In my practice, I add several tests to what is evaluated on a standard panel.

Most of the blood work I recommend is covered by traditional insurance plans, but some of the tests may lead to some out-of-pocket costs, depending on the specifics of your plan. When I opened my own clinic, I made the decision to step away from third-party payers, because I found myself increasingly restricted in how I could evaluate, diagnose, and treat my patients. That model simply wasn't serving the women I cared for. By creating an independent practice, I gained the autonomy to order all the labs I believe are necessary based on reported symptoms, risk factors, and clinical presentation. Ideally, you will be able to work with your own practitioner to get the same individualized form of care.

What follows is a list of the blood work I typically order for women in perimenopause to guide evidence-based, individualized care. (For a downloadable version of this list, visit thepauselife.com.)

Fasting Labs Commonly Ordered in Perimenopause

These labs are drawn in a fasting state to ensure accurate evaluation of metabolic, hormonal, and cardiovascular health. Each test provides critical insight into the physiologic changes occurring during the menopausal transition.

The following are typically checked as part of the standard annual wellness panel:

- **CBC with Differential and Platelets:** Evaluates for anemia, inflammation, and overall hematologic status. Heavy or irregular bleeding during perimenopause can lead to iron-deficiency anemia.

- **Comprehensive Metabolic Panel (CMP-14):** Measures glucose, kidney and liver function, and electrolyte balance. Metabolic changes during the transition make this a foundational test.

- **Hemoglobin A1C:** Indicates average blood glucose over the past two to three months. Insulin sensitivity often declines in perimenopause, increasing risk of diabetes.
- **Lipid Panel:** Standard screen for cholesterol levels and lipid metabolism. Estrogen loss negatively affects lipid profiles.
- **TSH:** The primary screening test for thyroid function. Thyroid changes are common in midlife and must be ruled out.
- **Vitamin D, 25-Hydroxy:** Evaluates vitamin D, essential for bone health, immune regulation, and mood—all affected by hormonal decline.
- **Gamma-Glutamyl Transferase (GGT):** Sensitive marker for liver health and oxidative stress. Hormonal shifts can affect liver metabolism.

To those labs, I will add . . .

- **Apolipoprotein B:** Assesses the number of atherogenic particles, offering a clearer picture of cardiovascular risk than LDL cholesterol alone. Important in perimenopause because of increased cardiovascular risk associated with hormonal shifts.
- **Lipoprotein(a):** Screens for inherited lipoprotein(a) levels, a significant but often-overlooked risk factor for cardiovascular disease. Levels don't fluctuate with lifestyle, so early detection matters.
- **High-Sensitivity CRP:** Detects low-grade systemic inflammation, which is associated with increased cardiovascular and metabolic risk—both of which rise in perimenopause.
- **Ferritin:** Reflects stored iron; helps detect iron deficiency or overload. Especially important in women with heavy or prolonged periods.
- **Homocysteine:** Elevated levels may signal cardiovascular risk or B-vitamin deficiencies. Levels tend to increase in midlife.

- **Fasting Insulin:** Provides insight into insulin resistance and early metabolic dysfunction, which become more common in the perimenopausal years.

- **HOMA-IR (Homeostatic Model Assessment for Insulin Resistance):** A calculated score using fasting insulin and glucose to estimate insulin resistance. This is particularly relevant in perimenopause, when metabolic shifts can increase the risk of developing prediabetes and type 2 diabetes.

- **Iron, Total and TIBC:** Further evaluates iron status and binding capacity. Useful in identifying causes of fatigue and supporting energy levels.

- **Lactate Dehydrogenase (LD):** Non-specific marker of tissue turnover or damage. Can help rule out other causes of symptoms.

- **Magnesium:** Critical for muscle function, sleep regulation, and cardiovascular health. Magnesium needs may rise during hormonal transition.

- **Phosphate:** Assesses bone metabolism and renal function. Important for evaluating skeletal health in the context of estrogen loss.

- **T3 Uptake:** Older measure related to thyroid hormone binding capacity; included as part of comprehensive thyroid evaluation. Thyroid dysfunction can mimic perimenopausal symptoms.

- **Uric Acid:** Elevated levels may be associated with gout or metabolic syndrome, both of which can be influenced by hormonal shifts.

- **Estradiol, Extraction Method:** Provides an accurate measure of circulating estradiol, particularly important in perimenopause when levels fluctuate. While a single estradiol level isn't diagnostic of perimenopause, very low levels are consistent with postmenopause. In women who don't have regular periods, who have had a hysterectomy, or who are using a hormonal IUD, pairing estradiol with FSH can provide valuable insight into menopausal staging.

(Note: You may need to emphasize that you would like high-sensitivity estradiol measurement rather than standard estradiol; this may cost you a bit of extra money but not much.)

- **FSH:** Assesses pituitary signaling to the ovaries; often elevated in later perimenopause. Helps confirm hormonal transition.

- **Sedimentation Rate:** A non-specific test for systemic inflammation. Can help evaluate unexplained fatigue, aches, or pain.

- **Free T3:** Active form of thyroid hormone; important in evaluating thyroid performance. Fatigue and weight changes may be thyroid related.

- **Free T4:** Unbound thyroxine level; used alongside TSH for thyroid assessment. Offers a full picture of thyroid function.

- **Testosterone, Free and Total:** Evaluates androgen status, relevant for libido, energy, and muscle maintenance. Levels often decline in midlife.

- **TPO and TG Antibodies:** Screens for autoimmune thyroid disorders, such as Hashimoto's. Autoimmunity tends to peak in midlife.

- **Vitamin B12 and Folate:** Essential for cognitive health, energy production, and red blood cell function. Deficiencies can mimic perimenopausal symptoms.

You Are Ready (and You Are Not Alone)

One of the most common sources of frustration in perimenopause is being dismissed and denied access to clinical support or a discussion of treatment options. I hope that the information provided in this chapter empowers you to get the assessment and answers you need. I also encourage you to connect with me on social media, where I often host live segments and AMAs—I don't get to all the questions submitted, but I do try to cover a lot of the most frequently asked ones. You can find me as Dr.

Mary Claire on all platforms. And don't be shy in the comments—the modern menopause era is defined by women who will not be shamed into silent suffering. My followers and those I see commenting on my colleagues' posts are engaged, they are active and outspoken, and they are eager to share what has worked or not worked for them in their search for better clinical care. All you have to do is log on and become part of the conversation. We will be waiting for you.

CONCLUSION

What I Wish I'd Known at Thirty-Five

I want to close this book with a roundup of what I wish I'd known when I was younger, a letter that shares with my thirty-five-year-old self an awareness of what is to come, insight into how to adapt, and motivation to take preventative steps to support my future health. I wrote this to myself, but it's for you—take the words to heart and use them as your guide in the years to come.

Dear Mary Claire,

You're thirty-five. You're in the thick of it: motherhood, marriage, and medicine. You're building a career, raising children, balancing patients and a home, and trying to do it all perfectly. You're thriving and exhausted all at once. You believe in science, in structure, in data. You think you're prepared for anything. But let me tell you something with love:
You are not prepared for menopause.
Not because you aren't capable, but because you haven't been taught. Like so many other physicians, you've been trained in a system that teaches you to value thinness over strength, to overlook the signs of hormonal change, and to underestimate the sheer force of midlife transformation. You've been subtly conditioned to believe that menopause is a blip, a whisper of inconvenience. You think you'll be one of the lucky ones who barely feels it.
But when it hits, it won't be a whisper. It will be a storm. And you will, for a time, gaslight yourself. You'll doubt your symptoms: your sleep disruptions, your anxiety, the aching in your joints, the way your body sud-

denly feels foreign. You'll blame stress, your schedule—just about anything but hormones. You'll do what many women have done and still do: suffer silently, push through, and pretend it's normal.

But here's the thing: *You'll fight your way through that fog.* And you'll emerge with clarity and an unshakable calling. You'll change everything—your practice, your priorities, and your platform—all because you'll realize that women deserve better.

So, Mary Claire, while you're holding babies and fielding pages, take a moment. Listen to me. Here's what I need you to know:

1. **Shift from thin to strong.** Stop chasing the number on the scale. It will never love you back. Shift your focus to strength: muscle, stamina, resilience. It will carry you through the storm.

    Strength training will become one of your most meaningful allies. It will support your bones, your brain, and your balance. It will make you feel powerful, not because of how you *look,* but because of what you can *do.*

2. **Focus on nutrition over calories.** You've counted calories. Now it's time to *count nutrients.* Feed your body what it needs: fiber, protein, antioxidants, healthy fats. Food is more than just fuel; it's information that tells your body how to function, how to fight inflammation, and how to age well. This philosophy will become the foundation of *The Galveston Diet.* You'll teach it to thousands, but first you'll have to learn it yourself.

3. **Educate yourself about menopause.** You're an incredible physician, but your knowledge has a blind spot when it comes to menopause. It's not your fault—you were taught next to nothing about menopause. And you're not alone. Menopause education in medicine is shockingly inadequate. So, I'm telling you now—learn everything you can and then teach it to others so you learn it twice. Share what you learn widely and loudly. The more you understand biology, the more you'll honor what your body is telling you—and what your patients have been trying to say all along.

And this will come as a big surprise to you, but it's major: Hormone therapy isn't the enemy or the last resort as you were taught.

4. **Consider aging a privilege.** You'll lose people, some of those closest to you: Your brothers and your father will go first. You'll grieve deeply. And it will teach you this: *Aging isn't a curse; it's a gift.*

    In your fifties, you'll pivot your entire career. You'll grow more fearless, more authentic, and more alive. Don't fear the wrinkles or the gray. They come with wisdom, freedom, and clarity.

5. **Focus on function and longevity.** I know I've already said this, but it needs repeating (I've seen how often you step on the scale): Your health isn't your weight.

    Also, your success isn't your busyness. Invest in your future self. Preserve muscle, protect your heart, and keep moving—literally and figuratively. Longevity isn't just about living longer; it's about living better for as long as possible.

Mary Claire, enjoy these beautiful years. Your babies will grow and leave; your marriage will bend and stretch and come back stronger. Your job will evolve in ways you can't imagine. Don't forget yourself in the process. Not just your body, but your joy, your rest, and your voice.

Menopause will rock your world, but it will also shape your purpose. You will become the advocate you never had. The teacher your younger self needed. The voice for millions of women who've been silenced too long.

This isn't the end of something; it's the beginning.

With love and gratitude,
Yourself, a little older, a lot wiser,
and more powerful than ever

Acknowledgments

This book was not written alone. It rests on the shoulders of so many whose dedication, brilliance, and love carried me through late nights, hard days, and the moments when the finish line felt impossibly far away.

To my extraordinary staff—Deb Millard, Jen Pearson, Dawn Drogosch, Jamie Hadley, Margaret Walsh, Amy Chase, Jennifer Anderson, Tianna Miller-Donaldson, Melissa Dreyer, Zach Toth, Rachel Perry, Jackie Schaiper, Camilo Navarro, Kathy Champagne, Kristen Lewis, Sierra Sertass, Tammy Frelly, Sarah Lux, Lisa McDonald, Catherine Power, Dayle Harris, Ariel Margolis, Chris Haver, Katie Lemaire, Angie Parker, Susan Dreling, Molly McPhearson, and Gabi Anderson—thank you for keeping the wheels turning and the mission alive, and for believing in this work every single day.

To my clinic family—Dr. Sharon McCloskey, Joan Moss, Stacy Lord, Mary Turner, Samantha Green, Kennedy Harrington, Deann Maddox, and Cheryl Mills—your dedication to our patients and to the science of menopause care is the heartbeat of what we do.

To my friends and family—Christopher Haver, Katherine Haver, Madeline Haver, Leah Pastor Rion, Mary (Maugie) Landry Pastor, Carolyn Mahtook, Heidi Seigel, Pamela Gabriel, Erica K, Cara Koza, Donna Girouard, Dr. Erica Kelly, Dr. Lisa Farmer, my brothers, and my father in heaven—your love and encouragement have sustained me more than I can say.

To the brilliant, fearless Menoposse—Dr. Kelly Casperson; Dr. Suzanne Gilberg; Dr. Jackie Piasta; Dr. Corinne Menn; Dr. Vonda Wright; Dr. Natalie Crawford; Dr. Heather Hirsch; Dr. Sharon Malone; Dr. Avrum Bluming; Dr. Carol Tavris; Dr. Gabrielle Lyon; Dr. Rocio Salas-Whalen; Tamsen Fadal; Dr. Kate White; Dr. Lisa Mosconi; Dr. Aoife O'Sullivan; Dr. Alicia

Robbins; Dr. Andrea Matsumura; Dr. Ceri Cashel; Dr. Louise Newson; Dr. Fatima Kahn; Dr. Sarah Glynne; Dr. Sheila Deliz; Dr. Heidi Flagg; Dr. Shieva Ghofrany; Dr. Judith Johnson; Dr. Jill Krapf; Dr. Jayne Morgan; Dr. Heather Quaile; Dr. Jessica Shepard; Dr. Noor Al-Humaidhi; Rachel Frankenthal, PA-C; Dr. Lauren Streicher; Dr. Lisa Larkin; Dr. Jim Simon; and Dr. Rachel Rubin, thank you for standing shoulder-to-shoulder in this fight, sharing your voices, expertise, and courage.

To my publishing partners—my friend and fantastic collaborator Gretchen Lees; Heather Jackson, my wise and steadfast agent; Marnie Cochran, my insightful and generous editor; Cindy Murray, whose vision and support have been invaluable; and the incredible team at Rodale—thank you for helping me shape this book into something worthy of the women it serves.

To Anna Doherty, Mally Roncal, Sima Sistani, Maria Shriver, Katie Couric, Oprah Winfrey, Naomi Watts, Amy Griffin, Leanne Morgan, Mel Robbins, Dr. Andrew Huberman, Steven Bartlett, Alisa Volkman, and Monica Lewinsky—your inspiration and willingness to help share this message far and wide have made an indelible mark on this journey.

And finally, to every woman who has ever shared her story with me, in clinic, at a conference, or across the vast space of the internet, you are the reason this book exists. Your questions, your struggles, and your determination to be heard are the heart of *The New Perimenopause*.

APPENDIX A

Selected Resources

A Citizen's Guide to Menopause Advocacy: thepauselife.com/pages/menopause-advocacy.

The Musculoskeletal Syndrome of Menopause: The study conducted by Dr. Vonda Wright et al. can be accessed here: doi.org/10.1080/13697137.2024.2380363.

The American Urological Association 2025 Guideline on the Genitourinary Syndrome of Menopause: I'm including the text and table here so that you can share this information with your practitioner, if necessary.

The AUA made the following guideline statements:

SHARED DECISION-MAKING

- Clinicians and patients should engage in shared decision-making, taking into consideration the best available evidence and the patient's expressed values, preferences, and goals of GSM care.

SCREENING AND DIAGNOSIS

- Screen all at-risk patients with a focused medical, sexual, and psychosocial history.
- Conduct a genitourinary exam in all symptomatic patients.
- Educate patients on the hormonal origins of GSM symptoms.
- Evaluate for other genitourinary conditions and refer when necessary.
- Consider referrals to licensed therapists for sexual or psychosocial concerns.
- Refer to pelvic floor physical therapists when dysfunction is present.

HORMONAL THERAPIES

- Offer local low-dose vaginal estrogen to improve dryness, discomfort, and dyspareunia.
- Offer vaginal DHEA for similar symptoms.
- Consider ospemifene as an oral option for vulvovaginal discomfort.
- Offer local estrogen or DHEA even to patients already on systemic estrogen.
- Use local estrogen to treat GSM in patients with co-morbid conditions like overactive bladder or recurrent urinary tract infections.

NON-HORMONAL THERAPY

- Recommend vaginal moisturizers and lubricants alone or alongside other treatments.
- Counsel patients that supplements have no proven benefit for GSM.
- Advise avoiding irritants and harsh cleansers that may worsen symptoms.

ENERGY-BASED THERAPIES

- Inform patients that CO_2 laser, ER:YAG laser, or radiofrequency devices for treating GSM are not supported by current evidence.
- If used, they should be offered only with full disclosure and to patients who cannot use or prefer to avoid FDA-approved treatments.

CANCER CONSIDERATIONS

- Local vaginal estrogen does not increase the risk of breast or endometrial cancer.
- Vaginal DHEA and ospemifene also show no increased cancer risk.
- Local vaginal estrogen may be used in breast cancer survivors after shared decision-making with their care team.
- Routine endometrial surveillance is not required for patients using local therapies or ospemifene.

FOLLOW-UP

- Reassess treatment response regularly.
- Prepare patients for the potential need for long-term therapy and monitoring.

FDA-Approved Treatments for GSM

CATEGORY	COMPOSITION	COMMONLY USED STARTING DOSE	COMMONLY USED MAINTENANCE DOSE	TYPICAL SERUM ESTRADIOL LEVEL (PG/ML)
VAGINAL CREAMS	17β-estradiol 0.01% (0.1 mg active ingredient/g)	0.5-1 gram daily for 2 weeks	0.5-1 gram 1-3 times/week	Variable, 3-5a
	Conjugated estrogen (0.625 mg active ingredient/g)	0.5-1 gram daily for 2 weeks	0.5 grams 1-3 times/week	Variable
VAGINAL INSERTS	17β-estradiol inserts	4 or 10 µg/d for 2 weeks	1 insert twice/week	3.6 (4 µg) 4.6 (10 µg)
	Estradiol hemihydrate tablets	4 or 10 µg/d for 2 weeks	1 insert twice/week	5.5
	Prasterone (DHEA) inserts	6.5mg/day	1 insert/day	5
VAGINAL RINGS	Silicone polymer with a core containing 2mg estradiol	7.5 mcg/day for 3 months	1 ring/three months	8
ORAL TABLETS	Ospemifene	60 mg/day	1 tablet by mouth/day	N/A

The American Urological Society 2025 Guidelines for Hormonal Interventions for genitourinary syndrome of menopause (GSM)

APPENDIX B

The New Perimenopause Five-Day Meal Plan

RECIPES

DAY ONE

• MEAL ONE •

THE MENOPAUSE POWER SHAKE

(1 SERVING)

INGREDIENTS

¾ cup plain Siggi's Skyr or other high-protein yogurt

1 scoop The 'Pause Nutrition (TPN) Protein + Creatine

1 tbsp chia seeds

1 tbsp ground flaxseeds

1 tbsp hemp hearts

1 cup frozen berries of your choice

2 scoops TPN Skin & Bone Collagen, unflavored

1 scoop TPN Fiber GDX, unflavored

water, to desired consistency (optional)

ice (optional)

DIRECTIONS

1. Place all ingredients in a high-powered blender and process until smooth.

• MEAL TWO •

TPN DENSE BEAN SALAD WITH ROTISSERIE CHICKEN
(1 SERVING)

INGREDIENTS

1 cup TPN Dense Bean Salad (see recipe below)

3 oz rotisserie chicken

DIRECTIONS

1. Combine ingredients and enjoy warmed in the microwave for 1 minute or cold out of the refrigerator.

TPN DENSE BEAN SALAD MEAL PREP RECIPE (10 1-CUP SERVINGS)

INGREDIENTS

1 can cannellini beans, rinsed and drained

1 can red kidney beans, rinsed and drained

1 can chickpeas, rinsed and drained

1 can butter beans, rinsed and drained

½ medium yellow onion, diced

1 cup olive oil

6 tbsp white wine vinegar

1 long English cucumber, diced

¼ cup sunflower seeds

¼ cup pine nuts

1 cup cilantro, chopped

2 cups parsley, chopped

½ cup feta cheese, crumbled

10 green onions, tops only

DIRECTIONS

1. Combine all ingredients in a large airtight container and allow to marinate in the refrigerator several hours to overnight.

2. Enjoy alone or with added protein of your choice.

NOTE: Use this recipe as a guide and add or replace ingredients to suit your preferences.

• MEAL THREE •

HOT HONEY TURKEY BOWL
(4 servings)

INGREDIENTS

- 16 oz lean ground turkey (93%/7%)
- 2 cups brown rice, steamed
- 2 cups broccoli, steamed from fresh or frozen
- 1 medium sweet potato, baked
- 2 oz cheddar cheese, shredded
- 4 tbsp hot honey

DIRECTIONS

1. In a large skillet over medium-high heat, cook turkey, breaking up with a wooden spoon, until browned and cooked through. (Note: Add any seasonings you desire.)
2. Once turkey is cooked through, assemble ½ cup brown rice, ½ cup steamed broccoli, ¼ sweet potato, ½ oz cheese, and 4 oz cooked turkey in each of 4 bowls.
3. Top each bowl with 1 tbsp of hot honey.

• SNACK ONE •

GUACAMOLE WITH CARROT STICKS

INGREDIENTS

- 2 tbsp store-bought or homemade guacamole
- 5 baby carrots

DIRECTIONS

1. Enjoy!

• SNACK TWO •

MOZZARELLA CHEESE

INGREDIENTS

1 part-skim mozzarella cheese stick

DIRECTIONS

1. Enjoy!

DAY ONE MACROS

Calories: 1844

Protein: 147 grams

Fiber: 41 grams

DAY TWO

• MEAL ONE •

OVERNIGHT OATS

(1 SERVING, BASE RECIPE)

INGREDIENTS

½ cup rolled oats

1 scoop TPN Protein + Creatine

½ tbsp chia seeds

½ cup milk of your choice (dairy or plant-based)

¼ cup plain Siggi's Skyr or other high-protein yogurt

¼ cup raspberries or berries of your choice

DIRECTIONS

1. Combine oats, TPN Protein, and chia seeds in a glass container with a lid.
2. Add milk and yogurt and stir until thoroughly combined.
3. Place the lid on the container and refrigerate the oat mixture for at least 5 hours or overnight.
4. Top with berries prior to serving, stir, and enjoy.

NOTE: Add any fruit or additional toppings you'd like, including unsweetened nut or seed butter and cinnamon or other spices, and enjoy warm, room temperature, or cold.

• MEAL TWO •

CHICKEN AVOCADO WRAP
(1 SERVING)

INGREDIENTS

4 oz rotisserie chicken breast

1 Joseph's Flax, Oat Bran & Whole Wheat lavash bread or Joseph's Flax, Oat Bran & Whole Wheat wrap

2 large romaine lettuce leaves

½ avocado, sliced

1 tbsp Primal Kitchen Ranch, Caesar, or Greek Vinaigrette dressing

DIRECTIONS

1. Heat chicken if desired or enjoy cold or at room temperature.
2. Lay bread or wrap flat on a cutting board.
3. Lay lettuce leaves down the center of the bread or wrap.
4. Add sliced avocado and chicken.
5. Drizzle dressing over the chicken, and if making a wrap, roll the sides in to cover the chicken. Enjoy!

• MEAL THREE •

PECAN-CRUSTED SALMON
(4 SERVINGS)

INGREDIENTS

1 tbsp salted butter

2 cups brown rice

16 oz salmon fillet

1 tbsp + 1 tsp olive oil, divided
½ cup pecans, chopped
4 cups brussels sprouts, halved lengthwise

DIRECTIONS

1. Cook brown rice according to package directions, adding butter to water before adding rice. Preheat the oven to 375°F.
2. Lay salmon in the center of a sheet pan. Top with 1 tsp olive oil and pecans.
3. Toss halved brussels sprouts with 1 tbsp olive oil and place them around the salmon.
4. Roast in the oven for 20–25 minutes or until fish flakes easily with a fork and vegetables are fork-tender.

• SNACK ONE •

HUMMUS AND FLACKERS

INGREDIENTS

2 tbsp store-bought or homemade hummus, flavor of your choice
1 oz (~30 grams) Flackers flaxseed crackers, flavor of your choice

DIRECTIONS

1. Dunk Flackers in hummus or spread hummus over Flackers and enjoy.

• SNACK TWO •

CELERY AND NUT BUTTER BOAT

INGREDIENTS

1 large celery stalk, rinsed and dried
1 tbsp unsweetened nut or seed butter of your choice

DIRECTIONS

1. Fill the cavity of the celery stalk with nut or seed butter and enjoy.

DAY TWO MACROS

    Calories: 1825

    Protein: 136 grams

    Fiber: 48 grams

DAY THREE

• MEAL ONE •

THE MENOPAUSE POWER SHAKE
(1 SERVING)

See recipe on page 289.

• MEAL TWO •

CHICKEN HUMMUS BOWL
(1 SERVING)

INGREDIENTS

    1 cup romaine lettuce, chopped

    ¼ cup store-bought or homemade hummus

    4 cherry tomatoes, halved or quartered

    1 small cucumber, diced

    red onion to taste, thinly sliced

    3 oz rotisserie chicken breast, diced

    2 tbsp Primal Kitchen Greek Vinaigrette dressing

DIRECTIONS

1. Add romaine to a bowl and top with hummus, tomatoes, cucumber, and red onion.
2. Add chicken and top with Greek Vinaigrette dressing.

NOTE: Add olives, crumbled feta, sunflower seeds, or pine nuts to your bowl to make it your own.

• MEAL THREE •

SHEET PAN STEAK FAJITAS
(4 SERVINGS)

INGREDIENTS

16 oz flank steak

1 large red bell pepper, sliced into strips

1 large green bell pepper, sliced into strips

1 large yellow onion, sliced

¼ cup avocado oil

2 garlic cloves, diced

1 tbsp chili powder

1 tsp oregano

1 tsp cumin

1 tbsp lime juice

4 Joseph's Flax, Oat Bran & Whole Wheat lavash bread or Joseph's Flax, Oat Bran & Whole Wheat wraps

½ cup store-bought or homemade guacamole

DIRECTIONS

1. Preheat the oven to 400°F.
2. Slice steak into thin strips, going against the grain, about ¼ inch thick.
3. Add steak, sliced peppers and onions, avocado oil, garlic, seasoning, and lime juice to a large mixing bowl. Toss well to combine.
4. Transfer steak and vegetables to a large sheet pan and spread into an even layer.
5. Roast steak and vegetables in the oven for 15–18 minutes, until steak is browned and vegetables are tender.
6. Serve with warmed lavash bread or wraps and guacamole.

THE NEW PERIMENOPAUSE FIVE-DAY MEAL PLAN

• SNACK ONE •

COTTAGE CHEESE CUP

INGREDIENTS

½ cup cottage cheese (your choice: 1%, 2%, or 4% fat)

1 small cucumber, diced

½ tsp everything bagel seasoning

1 tbsp ground flaxseeds

DIRECTIONS

1. To a small bowl add cottage cheese.
2. Top with cucumber, everything bagel seasoning, and ground flaxseeds.
3. Layer as a parfait or stir to combine ingredients thoroughly.

• SNACK TWO •

BERRY AND NUT BOWL

INGREDIENTS

½ cup berries of your choice

2 tbsp walnuts, chopped

cinnamon (optional)

DIRECTIONS

1. To a small bowl add berries and walnuts.
2. Top with a pinch of cinnamon if desired.

DAY THREE MACROS

Calories: 1663

Protein: 141 grams

Fiber: 43 grams

DAY FOUR

• MEAL ONE •

OVERNIGHT OATS
(1 SERVING, BASE RECIPE)

See recipe on page 292.

• MEAL TWO •

TPN DENSE BEAN SALAD WITH TUNA
(1 SERVING)

INGREDIENTS

½ cup TPN Dense Bean Salad (page 290)

1 3.5-oz can tuna packed in water

DIRECTIONS

1. Combine ingredients and enjoy.

• MEAL THREE •

EGG ROLL IN A BOWL
(3 SERVINGS)

INGREDIENTS

16 oz lean ground turkey (93%/7%)

salt and pepper (optional)

1 small yellow onion, chopped

2 garlic cloves, minced

1 tbsp fresh ginger, grated

1 12-oz package broccoli slaw mix

1 12-oz package cauliflower rice, thawed if frozen

¼ cup coconut aminos

1 tbsp toasted sesame oil

1 tbsp sriracha

2 green onions, chopped

1 tbsp sesame seeds

DIRECTIONS

1. In a large skillet over medium-high heat, cook turkey, breaking up with a wooden spoon, until no longer pink, about 5–6 minutes. Season with salt and pepper if desired.

2. Add yellow onion, garlic, ginger, broccoli slaw mix, cauliflower rice, coconut aminos, toasted sesame oil, and sriracha to the skillet. Cook for another 5 minutes or so, until broccoli slaw is tender. Taste and add more coconut aminos or sriracha if desired.

3. Portion mixture into bowls and top with green onions and sesame seeds. Serve with additional coconut aminos or sriracha if desired.

• SNACK ONE •

CELERY AND NUT BUTTER BOAT

See recipe on page 294.

• SNACK TWO •

HUMMUS AND FLACKERS

See recipe on page 294.

DAY FOUR MACROS

Calories: 1722

Protein: 137 grams

Fiber: 44 grams

DAY FIVE

• MEAL ONE •

COTTAGE CHEESE SCRAMBLED EGGS WITH EZEKIEL TOAST
(1 SERVING)

INGREDIENTS

1 slice Ezekiel bread

olive oil spray

1 cup spinach

2 large eggs

¼ cup cottage cheese (your choice 1%, 2%, or 4% fat)

salt and pepper (optional)

1 cup raspberries or berries of your choice

DIRECTIONS

1. Heat a small pan over medium heat, and put Ezekiel bread in the toaster to toast to desired doneness.
2. Spray pan with olive oil and add spinach. Cover and allow spinach to wilt.
3. Meanwhile, in a small bowl, whisk together eggs and cottage cheese and set aside.
4. When spinach is wilted, add egg and cottage cheese mixture to the pan and season with salt and pepper to taste if desired.
5. Use a rubber spatula to break egg mixture into pieces and cook to desired doneness, then transfer egg, cottage cheese, and spinach mixture to a plate.
6. Remove bread from the toaster, add berries to a small bowl, and enjoy.

• MEAL TWO •

THE MENOPAUSE POWER SHAKE
(1 SERVING)

See recipe on page 289.

• MEAL THREE •

CHICKEN CRUST PIZZA WITH SIDE SALAD
(4 SERVINGS)

PIZZA INGREDIENTS

16 oz ground chicken breast

2 large eggs

¼ cup parmesan cheese, grated

1 tsp garlic powder

1 tsp Italian seasoning

¼ cup marinara or pizza sauce

1 cup mozzarella cheese, shredded

DIRECTIONS

1. Preheat the oven to 400°F and line a large baking sheet with parchment paper.
2. To a large bowl, add chicken, eggs, parmesan, garlic powder, and Italian seasoning, and mix well.
3. Transfer chicken mixture to the lined baking sheet and press down into a large pizza shape.
4. Bake for 20 minutes, then remove from the oven and let rest for 5 minutes.
5. Spread marinara or pizza sauce on the crust and top with mozzarella and any other toppings of your choice.
6. Return to the oven and bake for an additional 8–10 minutes or until desired doneness.

SALAD INGREDIENTS

1½ cups mixed lettuce, chopped

½ cup Roma tomato, chopped

1 tbsp ground flaxseeds

1 tbsp chia seeds

1 tbsp hemp hearts

4 tbsp Primal Kitchen Ranch, Caesar, or Greek Vinaigrette dressing

DIRECTIONS

1. In a small bowl combine all ingredients and enjoy.

• SNACK ONE •

MOZZARELLA CHEESE

INGREDIENTS

1 part-skim mozzarella cheese stick or 1 oz mozzarella cheese, shredded, remaining from Chicken Crust Pizza

DIRECTIONS

1. Enjoy!

• SNACK TWO

BERRY AND NUT BOWL

See recipe on page 297.

DAY FIVE MACROS

Calories: 1711

Protein: 141 grams

Fiber: 42 grams

MEAL PLAN

DAY	MEAL 1	MEAL 2	MEAL 3	SNACK 1	SNACK 2	MACROS
DAY 1	The Menopause Power Shake	TPN Dense Bean Salad w/ Rotisserie Chicken	Hot Honey Turkey Bowl	Guacamole w/Carrot Sticks	Mozzarella Cheese	Cals: 1844 Protein: 147g Fiber: 41g
DAY 2	Overnight Oats (base recipe)	Chicken Avocado Wrap	Pecan-Crusted Salmon	Hummus and Flackers	Celery and Nut Butter Boat	Cals: 1825 Protein: 136g Fiber: 48g
DAY 3	The Menopause Power Shake	Chicken Hummus Bowl	Sheet Pan Steak Fajitas	Cottage Cheese Cup	Berry and Nut Bowl	Cals: 1663 Protein: 141g Fiber: 43g
DAY 4	Overnight Oats (base recipe)	TPN Dense Bean Salad w/Tuna	Egg Roll in a Bowl	Celery and Nut Butter Boat	Hummus and Flackers	Cals: 1722 Protein: 137g Fiber: 44g
DAY 5	Cottage Cheese Scrambled Eggs w/ Ezekiel Toast	The Menopause Power Shake	Chicken Crust Pizza w/Side Salad	Mozzarella Cheese	Berry and Nut Bowl	Cals: 1711 Protein: 141g Fiber: 42g

SHOPPING LIST

Produce	
1	avocado
1	bell pepper, green
1	bell pepper, red
2.5 cups	berries of choice
1 large head (or one bag frozen)	broccoli
12-oz bag	broccoli slaw
4 cups	brussels sprouts
1 small bag	carrots, baby
12-oz bag	cauliflower rice
1 small head	celery
1 bunch	cilantro
1 long	cucumber, English
2 small	cucumbers, traditional
4 cloves	garlic cloves
1 root	ginger root
12	green onions
1 small container	guacamole
1 container	hummus
1	lime
1 container	mixed lettuce
1	onion, red
3	onions, yellow
1 bunch	parsley
1 head/1 bag	romaine lettuce
5-oz bag	spinach
1 medium	sweet potato
1	tomato, Roma
1 small container	tomatoes, cherry or grape

Pantry Items	
1 small bottle	avocado oil
1 can	butter beans
1 can	cannellini beans
1 can	red kidney beans
1 bag	brown rice
1 can	chickpeas
1 small bottle	coconut aminos
1 bottle	dressing, Primal Kitchen Ranch, Caesar, or Greek Vinaigrette
1 box	Flackers
1 small bottle	hot honey
1 package	lavash/wraps, Joseph's Flax, Oat Bran & Whole Wheat
1 small jar	marinara/pizza sauce
1 small container	oats, rolled
1 small bottle	olive oil
1 small bottle	sriracha
1 small bottle	toasted sesame oil
3.5-oz can	tuna in water
1 small bottle	white wine vinegar
The 'Pause Nutrition Supplements	
1 pouch	Creatine
1 pouch	Fiber GDX, unflavored
1 pouch	Protein
1 pouch	Skin & Bone Collagen, unflavored

SHOPPING LIST

Nuts/Seeds	
1 small bag	chia seeds
1 small bag	flaxseeds, ground
1 small bag	hemp hearts, hulled
1 jar	nut or seed butter, unsweetened
1 small bag	pecans
1 small bag	pine nuts
1 small container	sesame seeds
1 small bag	sunflower seeds
1 small bag	walnuts

Meat/Poultry/Eggs	
16 oz	chicken breast, ground
1	chicken, rotisserie
½ dozen	eggs
16 oz	salmon, fillet
16 oz	steak, flank
32 oz	turkey, ground (93%/7%)

Seasonings	
1 small jar	chili powder
1 small jar	cumin
1 small jar	everything bagel
1 small jar	garlic powder
1 small jar	Italian
1 small jar	oregano

Dairy	
1 stick	butter, salted
1 block	cheddar
6-oz container	cottage cheese (1%, 2%, or 4% fat)
1 small container	feta
1 pint	milk of choice
5-oz bag	mozzarella, shredded
1 small bag	mozzarella string cheese
1 small container	parmesan, grated
1 large container (at least 3 cups)	plain yogurt, Siggi's Skyr or other high-protein brand

Frozen Foods	
1 large bag	berries of choice
1 loaf	Ezekiel sprouted grain bread

References

CHAPTER 1: THE STATUS QUO EXPERIENCE OF PERIMENOPAUSE

"ACOG Practice Bulletin No. 141: Management of Menopausal Symptoms," *Obstetrics & Gynecology* 123, no. 1 (2014): 202–16, doi.org/10.1097/01.AOG.0000441353.20693.78.

Rita Rubin, "It Takes an Average of 17 Years for Evidence to Change Practice: The Burgeoning Field of Implementation Science Seeks to Speed Things Up," *JAMA* 329, no. 16 (2023): 1333–36, doi.org/10.1001/jama.2023.4387.

National Academies of Sciences, Engineering, and Medicine, *A New Vision for Women's Health Research: Transformative Change at the National Institutes of Health*, ed. Sheila P. Burke, Alina Salganicoff, and Amy Geller (National Academies Press, 2025), https://doi.org/10.17226/28586.

"The Evernow Menopause Study," Evernow, evernow.com/menopause-study.

"Antidepressants and Menopause," The Menopause Charity, last modified October 2022, themenopausecharity.org/information-and-support/what-can-help/treatment-options/hormone-replacement-therapy/antidepressants-and-menopause.

Qingfang He et al., "Determining the Status of Small Dense Low-Density Lipoprotein Cholesterol Level in Women Undergoing Menopausal Transition," *Frontiers in Endocrinology* 15 (2025), doi.org/10.3389/fendo.2024.1500712.

Jianheng Hao et al., "Blood-Detected Mitochondrial Biomarker NSUN4: A Potential Indicator of Ovarian Aging," *Experimental Gerontology* 208 (2025): 112825, doi.org/10.1016/j.exger.2025.112825.

World Economic Forum with McKinsey Health Institute, *Closing the Women's Health Gap: A $1 Trillion Opportunity to Improve Lives and Economies* (World Economic Forum, January 2024), 5, mckinsey.com/mhi/our-insights/closing-the-womens-health-gap-a-1-trillion-dollar-opportunity-to-improve-lives-and-economies.

CHAPTER 2: THE ZONE OF CHAOS

Pliny the Elder, *The Natural History,* trans. John Bostock and H. T. Riley (Taylor and Francis, 1855), 18.23, perseus.tufts.edu/hopper/text?doc=Perseus%3Atext%3A1999.02.0137%3Abook%3D28%3Achapter%3D23.

Maureen C. McHugh, "Menstrual Shame: Exploring the Role of 'Menstrual Moaning,'" in *The Palgrave Handbook of Critical Menstruation Studies,* ed. Chris Bobel et al. (Palgrave Macmillan, 2020), 409–22, doi.org/10.1007/978-981-15-0614-7_32.

Christina A. Metcalf et al., "Cognitive Problems in Perimenopause: A Review of Recent Evidence," *Current Psychiatry Reports* 25 (2023): 501–11, doi.org/10.1007/s11920-023-01447-3.

Liisa Hantsoo et al., "The Role of the Hypothalamic-Pituitary-Adrenal Axis in Depression Across the Female Reproductive Lifecycle: Current Knowledge and Future Directions," *Frontiers in Endocrinology* 14 (2023), doi.org/10.3389/fendo.2023.1295261.

Tiziana Fidecicchi et al., "Neuroendocrine Mechanisms of Mood Disorders During Menopause Transition: A Narrative Review and Future Perspectives," *Maturitas* 188 (2024), doi.org/10.1016/j.maturitas.2024.108087.

N. Santoro et al., "Characterization of Reproductive Hormonal Dynamics in the Perimenopause," *Journal of Clinical Endocrinology & Metabolism* 81, no. 4 (1996): 1495–501, doi.org/10.1210/jcem.81.4.8636357.

Kathleen A. O'Connor, Darryl J. Holman, and James W. Wood, "Menstrual Cycle Variability and the Perimenopause," *American Journal of Human Biology* 13, no. 4 (2001): 465–78, doi.org/10.1002/ajhb.1078.

Henry G. Burger et al., "Cycle and Hormone Changes During Perimenopause: The Key Role of Ovarian Function," *Menopause* 15, no. 4 (2008): 603–12, doi.org/10.1097/gme.0b013e318174ea4d.

Lauren P. Klosinski et al., "White Matter Lipids as a Ketogenic Fuel Supply in Aging Female Brain: Implications for Alzheimer's Disease," *EBioMedicine* 2, no. 12 (2015): 1888–1904, doi.org/10.1016/j.ebiom.2015.11.002.

"Committee Opinion No. 589: Female Age-Related Fertility Decline," *Obstetrics & Gynecology* 123, no. 3 (2014): 719–21, doi.org/10.1097/01.AOG.0000444440.96486.61.

M. J. Faddy et al., "Accelerated Disappearance of Ovarian Follicles in Mid-life: Implications for Forecasting Menopause," *Human Reproduction* 7, no. 10 (1992): 1342–46, doi.org/10.1093/oxfordjournals.humrep.a137570.

Rachel Ann Tee-Melegrito, "How many eggs does a woman have?" *Medical News Today,* medicalnewstoday.com/articles/how-many-eggs-does-a-woman-have.

CHAPTER 3: THE TROUBLING PATTERN OF MISDIAGNOSIS (AND GASLIGHTING)

"Gendered Pain: A Call for Recognition and Health Equity," *eClinicalMedicine* 69 (2024), doi.org/10.1016/j.eclinm.2024.102558.

Darcy Banco et al., "Sex and Race Differences in the Evaluation and Treatment of Young Adults Presenting to the Emergency Department with Chest Pain," *Journal of the American Heart Association* 11, no. 10 (2022), doi.org/10.1161/JAHA.121.024199.

Linda Brubaker et al., "Forming Consensus to Advance Urobiome Research," mSystems 6, no. 4 (2021): e0137120, doi.org/10.1128/mSystems.01371-20.

Yuko M. Komesu et al., "Defining the Relationship Between Vaginal and Urinary Microbiomes," *American Journal of Obstetrics & Gynecology* 222, no. 2 (2020): 154.e1–154.e10, doi.org/10.1016/j.ajog.2019.08.011.

Christian Temml et al., "Prevalence and Correlates for Interstitial Cystitis Symptoms in Women Participating in a Health Screening Project," *European Urology* 51, no. 3 (2007): 803–9, doi.org/10.1016/j.eururo.2006.08.028.

Krystal Thomas-White et al., "Vaginal Estrogen Therapy Is Associated with Increased *Lactobacillus* in the Urine of Postmenopausal Women with Overactive Bladder Symptoms," *American Journal of Obstetrics & Gynecology* 223, no. 5 (2020), doi.org/10.1016/j.ajog.2020.08.006.

C. Neill Epperson et al., "Impact of Atomoxetine on Subjective Attention and Memory Difficulties in Perimenopausal and Postmenopausal Women," *Menopause* 18, no. 5 (2011): 542–48, doi.org/10.1097/gme.0b013e3181fcafd6.

C. Neill Epperson et al., "New Onset Executive Function Difficulties at Menopause: A Possible Role for Lisdexamfetamine," *Psychopharmacology* 232 (2015): 3091–100, doi.org/10.1007/s00213-015-3953-7.

Devon Kardel and Sarah Weber, "The Effect of Perimenopause on Women's Executive Functioning: A Systematic Review," *Archives of Clinical Neuropsychology* 39, no. 7 (2024), doi.org/10.1093/arclin/acae067.235.

J. S. Kooij, "ADHD in a Woman During (Peri)menopause: Missed Diagnoses and Cardiac Complaints," *European Psychiatry* 67 (2024), doi.org/10.1192/j.eurpsy.2024.1666.

Jeanette Wasserstein, Gerry A. Stefanatos, and Mary V. Solanto, "Perimenopause, Menopause and ADHD," *Journal of the International Neuropsychological Society* 29 (2023): 881, doi.org/10.1017/s1355617723010846.

Jim Russell et al., "Number of ADHD Patients Rising, Especially Among Women," Epic Research, March 30, 2023, epicresearch.org/articles/number-of-adhd-patients-rising-especially-among-women.

Sarah M. Andres, Jesse M. Galina, and Sarah L. Berga, "Iatrogenic Cushing Syndrome and Adrenal Suppression Presenting as Perimenopause," *JCEM Case Reports* 2, no. 11 (2024), doi.org/10.1210/jcemcr/luae183.

Jennifer L. Gordon et al., "Naturally Occurring Changes in Estradiol Concentrations in the Menopause Transition Predict Morning Cortisol and Negative Mood in Perimenopausal Depression," *Clinical Psychological Science* 4, no. 5 (2016): 919–35, doi.org/10.1177/2167702616647924.

Paul Newhouse and Kimberly Albert, "Estrogen, Stress, and Depression: A Neurocognitive Model," *JAMA Psychiatry* 72, no. 7 (2015): 727–29, doi.org/10.1001/jamapsychiatry.2015.0487.

Tianna Sauer et al., "Perimenopausal Vasomotor Symptoms and the Cortisol Awakening Response," *Menopause* 27, no. 11 (2020): 1322–27, doi.org/10.1097/GME.0000000000001588.

Isabelle Rodrigues-Santos, Bruna Kalil-Cutti, and Janete Aparecida Anselmo-Franci, "Low Corticosterone Response to Stress in a Perimenopausal Rat Model Is Associated with the Hypoactivation of PaMP Region of the Paraventricular Nucleus and Can Be Corrected by Exogenous Progesterone Supplementation," *Neuroendocrinology* 112, no. 5 (2022): 467–80, doi.org/10.1159/000518336.

Stuart Stewart et al., "Menopause Symptom Prevalence in Three Post-COVID-19 Syndrome Clinics in England: A Cross-Sectional Analysis," *IJID Regions* 12 (2024), doi.org/10.1016/j.ijregi.2024.100405.

Jack Waxman and Susan McSherry Zatzkis, "Fibromyalgia and Menopause: Examination of the Relationship," *Postgraduate Medicine* 80, no. 4 (1986): 165–71, doi.org/10.1080/00325481.1986.11699544.

J. Ben Shimol, "Perimenopause in Women with Rheumatologic Diseases: A Spotlight on an Under-Addressed Transition," *Climacteric* 27, no. 2 (2024): 115–21, doi.org/10.1080/13697137.2023.2276201.

Ö. N. Pamuk and N. Çakir, "The Variation in Chronic Widespread Pain and Other Symptoms in Fibromyalgia Patients: The Effects of Menses and Menopause," *Clinical and Experimental Rheumatology* 23, no. 6 (2005): 778–82, clinexprheumatol.org/abstract.asp?a=2740.

Ciro Conversano et al., "Psychological and Physical Interdependence Between Fibromyalgia Syndrome and Menopause: A Review of the Literature," *Mediterranean Journal of Clinical Psychology* 7, no. 3 (2019), doi.org/10.6092/2282-1619/2019.7.2279.

Alma Rus et al., "Effect of Menopause on Circulating Amino Acid Concentrations in Women with Fibromyalgia and Healthy Women," *Maturitas* 193 (2025), doi.org/10.1016/j.maturitas.2024.108171.

M. Martínez-Jauand et al., "Age-of-Onset of Menopause Is Associated with Enhanced Painful and Non-Painful Sensitivity in Fibromyalgia," *Clinical Rheumatology* 32 (2013): 975–81, doi.org/10.1007/s10067-013-2212-8.

E. Hysa et al., "Fibromyalgia and Body Mass Composition in Post-Menopausal Women: Preliminary Results from a Cross-Sectional Monocentric Study," *Annals of the Rheumatic Diseases* 81 (2022), doi.org/10.1136/annrheumdis-2022-eular.4583.

Rejane Camila Alvarenga Dias et al., "Fibromyalgia, Sleep Disturbance and Menopause: Is There a Relationship? A Literature Review," *International Journal of Rheumatic Diseases* 22, no. 11 (2019): 1961–71, doi.org/10.1111/1756-185X.13713.

Vonda J. Wright et al., "The Musculoskeletal Syndrome of Menopause," *Climacteric* 27, no. 5 (2024): 466–72, doi.org/10.1080/13697137.2024.2380363.

Stephanie S. Faubion et al., "The 2020 Genitourinary Syndrome of Menopause Position Statement of the North American Menopause Society," *Menopause* 27, no. 9 (2020): 976–92, doi.org/10.1097/GME.0000000000001609.

CHAPTER 4: THIS IS YOUR BRAIN ON PERIMENOPAUSE

Sandra Zárate, Tinna Stevnsner, and Ricardo Gredilla, "Role of Estrogen and Other Sex Hormones in Brain Aging, Neuroprotection and DNA Repair," *Frontiers in Aging Neuroscience* 9 (2017), doi.org/10.3389/fnagi.2017.00430.

Rachel E. Gross, "Sex Hormones Are Brain Hormones: What Does This Mean for Treating Brain Diseases?" *New York Times,* April 22, 2025, nytimes.com/2025/04/22/health/neuroscience-estrogen-hormones.html.

J. Bancroft, "The Endocrinology of Sexual Arousal," *Journal of Endocrinology* 186, no. 3 (2005): 411–27, doi.org/10.1677/JOE.1.06233.

Catherine de Bournonville, Aiden McGrath, and Luke Remage-Healey, "Testosterone Synthesis in the Female Songbird Brain," *Hormones and Behavior* 121 (2020), doi.org/10.1016/j.yhbeh.2020.104716.

Susan R. Davis et al., "Androgens and Female Sexual Function and Dysfunction: Findings from the Fourth International Consultation of Sexual Medicine," *The Journal of Sexual Medicine* 13, no. 2 (2016): 168–78, doi.org/10.1016/j.jsxm.2015.12.033.

Abdel Mouman Ghoumari et al., "Roles of Progesterone, Testosterone and Their Nuclear Receptors in Central Nervous System Myelination and Remyelination," *International Journal of Molecular Sciences* 21, no. 9 (2020), doi.org/10.3390/ijms21093163.

Lydia Kogler et al., "Testosterone and the Amygdala's Functional Connectivity in Women and Men," *Journal of Clinical Medicine* 12, no. 20 (2023), doi.org/10.3390/jcm12206501.

Elisa Maseroli and Linda Vignozzi, "Are Endogenous Androgens Linked to Female Sexual Function? A Systemic Review and Meta-Analysis," *The Journal of Sexual Medicine* 19, no. 4 (2022): 553–68, doi.org/10.1016/j.jsxm.2022.01.515.

Małgorzata Stefaniak et al., "Progesterone and Its Metabolites Play a Beneficial Role in Affect Regulation in the Female Brain," *Pharmaceuticals* 16, no. 4 (2023), doi.org/10.3390/ph16040520.

Peter Höfer, Rupert Lanzenberger, and Siegfried Kasper, "Testosterone in the Brain: Neuroimaging Findings and the Potential Role for Neuropsychopharmacology," *European Neuropsychopharmacology* 23, no. 2 (2013): 79–88, doi.org/10.1016/j.euroneuro.2012.04.013.

Oscar González-Flores et al., "Cellular and Molecular Mechanisms of Action of Ovarian Steroid Hormones: Regulation of Central Nervous System Function," *Neuroscience & Biobehavioral Reviews* 167 (2024), doi.org/10.1016/j.neubiorev.2024.105937.

C. Finocchi and M. Ferrari, "Female Reproductive Steroids and Neuronal Excitability," *e32* (2011): 31–35, doi.org/10.1007/s10072-011-0532-5.

Jaideep Kapur and Suchitra Joshi, "Progesterone Modulates Neuronal Excitability Bidirectionally," *Neuroscience Letters* 744 (2021), doi.org/10.1016/j.neulet.2020.135619.

Etienne-Emile Baulieu and Michael Schumacher, "Progesterone as a Neuroactive Neurosteroid, with Special Reference to the Effect of Progesterone on Myelination," *Steroids* 65 (2000): 605–12, doi.org/10.1016/S0039-128X(00)00173-2.

S. K. Chaudhuri et al., "Effects of Progesterone on Some Brain Neurotransmitters in Intact Rats," *Indian Journal of Physiology and Pharmacology* 36, no. 4 (1992): 255–58, pubmed.ncbi.nlm.nih.gov/1363321.

R. Guennoun et al., "Progesterone and Allopregnanolone in the Central Nervous System: Response to Injury and Implication for Neuroprotection," *The Journal of Steroid Biochemistry and Molecular Biology* 146 (2015): 48–61, doi.org/10.1016/j.jsbmb.2014.09.001.

Rachida Guennoun, "Progesterone in the Brain: Hormone, Neurosteroid and Neuroprotectant," *International Journal of Molecular Sciences* 21, no. 15 (2020), doi.org/10.3390/ijms21155271.

M. Schumacher et al., "Revisiting the Roles of Progesterone and Allopregnanolone in the Nervous System: Resurgence of the Progesterone Receptors," *Progress in Neurobiology* 113 (2014): 6–39, doi.org/10.1016/j.pneurobio.2013.09.004.

Juan Pablo Del Río et al., "Steroid Hormones and Their Action in Women's Brains: The Importance of Hormonal Balance," *Frontiers in Public Health* 6 (2018), doi.org/10.3389/fpubh.2018.00141.

"Perimenopause Symptoms, Treatment & Online Care," Evernow, evernow.com/care/perimenopause.

Zhaoyuan Gong et al., "Lower Myelin Content Is Associated with More Rapid Cognitive Decline Among Cognitively Unimpaired Individuals," *Alzheimer's and Dementia* 19, no. 7 (2023): 3098–107, doi.org/10.1002/alz.12968.

CHAPTER 5: THE MENTAL HEALTH CHANGES YOU MAY NOTICE

Erika Comasco, C. Neill Epperson, and Jayashri Kulkarni, "Psychiatric Symptoms on the Ovarian Hormone Roller-Coaster," *The British Journal of Psychiatry* 226 (2025): 329–30, doi.org/10.1192/bjp.2025.10298.

Megan Herson and Jayashri Kulkarni, "Hormonal Agents for the Treatment of Depression Associated with the Menopause," *Drugs & Aging* 39 (2022): 607–18, doi.org/10.1007/s40266-022-00962-x.

Lee S. Cohen et al., "Risk for New Onset of Depression During the Menopausal Transition: The Harvard Study of Moods and Cycles," *Archives of General Psychiatry* 63, no. 4 (2006): 385–90, doi.org/10.1001/archpsyc.63.4.385.

Claudio N. Soares, "Depression in Peri- and Postmenopausal Women: Prevalence, Pathophysiology and Pharmacological Management," *Drugs & Aging* 30 (2013): 677–85, doi.org/10.1007/s40266-013-0100-1.

Jennifer L. Gordon et al., "Ovarian Hormone Fluctuation, Neurosteroids, and HPA Axis Dysregulation in Perimenopausal Depression: A Novel Heuristic Model," *American Journal of Psychiatry* 172, no. 3 (2015): 227–36, doi.org/10.1176/appi.ajp.2014.14070918.

Marija Kundakovic and Devin Rocks, "Sex Hormone Fluctuation and Increased Female Risk for Depression and Anxiety Disorders: From Clinical Evidence to Molecular Mechanisms," *Frontiers in Neuroendocrinology* 66 (2022), doi.org/10.1016/j.yfrne.2022.101010.

Anouk E. de Wit et al., "Predictors of Irritability Symptoms in Mildly Depressed Perimenopausal Women," *Psychoneuroendocrinology* 126 (2021), doi.org/10.1016/j.psyneuen.2021.105128.

Robin Green, Christina A. Metcalf, and Nanette Santoro, "Mental Well-Being in Menopause," *Obstetrics and Gynecology Clinics of North America* 52, no. 1 (2025): 51–66, doi.org/10.1016/j.ogc.2024.10.002.

Elena Toffol, Oskari Heikinheimo, and Timo Partonen, "Hormone Therapy and Mood in Perimenopausal and Postmenopausal Women: A Narrative Review," *Menopause* 22, no. 5 (2015): 564–78, doi.org/10.1097/GME.0000000000000323.

Serena Lozza-Fiacco et al., "Baseline Anxiety-Sensitivity to Estradiol Fluctuations Predicts Anxiety Symptom Response to Transdermal Estradiol Treatment in Perimenopausal Women: A Randomized Clinical Trial," *Psychoneuroendocrinology* 143 (2022), doi.org/10.1016/j.psyneuen.2022.105851.

Xin Liu et al., "Efficacy of Manual Acupuncture vs. Placebo Acupuncture for Generalized Anxiety Disorder (GAD) in Perimenopausal Women: A Randomized,

Single-Blinded Controlled Trial," *Frontiers in Psychiatry* 14 (2023), doi.org/10.3389/fpsyt.2023.1240489.

Sophie Schweizer-Schubert et al., "Steroid Hormone Sensitivity in Reproductive Mood Disorders: On the Role of the $GABA_A$ Receptor Complex and Stress During Hormonal Transitions," *Frontiers in Medicine* 7 (2020), doi.org/10.3389/fmed.2020.479646.

Kayla McElhany et al., "Protective and Harmful Social and Psychological Factors Associated with Mood and Anxiety Disorders in Perimenopausal Women: A Narrative Review," *Maturitas* 190 (2024), doi.org/10.1016/j.maturitas.2024.108118.

Shahenda A. Saleh et al., "Exploring the Intersection of Depression, Anxiety, and Sexual Health in Perimenopausal Women," *International Journal of Women's Health* 16 (2024): 1315–27, doi.org/10.2147/IJWH.S464129.

CHAPTER 6: STRANGE COGNITION: THE RISE OF BRAIN FOG AND ADHD-LIKE SYMPTOMS

C. Kawas et al., "Age-Specific Incidence Rates of Alzheimer's Disease: The Baltimore Longitudinal Study of Aging," *Neurology* 54, no. 11 (2000): 2072–77, doi.org/10.1212/WNL.54.11.2072.

"2015 Alzheimer's Disease Facts and Figures," *Alzheimer's & Dementia* 11, no. 3 (2015): 332–84, doi.org/10.1016/j.jalz.2015.02.003.

Gabriella Conti et al., "The Menopause 'Penalty,'" *CESifo Working Papers*, no. 11761, March 1, 2025, doi.org/10.2139/ssrn.5200582.

Kayt Sukel, "Lifting the Fog," *New Scientist* 254, no. 3390 (2022): 38–41, doi.org/10.1016/S0262-4079(22)01024-7.

Lisa Mosconi et al., "In Vivo Brain Estrogen Receptor Density by Neuroendocrine Aging and Relationships with Cognition and Symptomatology," *Scientific Reports* 14 (2024), doi.org/10.1038/s41598-024-62820-7.

Gabriela Briceno Silva et al., "Influence of the Onset of Menopause on the Risk of Developing Alzheimer's Disease," *Cureus* 16, no. 9 (2024), doi.org/10.7759/cureus.69124.

Stephanie S. Faubion et al., "Impact of Menopause Symptoms on Women in the Workplace," *Mayo Clinic Proceedings* 98, no. 6 (2023): 833–45, doi.org/10.1016/j.mayocp.2023.02.025.

Devon Kardel and Sarah Weber, "The Effect of Perimenopause on Women's Executive Functioning: A Systematic Review," *Archives of Clinical Neuropsychology* 39, no. 7 (2024), doi.org/10.1093/arclin/acae067.235.

N. G. Jaff and P. M. Maki, "Scientific Insights into Brain Fog During the Menopausal Transition," *Climacteric* 24, no. 4 (2021): 317–18, doi.org/10.1080/13697137.2021.1942700.

Jason K. Russell, Carrie K. Jones, and Paul A. Newhouse, "The Role of Estrogen in Brain and Cognitive Aging," *Neurotherapeutics* 16, no. 3 (2019): 649–65, doi.org/10.1007/s13311-019-00766-9.

Hadine Joffe et al., "Estrogen Therapy Selectively Enhances Prefrontal Cognitive Processes: A Randomized, Double-Blind, Placebo-Controlled Study with Functional Magnetic Resonance Imaging in Perimenopausal and Recently Postmenopausal Women," *Menopause* 13, no. 3 (2006): 411–22, doi.org/10.1097/01.gme.0000189618.48774.7b.

Janet E. Shepherd, "Effects of Estrogen on Cognition, Mood, and Degenerative Brain Diseases," *Journal of the American Pharmaceutical Association* 41, no. 2 (2001): 221–28, doi.org/10.1016/S1086-5802(16)31233-5.

Swati Chaurasia, Meenakshi Gupta, and Nazia Ishrat, "Effect of Change in Estrogen Levels on Cognitive Functions in Premenopausal, Early Perimenopausal and Late Perimenopausal Females: A Hospital Based Cross-Sectional Study," *International Journal of Scientific Research* 11, no. 9 (2022): 36–38, doi.org/10.36106/ijsr/9003812.

Pauline M. Maki and Nicole G. Jaff, "Menopause and Brain Fog: How to Counsel and Treat Midlife Women," *Menopause* 31, no. 7 (2024): 647–49, doi.org/10.1097/GME.0000000000002382.

T. Duka, R. Tasker, and J. F. McGowan, "The Effects of 3-Week Estrogen Hormone Replacement on Cognition in Elderly Healthy Females," *Psychopharmacology* 149 (2000): 129–39, doi.org/10.1007/s002139900324.

Roberta D. Brinton et al., "Perimenopause as a Neurological Transition State," *Nature Reviews Endocrinology* 11 (2015): 393–405, doi.org/10.1038/nrendo.2015.82.

C. Neill Epperson et al., "Impact of Atomoxetine on Subjective Attention and Memory Difficulties in Perimenopausal and Postmenopausal Women," *Menopause* 18, no. 5 (2011): 542–48, doi.org/10.1097/gme.0b013e3181fcafd6.

C. Neill Epperson et al., "New Onset Executive Function Difficulties at Menopause: A Possible Role for Lisdexamfetamine," *Psychopharmacology* 232 (2015): 3091–100, doi.org/10.1007/s00213-015-3953-7.

Stephanie Mulhall, Ross Andel, and Kaarin J. Anstey, "Variation in Symptoms of Depression and Anxiety in Midlife Women by Menopausal Status," *Maturitas* 108 (2018), 7–12, doi.org/10.1016/j.maturitas.2017.11.005.

Buket Belkiz Gungor et al., "The Effect of Perimenopausal Estrogen Levels on Depression and Anxiety: A Pilot Study," *The European Research Journal* (2015): 8–13, doi.org/10.18621/eurj.2015.1.1.8.

Chen Zhu et al., "Evaluation of the Everyday Memory Questionnaire—Revised in a Menopausal Population: Understanding the Brain Fog During Menopause," *Menopause* 30, no. 11 (2023): 1147–56, doi.org/10.1097/GME.0000000000002256.

Chen Zhu et al., "Cut-Off Point Development for the Everyday Memory Questionnaire—Revised in Perimenopausal Women," *Climacteric* 28, no. 1 (2025): 51–60, doi.org/10.1080/13697137.2024.2401369.

Jasper F. E. Crockford et al., "Cognitive and Behavioral Decline Predicted by Perimenopausal Symptoms: A CAN-PROTECT Study," *Alzheimer's & Dementia* 20 (2024), doi.org/10.1002/alz.092052.

Gail A. Greendale, Carol A. Derby, and Pauline M. Maki, "Perimenopause and Cognition," *Obstetrics and Gynecology Clinics of North America* 38, no. 3 (2011): 519–35, doi.org/10.1016/j.ogc.2011.05.007.

Claudio Mencacci, Paola Landi, and Roberta Anniverno, "Depression and Cognitive Functions in Perimenopause," *Journal of Sex- and Gender-Specific Medicine* 6, no. 2 (2020): 64–67, doi.org/10.1723/3351.33222.

S. Shrividya and Molly Joy, "Brain Fog Among Perimenopausal Women: A Comparative Study," *Journal of International Women's Studies* 22, no. 6 (2021), vc.bridgew.edu/jiws/vol22/iss6/3.

Pauline M. Maki and Julie Dumas, "Mechanisms of Action of Estrogen in the Brain: Insights from Human Neuroimaging and Psychopharmacologic Studies," *Seminars in Reproductive Medicine* 27, no. 3 (2009): 250–59, doi.org/10.1055/s-0029-1216278.

Christina A. Metcalf et al., "Cognitive Problems in Perimenopause: A Review of Recent Evidence," *Current Psychiatry Reports* 25 (2023): 501–11, doi.org/10.1007/s11920-023-01447-3.

Yuko Hara et al., "Estrogen Effects on Cognitive and Synaptic Health over the Lifecourse," *Physiological Reviews* 95, no. 3 (2015): 785–807, doi.org/10.1152/physrev.00036.2014.

Eef Hogervorst and Stephan Bandelow, "Sex Steroids to Maintain Cognitive Function in Women After the Menopause: A Meta-Analysis of Treatment Trials," *Maturitas* 66, no. 1 (2010): 56–71, doi.org/10.1016/j.maturitas.2010.02.005.

Barbara B. Sherwin, "Estrogen and Cognitive Functioning in Women," *Endocrine Reviews* 24, no. 2 (2003): 133–51, doi.org/10.1210/ER.2001-0016.

J. S. Kooij, "ADHD in a Woman During (Peri)menopause: Missed Diagnoses and Cardiac Complaints," *European Psychiatry* 67 (2024), doi.org/10.1192/j.eurpsy.2024.1666.

Jeanette Wasserstein, Gerry A. Stefanatos, and Mary V. Solanto, "Perimenopause, Menopause and ADHD," *Journal of the International Neuropsychological Society* 29 (2023): 881, doi.org/10.1017/s1355617723010846.

CHAPTER 7: PERIMENOPAUSE AND METABOLIC SYNDROME

Sherry Sherman, "Defining the Menopausal Transition," *The American Journal of Medicine* 118, no. 12 (2005): 1405, doi.org/10.1016/j.amjmed.2005.10.006.

"Liver Function Tests," Mayo Clinic, January 18, 2025, mayoclinic.org/tests-procedures/liver-function-tests/about/pac-20394595.

Qingfang He et al., "Determining the Status of Small Dense Low-Density Lipoprotein Cholesterol Level in Women Undergoing Menopausal Transition," *Frontiers in Endocrinology* 15 (2025), doi.org/10.3389/fendo.2024.1500712.

Luana Ferreira Campos et al., "Effect of Hormone Therapy on Blood Pressure and Hypertension in Postmenopausal Women: A Systematic Review and Meta-Analysis," *Menopause* 31, no. 6 (2024): 556–62, doi.org/10.1097/GME.0000000000002359.

Georgios E. Papadakis et al., "Menopausal Hormone Therapy Is Associated with Reduced Total and Visceral Adiposity: The OsteoLaus Cohort," *The Journal of Clinical Endocrinology & Metabolism* 103, no. 5 (2018): 1948–57, doi.org/10.1210/jc.2017-02449.

Alessandro D. Genazzani et al., "Metabolic Syndrome, Insulin Resistance and Menopause: The Changes in Body Structure and the Therapeutic Approach," *Gynecological and Reproductive Endocrinology & Metabolism* 4 (2023): 86–91, doi.org/10.53260/grem.234026.

Samar R. El Khoudary et al., "Low-Density Lipoprotein Subclasses over the Menopausal Transition and Risk of Coronary Calcification and Carotid Atherosclerosis: The SWAN Heart and HDL Ancillary Studies," *Menopause* 30, no. 10 (2023): 1006–13, doi.org/10.1097/GME.0000000000002245.

Jari E. Karppinen et al., "Menopause Modulates the Circulating Metabolome: Evidence from a Prospective Cohort Study," *European Journal of Preventive Cardiology* 29, no. 10 (2022): 1448–59, doi.org/10.1093/eurjpc/zwac060.

Veronica Inaraja et al., "Lipid Profile Changes During the Menopausal Transition," *Menopause* 27, no. 7 (2020): 780–87, doi.org/10.1097/GME.0000000000001532.

Eun Jeung Cho et al., "Effects of the Transition from Premenopause to Postmenopause on Lipids and Lipoproteins: Quantification and Related Parameters," *The Korean Journal of Internal Medicine* 26, no. 1 (2011): 47–53, doi.org/10.3904/kjim.2011.26.1.47.

M. C. Carr et al., "Changes in LDL Density Across the Menopausal Transition," *Journal of Investigative Medicine* 48, no. 4 (2000): 245–50, pubmed.ncbi.nlm.nih.gov/10916282.

Ayaz Khurram Mallick et al., "Study of Lipid Profile During Late Reproductive Phase, Perimenopause and Postmenopause in North Indian Women," *International Journal of Medical Research & Review* 3, no. 1 (2015): 45–50, doi.org/10.17511/IJMRR.2015.I1.08.

Ouarda Taleb-Belkadi et al., "Lipid Profile, Inflammation, and Oxidative Status in Peri- and Postmenopausal Women," *Gynecological Endocrinology* 32, no. 12 (2016): 982–85, doi.org/10.1080/09513590.2016.1214257.

Koichi Fujita et al., "Systemic Oxidative Stress Is Associated with Visceral Fat Accumulation and the Metabolic Syndrome," *Circulation Journal* 70, no. 11 (2006): 1437–42, doi.org/10.1253/CIRCJ.70.1437.

Jacqueline R. Leachman et al., "Early Life Stress Exacerbates Obesity in Adult Female Mice via Mineralocorticoid Receptor-Dependent Increases in Adipocyte Triglyceride and Glycerol Content," *Life Sciences* 304 (2022), doi.org/10.1016/j.lfs.2022.120718.

P. Björntorp, "Do Stress Reactions Cause Abdominal Obesity and Comorbidities?" *Obesity Reviews* 2, no. 2 (2001): 73–86, doi.org/10.1046/j.1467-789x.2001.00027.x.

Per Björntorp, "Endocrine Abnormalities of Obesity," *Metabolism: Clinical and Experimental* 44 (no. S3) (1995): 21–23, doi.org/10.1016/0026-0495(95)90315-1.

Carol A. Shively, Thomas C. Register, and Thomas B. Clarkson, "Social Stress, Visceral Obesity, and Coronary Artery Atherosclerosis: Product of a Primate Adaptation," *American Journal of Primatology* 71, no. 9 (2009): 742–51, doi.org/10.1002/ajp.20706.

Kirstin Aschbacher et al., "Chronic Stress Increases Vulnerability to Diet-Related Abdominal Fat, Oxidative Stress, and Metabolic Risk," *Psychoneuroendocrinology* 46 (2014): 14–22, doi.org/10.1016/j.psyneuen.2014.04.003.

Ioannis Kyrou and Constantine Tsigos, "Stress Hormones: Physiological Stress and Regulation of Metabolism," *Current Opinion in Pharmacology* 9, no. 6 (2009): 787–93, doi.org/10.1016/j.coph.2009.08.007.

A. García-Sánchez et al., "The Effect of Visceral Abdominal Fat Volume on Oxidative Stress and Proinflammatory Cytokines in Subjects with Normal Weight, Overweight and Obesity," *Diabetes, Metabolic Syndrome and Obesity* 13 (2020): 1077–87, doi.org/10.2147/DMSO.S245494.

Kristin J. Speaker and Monika Fleshner, "Interleukin-1 Beta: A Potential Link Between Stress and the Development of Visceral Obesity," *BMC Physiology* 12 (2012), doi.org/10.1186/1472-6793-12-8.

Vonda J. Wright et al., "The Musculoskeletal Syndrome of Menopause," *Climacteric* 27, no. 5 (2024): 466–72, doi.org/10.1080/13697137.2024.2380363.

Cameron Gofton et al., "MAFLD: How Is It Different from NAFLD?" *Clinical and Molecular Hepatology* 29 (2023), doi.org/10.3350/cmh.2022.0367.

Seong-Ah Kim and Sangah Shin, "Red Meat and Processed Meat Consumption and the Risk of Dyslipidemia in Korean Adults: A Prospective Cohort Study Based on the Health Examinees (HEXA) Study," *Nutrition, Metabolism & Cardiovascular Diseases* 31, no. 6 (2021): 1714–27, doi.org/10.1016/j.numecd.2021.02.008.

Frank Qian et al., "Red and Processed Meats and Health Risks: How Strong Is the Evidence?" *Diabetes Care* 43, no. 2 (2020): 265–71, doi.org/10.2337/dci19-0063.

Hui Li, Erna Jia, and Jian Jiao, "Phytoestrogens in NAFLD: Potential Mechanisms of Action," *Hormone and Metabolic Research* 52, no. 2 (2020): 77–84, doi.org/10.1055/a-1089-7710.

Ralitsa Robeva et al., "The Interplay Between Metabolic Dysregulations and Non-Alcoholic Fatty Liver Disease in Women After Menopause," *Maturitas* 151 (2021): 22–30, doi.org/10.1016/j.maturitas.2021.06.012.

Masahiro Akishita and Jing Yu, "Hormonal Effects on Blood Vessels," *Hypertension Research* 35 (2012): 363–69, doi.org/10.1038/hr.2012.4.

Bulbul Ahmed, Rifat Sultana, and Michael W. Greene, "Adipose Tissue and Insulin Resistance in Obese," *Biomedicine & Pharmacotherapy* 137 (2021), doi.org/10.1016/j.biopha.2021.111315.

Julie Abildgaard et al., "Increased Systemic Inflammation and Altered Distribution of T-Cell Subsets in Postmenopausal Women," *PLoS One* 15, no. 6 (2020), doi.org/10.1371/journal.pone.0235174.

Julie Abildgaard et al., "Ectopic Lipid Deposition Is Associated with Insulin Resistance in Postmenopausal Women," *The Journal of Clinical Endocrinology & Metabolism* 103, no. 9 (2018): 3394–404, doi.org/10.1210/jc.2018-00554.

Supreeya Swarup et al., *Metabolic Syndrome* (StatPearls, 2025), ncbi.nlm.nih.gov/books/NBK459248.

Ranu Patni and Annil Mahajan, "The Metabolic Syndrome and Menopause," *Journal of Mid-Life Health* 9, no. 3 (2018): 111–12, doi.org/10.4103/0976-7800.241951.

João Paulo Camporez et al., "Anti-Inflammatory Effects of Oestrogen Mediate the Sexual Dimorphic Response to Lipid-Induced Insulin Resistance," *The Journal of Physiology* 597, no. 15 (2019): 3885–903, doi.org/10.1113/JP277270.

Elodie Riant et al., "Estrogens Protect Against High-Fat Diet-Induced Insulin Resistance and Glucose Intolerance in Mice," *Endocrinology* 150, no. 5 (2009): 2109–17, doi.org/10.1210/en.2008-0971.

Lin Zhu et al., "Estrogen Signaling Prevents Diet-Induced Hepatic Insulin Resistance in Male Mice with Obesity," *Endocrinology and Metabolism* 306, no. 10 (2014), doi.org/10.1152/ajpendo.00579.2013.

Ester S. Alves et al., "Hepatic Estrogen Receptor Alpha Overexpression Protects Against Hepatic Insulin Resistance and MASLD," *Pathophysiology* 32, no. 1 (2025), doi.org/10.3390/pathophysiology32010001.

Xiaona Gao et al., "Estrogen Receptor α Regulates Metabolic-Associated Fatty Liver Disease by Targeting NLRP3-GSDMD Axis-Mediated Hepatocyte Pyroptosis," *Journal of Agricultural and Food Chemistry* 69, no. 48 (2021): 14544–56, doi.org/10.1021/acs.jafc.1c05400.

João Paulo G. Camporez et al., "Cellular Mechanism by Which Estradiol Protects Female Ovariectomized Mice from High-Fat Diet-Induced Hepatic and Muscle

Insulin Resistance," *Endocrinology* 154, no. 3 (2013): 1021–28, doi.org/10.1210/en.2012-1989.

Mennatallah A. Ali and Maher A. Kamel, "Modulation of the Hepatic Expression of MiR-33 and MiR-34a Possibly Mediates the Metabolic Effects of Estrogen in Ovariectomized Female Rats," *European Journal of Pharmacology* 873 (2020), doi.org/10.1016/j.ejphar.2020.173006.

Lin Zhu et al., "Estrogen Treatment After Ovariectomy Protects Against Fatty Liver and May Improve Pathway-Selective Insulin Resistance," *Diabetes* 62, no. 2 (2013): 424–34, doi.org/10.2337/db11-1718.

Franck Mauvais-Jarvis, Deborah J. Clegg, and Andrea L. Hevener, "The Role of Estrogens in Control of Energy Balance and Glucose Homeostasis," *Endocrine Reviews* 34, no. 3 (2013): 309–38, doi.org/10.1210/er.2012-1055.

Rajamannar Thennati et al., "Once Weekly Utreglutide (GL0034), a Glucagon-Like Peptide-1 Receptor Agonist, at 4 × 450 Mg Doses Reduces Blood Pressure, Lipids, and Body Weight in Post-Menopausal Females: A Phase I Study," *Circulation* 150 (2024), doi.org/10.1161/crc.150.suppl_1.4116298.

Stefan Störk et al., "The Effect of 17beta-Estradiol on Endothelial and Inflammatory Markers in Postmenopausal Women: A Randomized, Controlled Trial," *Atherosclerosis* 165, no. 2 (2002): 301-7, doi.org/10.1016/s0021-9150(02)00242-3.

CHAPTER 8: OSTEOPOROSIS: THE DEBILITATING BONE DISEASE THAT STARTS SOONER THAN YOU THINK

Martyna Patalong-Wójcik et al., "Associations of Hormonal and Metabolic Parameters with Bone Mineralization in Young Adult Females," *Nutrients* 15, no. 11 (2023), doi.org/10.3390/nu15112482.

Bingru Lu et al., "Associations Between Hormones, Metabolic Markers, and Bone Mass in Perimenopausal and Postmenopausal Women," *Journal of Bone and Mineral Metabolism* 43 (2025): 392–401, doi.org/10.1007/s00774-025-01595-x.

Catherine W. Gillespie and Pamela E. Morin, "Trends and Disparities in Osteoporosis Screening Among Women in the United States, 2008–2014," *The American Journal of Medicine* 130, no. 3 (2017): 306–16, doi.org/10.1016/j.amjmed.2016.10.018.

Y. C. Lin et al., "Peak Spine and Femoral Neck Bone Mass in Young Women," *Bone* 32, no. 5 (2003): 546–53, doi.org/10.1016/s8756-3282(03)00062-0.

Jincheng Xu et al., "Effects of Exercise on Bone Status in Female Subjects, from Young Girls to Postmenopausal Women: An Overview of Systematic Reviews and Meta-Analyses," *Sports Medicine* 46 (2016): 1165–82, doi.org/10.1007/s40279-016-0494-0.

R. D. Chapurlat et al., "Longitudinal Study of Bone Loss in Pre- and Perimenopausal Women: Evidence for Bone Loss in Perimenopausal Women," *Osteoporosis International* 11 (2000): 493–98, doi.org/10.1007/s001980070091.

L. Nilas and C. Christiansen, "Rates of Bone Loss in Normal Women: Evidence of Accelerated Trabecular Bone Loss After the Menopause," *European Journal of Clinical Investigation* 18, no. 5 (1988): 529–34, doi.org/10.1111/j.1365-2362.1988.tb01052.x.

Arun S. Karlamangla et al., "Anti-Mullerian Hormone as Predictor of Future and Ongoing Bone Loss During the Menopause Transition," *Journal of Bone and Mineral Research* 37, no. 7 (2022): 1224–32, doi.org/10.1002/jbmr.4525.

H. G. Ahlborg et al., "Bone Loss in Relation to Menopause: A Prospective Study During 16 Years," *Bone* 28, no. 3 (2001): 327–31, doi.org/10.1016/s8756-3282(00)00451-8.

Joan C. Lo, Sherri-Ann M. Burnett-Bowie, and Joel S. Finkelstein, "Bone and the Perimenopause," *Obstetrics and Gynecology Clinics of North America* 38, no. 3 (2011): 503–17, doi.org/10.1016/j.ogc.2011.07.001.

Daria Lizneva et al., "Emerging Concepts in the Epidemiology, Pathophysiology, and Clinical Care of Osteoporosis Across the Menopausal Transition," *Matrix Biology* 71–72 (2018): 70–81, doi.org/10.1016/j.matbio.2018.05.001.

V. Seifert-Klauss et al., "Influence of Pattern of Menopausal Transition on the Amount of Trabecular Bone Loss: Results from a 6-Year Prospective Longitudinal Study," *Maturitas* 55, no. 4 (2006): 317–24, doi.org/10.1016/j.maturitas.2006.04.024.

Albert Shieh et al., "Estradiol and Follicle-Stimulating Hormone as Predictors of Onset of Menopause Transition–Related Bone Loss in Pre- and Perimenopausal Women," *Journal of Bone and Mineral Research* 34, no. 12 (2019): 2246–53, doi.org/10.1002/jbmr.3856.

Joel S. Finkelstein et al., "Bone Mineral Density Changes During the Menopause Transition in a Multiethnic Cohort of Women," *The Journal of Clinical Endocrinology & Metabolism* 93, no. 3 (2008): 861–68, doi.org/10.1210/jc.2007-1876.

J. C. Gallagher, "Moderation of the Daily Dose of HRT: Prevention of Osteoporosis," *Maturitas* 33 (1999): 57–63, doi.org/10.1016/S0378-5122(99)00064-X.

John C. Stevenson, "Justification for the Use of HRT in the Long-Term Prevention of Osteoporosis," *Maturitas* 51, no. 2 (2005): 113–26, doi.org/10.1016/j.maturitas.2005.01.012.

E. F. Eriksen, M. Kassem, and B. Langdahl, "European and North American Experience with HRT for the Prevention of Osteoporosis," *Bone* 19, no. 5 (1996): 179S–183S, sciencedirect.com/science/article/abs/pii/S8756328296002529.

Martin H. Birkhäuser, "Is HRT Still Indicated for the Primary Prevention of Osteoporosis?" *Gynecological Endocrinology* 25, no. 10 (2009): 629–33, doi.org/10.1080/09513590903056746.

Yu Z. Bagger et al., "Two to Three Years of Hormone Replacement Treatment in Healthy Women Have Long-Term Preventive Effects on Bone Mass and Osteoporotic Fractures: The PERF Study," *Bone* 34, no. 4 (2004): 728–35, doi.org/10.1016/j.bone.2003.12.021.

M. Dören and G. Samsioe, "Prevention of Postmenopausal Osteoporosis with Oestrogen Replacement Therapy and Associated Compounds: Update on Clinical Trials Since 1995," *Human Reproduction Update* 6, no. 5 (2000): 419–26, doi.org/10.1093/humupd/6.5.419.

Marco Gambacciani and Marco Levancini, "Hormone Replacement Therapy and the Prevention of Postmenopausal Osteoporosis," *Przegląd Menopauzalny* 13, no. 4 (2014): 213–20, doi.org/10.5114/pm.2014.44996.

M. Martiniakova, M. Babikova, and R. Omelka, "Pharmacological Agents and Natural Compounds: Available Treatments for Osteoporosis," *Journal of Physiology and Pharmacology* 71, no. 3 (2020): 307–20, doi.org/10.26402/jpp.2020.3.01.

A.W.C. Kung, S.S.C. Yeung, and L. W. Chu, "The Efficacy and Tolerability of Alendronate in Postmenopausal Osteoporotic Chinese Women: A Randomized Placebo-Controlled Study," *Calcified Tissue International* 67 (2000): 286–90, doi.org/10.1007/s0022330001142.

Kelly R. Ragucci and Sarah P. Shrader, "Osteoporosis Treatment: An Evidence-Based Approach," *Journal of Gerontological Nursing* 37, no. 7 (2011): 17–22, doi.org/10.3928/00989134-20110602-02.

Kristie N. Tu et al., "Osteoporosis: A Review of Treatment Options," *Pharmacy and Therapeutics* 43, no. 2 (2018): 92–104, pmc.ncbi.nlm.nih.gov/articles/PMC5768298.

Daniel W. Isenbarger and Barrett L. Chapin, "Osteoporosis: Current Pharmacologic Options for Prevention and Treatment," *Postgraduate Medicine* 101, no. 1 (1997): 129–42, doi.org/10.3810/PGM.1997.01.145.

Jonathan D. Adachi, "Alendronate for Osteoporosis: Safe and Efficacious Nonhormonal Therapy," *Canadian Family Physician* 44 (1998), pmc.ncbi.nlm.nih.gov/articles/PMC2277603.

O. Ström et al., "Real-World Effectiveness of Osteoporosis Treatment in the Oldest Old," *Osteoporosis International* 31 (2020): 1525–33, doi.org/10.1007/s00198-020-05380-6.

Kelvin Li et al., "The Good, the Bad, and the Ugly of Calcium Supplementation: A Review of Calcium Intake on Human Health," *Clinical Interventions in Aging* 13 (2018): 2443–52, doi.org/10.2147/CIA.S157523.

Iacopo Chiodini and Mark J. Bolland, "Calcium Supplementation in Osteoporosis: Useful or Harmful?" *European Journal of Endocrinology* 178, no. 4 (2018), doi.org/10.1530/EJE-18-0113.

Antonio Cano et al., "Calcium in the Prevention of Postmenopausal Osteoporosis: EMAS Clinical Guide," *Maturitas* 107 (2018): 7–12, doi.org/10.1016/j.maturitas.2017.10.004.

I. R. Reid, S. M. Bristow, and M. J. Bolland, "Calcium Supplements: Benefits and Risks," *Journal of Internal Medicine* 278, no. 4 (2015): 354–68, doi.org/10.1111/joim.12394.

Stephen L. Kopecky et al., "Lack of Evidence Linking Calcium with or Without Vitamin D Supplementation to Cardiovascular Disease in Generally Healthy Adults: A Clinical Guideline from the National Osteoporosis Foundation and the American Society for Preventive Cardiology," *Annals of Internal Medicine* 165, no. 12 (2016), doi.org/10.7326/M16-1743.

Grzegorz B. Wasilewski, Marc G. Vervloet, and Leon J. Schurgers, "The Bone-Vasculature Axis: Calcium Supplementation and the Role of Vitamin K," *Frontiers in Cardiovascular Medicine* 6 (2019), doi.org/10.3389/fcvm.2019.00006.

Gary C. Curhan et al., "Comparison of Dietary Calcium with Supplemental Calcium and Other Nutrients as Factors Affecting the Risk for Kidney Stones in Women," *Annals of Internal Medicine* 126, no. 7 (1997), doi.org/10.7326/0003-4819-126-7-199704010-00001.

J. C. Prior, "Progesterone for the Prevention and Treatment of Osteoporosis in Women," *Climacteric* 21, no. 4 (2018): 366–74, doi.org/10.1080/13697137.2018.1467400.

Muzahem Mohialdeen Taha, Ekhlass M. Taha, and Suhayla K. Mohammed, "The Role of Testosterone Level in Women with Osteopenia," *Baghdad Science Journal* 21, no. 2 (2024), doi.org/10.21123/bsj.2023.8140.

N. V. Mohamad, I. Soelaiman, and K. Chin, "A Concise Review of Testosterone and Bone Health," *Clinical Interventions in Aging* 11 (2016): 1317–24, doi.org/10.2147/CIA.S115472.

Sunil J. Wimalawansa, "Prevention and Treatment of Osteoporosis: Efficacy of Combination of Hormone Replacement Therapy with Other Antiresorptive Agents," *Journal of Clinical Densitometry* 3, no. 2 (2000): 187–201, doi.org/10.1385/JCD:3:2:187.

Hosam K. Kamel, Horace M. Perry III, and John E. Morley, "Hormone Replacement Therapy and Fractures in Older Adults," *Journal of the American Geriatrics Society* 49, no. 2 (2001): 179–87, doi.org/10.1046/j.1532-5415.2001.49040.x.

Christine M. Snow et al., "Long-Term Exercise Using Weighted Vests Prevents Hip Bone Loss in Postmenopausal Women," *The Journals of Gerontology, Series A* 55, no. 9 (2000), doi.org/10.1093/GERONA/55.9.M489.

Ryan M. Miller et al., "Incorporating Nutrition, Vests, Education, and Strength Training (INVEST) in Bone Health: Trial Design and Methods," *Contemporary Clinical Trials* 104 (2021), doi.org/10.1016/j.cct.2021.106326.

Tayebeh Roghani et al., "Effects of Short-Term Aerobic Exercise with and Without External Loading on Bone Metabolism and Balance in Postmenopausal Women with Osteoporosis," *Rheumatology International* 33 (2013): 291–98, doi.org/10.1007/s00296-012-2388-2.

Panagiota Klentrou et al., "Effects of Exercise Training with Weighted Vests on Bone Turnover and Isokinetic Strength in Postmenopausal Women," *Journal of Aging and Physical Activity* 15, no. 3 (2007): 287–99, doi.org/10.1123/JAPA.15.3.287.

Marina B. Pinheiro et al., "Evidence on Physical Activity and Osteoporosis Prevention for People Aged 65+ Years: A Systematic Review to Inform the WHO Guidelines on Physical Activity and Sedentary Behaviour," *International Journal of Behavioral Nutrition and Physical Activity* 17 (2020), doi.org/10.1186/s12966-020-01040-4.

Donatella Bonaiuti et al., "Exercise for Preventing and Treating Osteoporosis in Postmenopausal Women," *Cochrane Database of Systematic Reviews* (2002), doi.org/10.1002/14651858.cd000333.

Carol Hamilton Zehnacker and Anita Bemis-Dougherty, "Effect of Weighted Exercises on Bone Mineral Density in Post-Menopausal Women: A Systematic Review," *Journal of Geriatric Physical Therapy* 30, no. 2 (2007): 79–88, doi.org/10.1519/00139143-200708000-00007.

G. A. Greendale, S. H. Hirsch, and T. J. Hahn, "The Effect of a Weighted Vest on Perceived Health Status and Bone Density in Older Persons," *Quality of Life Research* 2 (1993): 141–52, doi.org/10.1007/BF00435733.

Gail A. Greendale et al., "Trabecular Bone Score Declines During the Menopause Transition: The Study of Women's Health Across the Nation (SWAN)," *The Journal of Clinical Endocrinology & Metabolism* 105, no. 4 (2020), doi.org/10.1210/clinem/dgz056.

Arun S. Karlamangla, Sherri-Ann M. Burnett-Bowie, and Carolyn J. Crandall, "Bone Health During the Menopause Transition and Beyond," *Obstetrics and Gynecology Clinics of North America* 45, no. 4 (2018): 695–708, doi.org/10.1016/j.ogc.2018.07.012.

Lisbeth Nilas and Claus Christiansen, "Bone Mass and Its Relationship to Age and the Menopause," *The Journal of Clinical Endocrinology & Metabolism* 65, no. 4 (1987): 697–702, doi.org/10.1210/JCEM-65-4-697.

Arun S. Karlamangla et al., "Anti-Mullerian Hormone as Predictor of Future and Ongoing Bone Loss During the Menopause Transition," *Journal of Bone and Mineral Research* 37, no. 7 (2022): 1224–32, doi.org/10.1002/jbmr.4525.

Gail A. Greendale et al., "Bone Mineral Density Loss in Relation to the Final Menstrual Period in a Multiethnic Cohort: Results from the Study of Women's Health Across the Nation (SWAN)," *Journal of Bone and Mineral Research* 27, no. 1 (2012): 111–18, doi.org/10.1002/jbmr.534.

R. Recker et al., "Characterization of Perimenopausal Bone Loss: A Prospective Study," *Journal of Bone and Mineral Research* 15, no. 10 (2000): 1965–73, doi.org/10.1359/jbmr.2000.15.10.1965.

Albert Shieh et al., "Urinary N-Telopeptide as Predictor of Onset of Menopause-Related Bone Loss in Pre- and Perimenopausal Women," *JBMR Plus* 3, no. 4 (2018), pmc.ncbi.nlm.nih.gov/articles/PMC6478585.

Albert Shieh et al., "Estradiol and Follicle-Stimulating Hormone as Predictors of Onset of Menopause Transition-Related Bone Loss in Pre- and Perimenopausal Women," *Journal of Bone and Mineral Research* 34, no. 12 (2019): 2246–53, doi.org/10.1002/jbmr.3856.

P. J. Ryan et al., "A Clinical Profile of Back Pain and Disability in Patients with Spinal Osteoporosis," *Bone* 15, no. 1 (1994): 27–30, doi.org/10.1016/8756-3282(94)90887-7.

Naohisa Miyakoshi, Michio Hongo, and Yoichi Shimada, "Prevalence of Back Pain in Postmenopausal Osteoporosis and Associations with Multiple Spinal Factors," in *Osteoporosis*, ed. Yannis Dionyssiotis (IntechOpen, 2012), doi.org/10.5772/30772.

T. Liu-Ambrose et al., "The Influence of Back Pain on Balance and Functional Mobility in 65- to 75-Year-Old Women with Osteoporosis," *Osteoporosis International* 13 (2002): 868–73, doi.org/10.1007/s001980200119.

P. Kann et al., "Backache and Osteoporosis in Perimenopausal Women," *Medizinische Klinik* 88, no. 1 (1993): 9–15, europepmc.org/article/med/8437532.

Stuart L. Silverman et al., "Relationship of Health Related Quality of Life to Prevalent and New or Worsening Back Pain in Postmenopausal Women with Osteoporosis," *The Journal of Rheumatology* 32, no. 12 (2005): 2405–9, jrheum.org/content/32/12/2405.long.

C. Roux et al., "A Clinical Tool to Determine the Necessity of Spine Radiography in Postmenopausal Women with Osteoporosis Presenting with Back Pain," *Annals of the Rheumatic Diseases* 66, no. 1 (2007): 81–85, doi.org/10.1136/ard.2006.051474.

T. Paolucci, V. Saraceni, and G. Piccinini, "Management of Chronic Pain in Osteoporosis: Challenges and Solutions," *Journal of Pain Research* 9 (2016): 177–86, doi.org/10.2147/JPR.S83574.

Bruce Ettinger, Harry K. Genant, and Christopher E. Cann, "Long-Term Estrogen Replacement Therapy Prevents Bone Loss and Fractures," *Annals of Internal Medicine* 102, no. 3 (1985): 319–24, doi.org/10.7326/0003-4819-102-3-319.

Panagiotis Anagnostis et al., "Estrogen and Bones After Menopause: A Reappraisal of Data and Future Perspectives," *Hormones* 20 (2021): 13–21, doi.org/10.1007/s42000-020-00218-6.

Gautam Khastgir et al., "Anabolic Effect of Estrogen Replacement on Bone in Postmenopausal Women with Osteoporosis: Histomorphometric Evidence in a Longitudinal Study," *The Journal of Clinical Endocrinology & Metabolism* 86, no. 1 (2001): 289–95, doi.org/10.1210/JCEM.86.1.7161.

Anna Gosset, Jean-Michel Pouillès, and Florence Trémollieres, "Menopausal Hormone Therapy for the Management of Osteoporosis," *Clinical Endocrinology & Metabolism* 35, no. 6 (2021), doi.org/10.1016/j.beem.2021.101551.

R. Lindsay and J. F. Tohme, "Estrogen Treatment of Patients with Established Postmenopausal Osteoporosis," *International Journal of Gynecology & Obstetrics* 34, no. 4 (1991), doi.org/10.1016/0020-7292(91)90647-N.

Jan J. Stepan, Hana Hrušková, and Miloslav Kverka, "Update on Menopausal Hormone Therapy for Fracture Prevention," *Current Osteoporosis Reports* 17 (2019): 465–73, doi.org/10.1007/s11914-019-00549-3.

C. Gennari et al., "Estrogen Preserves a Normal Intestinal Responsiveness to 1,25-Dihydroxyvitamin D3 in Oophorectomized Women," *Maturitas* 13, no. 3 (1991): 258–59, doi.org/10.1016/0378-5122(91)90212-9.

Kok-Yong Chin, "The Relationship Between Follicle-stimulating Hormone and Bone Health: Alternative Explanation for Bone Loss Beyond Oestrogen?" *International Journal of Medical Sciences* 15, no. 12 (2018) 1373–83, doi.org/10.7150/ijms.26571.

CHAPTER 9: SARCOPENIA: THE MUSCLE LOSS NO ONE WARNED YOU ABOUT

Marc F. Österdahl et al., "Systematic Review on the Relationship Between Menopausal Hormone Replacement Therapy, Sarcopenia, and Sarcopenia-Related Parameters," *Maturitas* 199 (2025), doi.org/10.1016/j.maturitas.2025.108609.

Brittany C. Collins, Eija K. Laakkonen, and Dawn A. Lowe, "Aging of the Musculoskeletal System: How the Loss of Estrogen Impacts Muscle Strength," *Bone* 123 (2019): 137–44, doi.org/10.1016/j.bone.2019.03.033.

Brittany C. Collins et al., "Estrogen Regulates the Satellite Cell Compartment in Females," *Cell Reports* 28, no. 2 (2019), doi.org/10.1016/j.celrep.2019.06.025.

Annabel J. Critchlow et al., "The Role of Estrogen in Female Skeletal Muscle Aging: A Systematic Review," *Maturitas* 178 (2023), doi.org/10.1016/j.maturitas.2023.107844.

Chengmei Zhang et al., "Research Progress on the Correlation Between Estrogen and Estrogen Receptor on Postmenopausal Sarcopenia," *Frontiers in Endocrinology* 15 (2024), doi.org/10.3389/fendo.2024.1494972.

Kazuhiro Ikeda, Kuniko Horie-Inoue, and Satoshi Inoue, "Functions of Estrogen and Estrogen Receptor Signaling on Skeletal Muscle," *The Journal of Steroid Biochemistry and Molecular Biology* 191 (2019), doi.org/10.1016/j.jsbmb.2019.105375.

Ayesha A. Javed et al., "Association Between Hormone Therapy and Muscle Mass in Postmenopausal Women," *JAMA Network Open* 2, no. 8 (2019), doi.org/10.1001/jamanetworkopen.2019.10154.

Mette Hansen, "Female Hormones: Do They Influence Muscle and Tendon Protein Metabolism?" *Proceedings of the Nutrition Society* 77, no. 1 (2017): 32–41, doi.org/10.1017/S0029665117001951.

Jiayi Yang et al., "A Nomogram to Predict Sarcopenia in Middle-Aged and Older Women: A Nationally Representative Survey in China," *Frontiers in Public Health* 13 (2025), doi.org/10.3389/fpubh.2025.1410895.

Marc Sim et al., "Sarcopenia Definitions and Their Associations with Mortality in Older Australian Women," *Journal of the American Medical Directors Association* 20, no. 1 (2019), doi.org/10.1016/j.jamda.2018.10.016.

Fanny Petermann-Rocha et al., "Factors Associated with Sarcopenia: A Cross-Sectional Analysis Using UK Biobank," *Maturitas* 133 (2020): 60–67, doi.org/10.1016/j.maturitas.2020.01.004.

Jongseok Hwang and Soonjee Park, "Gender-Specific Risk Factors and Prevalence for Sarcopenia Among Community-Dwelling Young-Old Adults," *International Journal of Environmental Research and Public Health* 19, no. 12 (2022), doi.org/10.3390/ijerph19127232.

Hunkyung Kim et al., "Incidence and Predictors of Sarcopenia Onset in Community-Dwelling Elderly Japanese Women: 4-Year Follow-Up Study," *Journal of the American Medical Directors Association* 16, no. 1 (2015), doi.org/10.1016/j.jamda.2014.10.006.

Maria Fernanda Carrillo-Vega et al., "Patterns of Muscle-Related Risk Factors for Sarcopenia in Older Mexican Women," *International Journal of Environmental Research and Public Health* 19, no. 16 (2022), doi.org/10.3390/ijerph191610239.

Jongseok Hwang and Soonjee Park, "Korean Nationwide Exploration of Sarcopenia Prevalence and Risk Factors in Late Middle-Aged Women," *Healthcare* 12, no. 3 (2024), doi.org/10.3390/healthcare12030362.

Maria Belén Zanchetta et al., "Postmenopausal Women with Sarcopenia Have Higher Prevalence of Falls and Vertebral Fractures," *Medicina* 81, no. 1 (2021): 47–53, pubmed.ncbi.nlm.nih.gov/33611244.

Anoohya Gandham et al., "Sarcopenia Definitions and Their Association with Fracture Risk in Older Swedish Women," *Journal of Bone and Mineral Research* 39, no. 4 (2024): 453–61, doi.org/10.1093/jbmr/zjae026.

Jennifer W. Bea et al., "Effect of Hormone Therapy on Lean Body Mass, Falls, and Fractures: 6-Year Results from the Women's Health Initiative Hormone Trials," *Menopause* 18, no. 1 (2011): 44–52, doi.org/10.1097/gme.0b013e3181e3aab1.

Barbara A. Gower and Lara Nyman, "Associations Among Oral Estrogen Use, Free Testosterone Concentration, and Lean Body Mass Among Postmenopausal Women," *The Journal of Clinical Endocrinology & Metabolism* 85, no. 12 (2000): 4476–80, doi.org/10.1210/JCEM.85.12.7009.

Zhao Chen et al., "Postmenopausal Hormone Therapy and Body Composition: A Substudy of the Estrogen Plus Progestin Trial of the Women's Health Initiative," *The American Journal of Clinical Nutrition* 82, no. 3 (2005): 651–56, pubmed.ncbi.nlm.nih.gov/16155280.

Adrian S. Dobs et al., "Differential Effects of Oral Estrogen Versus Oral Estrogen-Androgen Replacement Therapy on Body Composition in Postmenopausal Women," *The Journal of Clinical Endocrinology & Metabolism* 87, no. 4 (2002): 1509–16, doi.org/10.1210/JCEM.87.4.8362.

A. J. O'Sullivan et al., "The Route of Estrogen Replacement Therapy Confers Divergent Effects on Substrate Oxidation and Body Composition in Postmenopausal Women," *The Journal of Clinical Investigation* 102, no. 5 (1998): 1035–40, doi.org/10.1172/JCI2773.

Christian Hassager and Claus Christiansen, "Estrogen/Gestagen Therapy Changes Soft Tissue Body Composition in Postmenopausal Women," *Metabolism: Clinical and Experimental* 38, no. 7 (1989): 662–65, doi.org/10.1016/0026-0495(89)90104-2.

CHAPTER 10: DREAMING OF SLEEP IN PERIMENOPAUSE

Shazia Jehan et al., "Obstructive Sleep Apnea: Women's Perspective," *Journal of Sleep Medicine and Disorders* 3, no. 6 (2016), pmc.ncbi.nlm.nih.gov/articles/PMC5323064.

Colin A. Espie et al., "A Randomized, Placebo-Controlled Trial of Online Cognitive Behavioral Therapy for Chronic Insomnia Disorder Delivered via an Automated Media-Rich Web Application," *Sleep* 35, no. 6 (2012): 769–81, pubmed.ncbi.nlm.nih.gov/22654196.

Lee M. Ritterband et al., "Efficacy of an Internet-Based Behavioral Intervention for Adults with Insomnia," *Archives of General Psychiatry* 66, no. 7 (2009): 692–98, pubmed.ncbi.nlm.nih.gov/19581560.

"Somryst®," Digital Therapeutics Alliance, dtxalliance.org/products/somryst.

Sarra Nazem et al., "Efficacy of an Internet-Delivered Intervention for Improving Insomnia Severity and Functioning in Veterans: Randomized Controlled Trial," *JMIR Mental Health* 10 (2023), mental.jmir.org/2023/1/e50516.

"Sleepio," Big Health, bighealth.com/sleepio.

Howard M. Kravitz and Hadine Joffe, "Sleep During the Perimenopause: A SWAN Story," *Obstetrics and Gynecology Clinics of North America* 38, no. 3 (2011): 567–86, doi.org/10.1016/j.ogc.2011.06.002.

Jamie Coborn et al., "Disruption of Sleep Continuity During the Perimenopause: Associations with Female Reproductive Hormone Profiles," *The Journal of Clinical Endocrinology & Metabolism* 107, no. 10 (2022), doi.org/10.1210/clinem/dgac447.

Libera Troìa et al., "Sleep Disturbance and Perimenopause: A Narrative Review," *Journal of Clinical Medicine* 14, no. 5 (2025), doi.org/10.3390/jcm14051479.

Sneha Chenji et al. "Biopsychosocial Factors Intersecting with Weekly Sleep Difficulties in the Menopause Transition," *Maturitas* 189 (2024), doi.org/10.1016/j.maturitas.2024.108111.

Annika Haufe, Fiona C. Baker, and Brigitte Leeners, "The Role of Ovarian Hormones in the Pathophysiology of Perimenopausal Sleep Disturbances: A Systematic Review," *Sleep Medicine Reviews* 66 (2022), doi.org/10.1016/j.smrv.2022.101710.

Carmen Moreno-Frías, Nicté Figueroa-Vega, and Juan Manuel Malacara, "Relationship of Sleep Alterations with Perimenopausal and Postmenopausal Symptoms," *Menopause* 21, no. 9 (2014): 1017–22, doi.org/10.1097/GME.0000000000000206.

Paul J. Geiger et al., "Effects of Perimenopausal Transdermal Estradiol on Self-Reported Sleep, Independent of Its Effect on Vasomotor Symptom Bother and Depressive Symptoms," *Menopause* 26, no. 11 (2019): 1318–23, doi.org/10.1097/GME.0000000000001398.

Nanette Santoro, "Perimenopause: From Research to Practice," *Journal of Women's Health* 25, no. 4 (2016), doi.org/10.1089/jwh.2015.5556.

Massimiliano de Zambotti, Ian M. Colrain, and Fiona C. Baker, "Interaction Between Reproductive Hormones and Physiological Sleep in Women," *The Journal of Clinical Endocrinology & Metabolism* 100, no. 4 (2015): 1426–33, doi.org/10.1210/jc.2014-3892.

Qunyan Xu and Cathryne P. Lang, "Examining the Relationship Between Subjective Sleep Disturbance and Menopause: A Systematic Review and Meta-Analysis," *Menopause* 21, no. 12 (2014): 1301–18, doi.org/10.1097/GME.0000000000000240.

Fiona C. Baker et al., "Sleep Problems During the Menopausal Transition: Prevalence, Impact, and Management Challenges," *Nature and Science of Sleep* 10 (2018): 73–95, doi.org/10.2147/NSS.S125807.

Ellen W. Freeman et al., "Associations of Hormones and Menopausal Status with Depressed Mood in Women with No History of Depression," *Archives of General Psychiatry* 63, no. 4 (2006): 375–82, doi.org/10.1001/archpsyc.63.4.375.

M.W.L. Morssinkhof et al., "Associations Between Sex Hormones, Sleep Problems and Depression: A Systematic Review," *Neuroscience & Biobehavorial Reviews* 118 (2020): 669–80, doi.org/10.1016/j.neubiorev.2020.08.006.

Min-Ju Kim, Gyeyoon Yim, and Hyun-Young Park, "Vasomotor and Physical Menopausal Symptoms Are Associated with Sleep Quality," *PLoS One* 13, no. 2 (2018), doi.org/10.1371/journal.pone.0192934.

Jerilynn C. Prior et al., "Oral Micronized Progesterone for Perimenopausal Night Sweats and Hot Flushes: A Phase III Canada-Wide Randomized Placebo-Controlled 4 Month Trial," *Scientific Reports* 13 (2023), doi.org/10.1038/s41598-023-35826-w.

C. Silva et al., "Associations of Vasomotor Symptoms with Sleep Disturbances in Menopausal Women: A Systematic Review and Meta-Analysis," *Maturitas* 80, no. 3 (2015): 276–86.

L. Lamberg, "Sleep Disturbances Common During Menopause," *JAMA* 294, no. 5 (2005): 553–54, doi.org/10.1001/jama.294.5.553.

Helena Hachul et al., "Effects of Hormone Therapy with Estrogen and/or Progesterone on Sleep Pattern in Postmenopausal Women," *International Journal of Gynecology & Obstetrics* 103, no. 3 (2008): 207–12, doi.org/10.1016/j.ijgo.2008.07.009.

Elena Toffol et al., "Nighttime Melatonin Secretion and Sleep Architecture: Different Associations in Perimenopausal and Postmenopausal Women," *Sleep Medicine* 81 (2021): 52–61, doi.org/10.1016/j.sleep.2021.02.011.

I. Virtanen et al., "Effect of External Sleep Disturbance on Sleep Architecture in Perimenopausal and Postmenopausal Women," *Climacteric* 26, no. 2 (2023): 103–9, doi.org/10.1080/13697137.2022.2158727.

Nima Sahola et al., "Worse Sleep Architecture but Not Self-Reported Insomnia and Sleepiness Is Associated with Higher Cortisol Levels in Menopausal Women," *Maturitas* 187 (2024), doi.org/10.1016/j.maturitas.2024.108053.

Muhammed Furkan Dasdelen et al., "A Novel Theanine Complex, Mg-L-Theanine Improves Sleep Quality via Regulating Brain Electrochemical Activity," *Frontiers in Nutrition* 9 (2022), doi.org/10.3389/fnut.2022.874254.

Carl Langan-Evans et al., "Nutritional Modulation of Sleep Latency, Duration, and Efficiency: A Randomized, Repeated-Measures, Double-Blind Deception Study," *Medicine & Science in Sports & Exercise* 55, no. 2 (2023): 289–300, doi.org/10.1249/MSS.0000000000003040.

Monica Kazlausky Esquivel and Brittany Ghosn, "Current Evidence on Common Dietary Supplements for Sleep Quality," *American Journal of Lifestyle Medicine* 18, no. 3 (2024), doi.org/10.1177/15598276241227915.

Rafael M. Carlos et al., "The Effects of Melatonin and Magnesium in a Novel Supplement Delivery System on Sleep Scores, Body Composition and Metabolism in Otherwise Healthy Individuals with Sleep Disturbances," *Chronobiology International* 41, no. 6 (2024): 817–28, doi.org/10.1080/07420528.2024.2353225.

Gorica Djokic et al., "The Effects of Magnesium–Melatonin–Vit B Complex Supplementation in Treatment of Insomnia," *Open Access Macedonian Journal of Medical Sciences* 7, no. 18 (2019): 3101–5, doi.org/10.3889/oamjms.2019.771.

Vicky Chan and Kenneth Lo, "Efficacy of Dietary Supplements on Improving Sleep Quality: A Systematic Review and Meta-Analysis," *Postgraduate Medical Journal* 98 (2022): 285–93, doi.org/10.1136/postgradmedj-2020-139319.

Ji Won Yeom and Chul-Hyun Cho, "Herbal and Natural Supplements for Improving Sleep: A Literature Review," *Psychiatry Investigation* 21, no. 8 (2024): 810–21, doi.org/10.30773/pi.2024.0121.

Vimalkumar Patel, "Melatonin vs. Magnesium: Comparison," *International Journal of Science and Research* 10, no. 2 (2021): 1731–37, doi.org/10.21275/sr24314024820.

Arman Arab et al., "The Role of Magnesium in Sleep Health: A Systematic Review of Available Literature," *Biological Trace Element Research* 201 (2023): 121–28, doi.org/10.1007/s12011-022-03162-1.

Jasmine Mah and Tyler Pitre, "Oral Magnesium Supplementation for Insomnia in Older Adults: A Systematic Review & Meta-Analysis," *BMC Complementary Medicine and Therapies* 21 (2021), doi.org/10.1186/s12906-021-03297-z.

CHAPTER 11: WHEN DESIRE SHIFTS: PERIMENOPAUSE AND SEXUAL FUNCTION

"Female Sexual Function Index (FSFI)," National Vulvodynia Association, nva.org/wp-content/uploads/2015/01/FSFI-questionnaire2000.pdf.

Susan R. Davis et al., "Global Consensus Position Statement on the Use of Testosterone Therapy for Women," *The Journal of Clinical Endocrinology & Metabolism* 104, no. 10 (2019): 4660–66, doi.org/10.1210/jc.2019-01603.

Stephanie S. Faubion et al., "The 2022 Hormone Therapy Position Statement of the North American Menopause Society," *Menopause* 29, no. 7 (2022): 767–94, doi.org/10.1097/GME.0000000000002028.

Lisa Dawn Hamilton and Cindy M. Meston, "Chronic Stress and Sexual Function in Women," *The Journal of Sexual Medicine* 10, no. 10 (2013): 2443–54, doi.org/10.1111/jsm.12249.

Alfredo Nicolosi et al., "A Population Study of the Association Between Sexual Function, Sexual Satisfaction and Depressive Symptoms in Men," *Journal of Affective Disorders* 82, no. 2 (2004): 235–43, doi.org/10.1016/j.jad.2003.12.008.

Stacy Tessler Lindau et al., "A Study of Sexuality and Health Among Older Adults in the United States," *The New England Journal of Medicine* 357, no. 8 (2007), doi.org/10.1056/NEJMoa067423.

Edward O. Laumann, Anthony Paik, and Raymond C. Rosen, "Sexual Dysfunction in the United States: Prevalence and Predictors," *JAMA* 281, no. 6 (1999): 537–44, doi.org/10.1001/jama.281.6.537.

Sheryl A. Kingsberg and Terri Woodard, "Female Sexual Dysfunction: Focus on Low Desire," *Obstetrics & Gynecology* 125, no. 2 (2015): 477–86, doi.org/10.1097/AOG.0000000000000620.

David J. Portman and Margery L. S. Gass, "Genitourinary Syndrome of Menopause: New Terminology for Vulvovaginal Atrophy from the International Society for the Study of Women's Sexual Health and the North American Menopause Society," *Menopause* 21, no. 10 (2014): 1063–68, doi.org/10.1097/GME.0000000000000329.

Glenn D. Braunstein, "Androgen Insufficiency in Women: Summary of Critical Issues," *Fertility and Sterility* 77 (2002), doi.org/10.1016/s0015-0282(02)02962-x.

Susan R. Davis et al., "Testosterone for Low Libido in Postmenopausal Women Not Taking Estrogen," *The New England Journal of Medicine* 359, no. 19 (2008): 2005–17, doi.org/10.1056/NEJMoa0707302.

R. Rosen et al., "The Female Sexual Function Index (FSFI): A Multidimensional Self-Report Instrument for the Assessment of Female Sexual Function," *Journal of Sex & Marital Therapy* 26, no. 2 (2000): 191–208, doi.org/10.1080/009262300278597.

Lori A. Brotto, Rosemary Basson, and Mijal Luria, "A Mindfulness-Based Group Psychoeducational Intervention Targeting Sexual Arousal Disorder in Women," *The Journal of Sexual Medicine* 5, no. 7 (2008): 1646–59, doi.org/10.1111/j.1743-6109.2008.00850.x.

Emily Nagoski, *Come As You Are: The Surprising New Science That Will Transform Your Sex Life,* rev. ed. (Simon & Schuster, 2021).

Steven D. Solomon and Lorie J. Teagno, *Intimacy After Infidelity: How to Rebuild and Affair-Proof Your Marriage* (New Harbinger, 2006).

Andrea M. Isidori et al., "Development and Validation of a 6-Item Version of the Female Sexual Function Index (FSFI) as a Diagnostic Tool for Female Sexual Dysfunction," *The Journal of Sexual Medicine* 7, no. 3 (2010): 1139–46, doi.org/10.1111/j.1743-6109.2009.01635.x.

CHAPTER 12: FERTILITY CHANGES AND CHALLENGES: THE CLOCK IS REAL, BUT SO IS YOUR POWER

Gerson Weiss, "Understanding the Perimenopause," *Women's Health* 3, no. 4 (2007): 387–90, doi.org/10.2217/17455057.3.4.387.

Maureen K. Baldwin and Jeffrey T. Jensen, "Contraception During the Perimenopause," *Maturitas* 76, no. 3 (2013): 235–42, doi.org/10.1016/j.maturitas.2013.07.009.

Lauren Verrilli and Sarah L. Berga, "What Every Gynecologist Should Know About Perimenopause," *Clinical Obstetrics and Gynecology* 63, no. 4 (2020): 720–34, doi.org/10.1097/GRF.0000000000000578.

Maria G. Meyers, Lauren Vitale, and Kathryn Elenchin, "Perimenopause and the Use of Fertility Tracking: 3 Case Studies," *The Linacre Quarterly* 90, no. 1 (2021), doi.org/10.1177/00243639211050719.

Maria Meyers, Richard Jerome Fehring, and Mary Schneider, "Case Reports from Women Using a Quantitative Hormone Monitor to Track the Perimenopause Transition," *Medicina* 59, no. 10 (2023), doi.org/10.3390/medicina59101743.

Jerilynn C. Prior, "Perimenopause: The Complex Endocrinology of the Menopausal Transition," *Endocrine Reviews* 19, no. 4 (1998): 397–428, doi.org/10.1210/EDRV.19.4.0341.

Georgeanna Seegar Jones et al., "The Perimenopausal Patient in In Vitro Fertilization: The Use of Gonadotropin-Releasing Hormone," *Fertility and Sterility* 46, no. 5 (1986): 885–91, doi.org/10.1016/S0015-0282(16)49829-8.

David S. Guzick et al., "Efficacy of Superovulation and Intrauterine Insemination in the Treatment of Infertility," *The New England Journal of Medicine* 340, no. 3 (1999): 177–83, doi.org/10.1056/NEJM199901213400302.

W. Hamish, B. Wallace, and Thomas W. Kelsey, "Human Ovarian Reserve from Conception to the Menopause," *PLoS One* 5, no. 1 (2010), doi.org/10.1371/journal.pone.0008772.

Evelyn E. Telfer et al., "Making a Good Egg: Human Oocyte Health, Aging, and In Vitro Development," *Physiological Reviews* 103, no. 4 (2023): 2623–77, doi.org/10.1152/physrev.00032.2022.

CHAPTER 13: WHEN THE BLEEDING BECOMES A MYSTERY: UTERINE CHANGES IN PERIMENOPAUSE

"ACOG Committee Opinion No. 557: Management of Acute Abnormal Uterine Bleeding in Nonpregnant Reproductive-Aged Women," *Obstetrics & Gynecology* 121, no. 4 (2013): 891–896, doi.org/10.1097/01.AOG.0000428646.67925.9a.

Samar R. El Khoudary et al., "Patterns of Menstrual Cycle Length Over the Menopause Transition Are Associated with Subclinical Atherosclerosis After Menopause," *Menopause* 29, no. 1 (2021): 8–15, doi.org/10.1097/GME.0000000000001876.

Mary L. Marnach and Shannon K Laughlin-Tommaso, "Evaluation and Management of Abnormal Uterine Bleeding," *Mayo Clinic Proceedings* 94, no. 2 (2019): 326–335, doi.org/10.1016/j.mayocp.2018.12.012.

B. A. Mikes, E. S. Vadakekut, and P. B. Sparzak, *Abnormal Uterine Bleeding*, (StatPearls, 2025), ncbi.nlm.nih.gov/books/NBK532913.

J. V. Pinkerton et al, "Abnormal Uterine Bleeding," *MSD Manual Professional Version* (2023), msdmanuals.com/professional/gynecology-and-obstetrics/menstrual-abnormalities/abnormal-uterine-bleeding.

Mara Ulin et al., "Uterine Fibroids in Menopause and Perimenopause," *Menopause* 27, no. 2 (2020): 238–242, doi.org/10.1097/GME.0000000000001438.

CHAPTER 14: TREATING HORMONAL FLUCTUATION WITH HORMONES: A DEEP DIVE INTO MHT TO TREAT PERIMENOPAUSE

Preeyaporn Jirakittidul et al., "The Effectiveness of Quick Starting Oral Contraception Containing Nomegestrol Acetate and 17-β Estradiol on Ovulation Inhibition: A Randomized Controlled Trial," *Scientific Reports* 10 (2020), doi.org/10.1038/s41598-020-65642-5.

Saad Amer and Subul Bazmi, "HRT in Women Undergoing Pelvic Clearance for Endometriosis: A Case Report and a National Survey," *Journal of Clinical Medicine* 12, no. 1 (2023), doi.org/10.3390/jcm12010336.

L. C. Gemmell et al., "The Management of Menopause in Women with a History of Endometriosis: A Systematic Review," *Human Reproduction Update* 23, no. 4 (2017): 481–500, doi.org/10.1093/humupd/dmx011.

Hee Joong Lee et al., "Hormone Replacement Therapy and Risks of Various Cancers in Postmenopausal Women with De Novo or a History of Endometriosis," *Cancers* 16, no. 4 (2024), doi.org/10.3390/cancers16040809.

Roberto Matorras et al., "Recurrence of Endometriosis in Women with Bilateral Adnexectomy (with or Without Total Hysterectomy) Who Received Hormone Replacement Therapy," *Fertility and Sterility* 77, no. 2 (2002): 303–8, doi.org/10.1016/S0015-0282(01)02981-8.

Rosemary Howell et al., "Gonadotropin-Releasing Hormone Analogue (Goserelin) Plus Hormone Replacement Therapy for the Treatment of Endometriosis: A Randomized Controlled Trial," *Fertility and Sterility* 64, no. 3 (1995): 474–81, doi.org/10.1016/S0015-0282(16)57779-6.

N. F. Soliman and T. C. Hillard, "Hormone Replacement Therapy in Women with Past History of Endometriosis," *Climacteric* 9, no. 5 (2006): 325–35, doi.org/10.1080/13697130600868711.

Margherita Zanello et al., "Hormonal Replacement Therapy in Menopausal Women with History of Endometriosis: A Review of Literature," *Medicina* 55, no. 8 (2019), doi.org/10.3390/medicina55080477.

Nilüfer Akgün and Ertan Sarıdoğan, "Management of Menopause in Women with a History of Endometriosis," *Journal of the Turkish-German Gynecological Association* 25, no. 2 (2024): 107–11, doi.org/10.4274/jtgga.galenos.2024.2023-11-4.

Vrunda C. Karanjgaokar et al., "Malignant Transformation of Residual Endometriosis After Hysterectomy: A Case Series," *Fertility and Sterility* 92, no. 6 (2009), doi.org/10.1016/j.fertnstert.2009.08.012.

W. Hamish B. Wallace and Thomas W. Kelsey, "Human Ovarian Reserve from Conception to the Menopause," *PLoS One* 5, no. 1 (2010), doi.org/10.1371/journal.pone.0008772.

A. Bilge Şener et al., "The Effects of Hormone Replacement Therapy on Uterine Fibroids in Postmenopausal Women," *Fertility and Sterility* 65, no. 2 (1996): 354–57, doi.org/10.1016/S0015-0282(16)58098-4.

C. H. Yang et al., "Effect of Hormone Replacement Therapy on Uterine Fibroids in Postmenopausal Women: A 3-Year Study," *Maturitas* 43, no. 1 (2002): 35–39, doi.org/10.1016/S0378-5122(02)00159-7.

Elisa Moro et al., "The Impact of Hormonal Replacement Treatment in Postmenopausal Women with Uterine Fibroids: A State-of-the-Art Review of the Literature," *Medicina* 55, no. 9 (2019), doi.org/10.3390/medicina55090549.

W. C. Ang, E. Farrell, and B. Vollenhoven, "Effect of Hormone Replacement Therapies and Selective Estrogen Receptor Modulators in Postmenopausal Women with Uterine Leiomyomas: A Literature Review," *Climacteric* 4, no. 4 (2001): 284–92, doi.org/10.1080/cmt.4.4.284.292.

Eva M. Sommer et al., "Effects of Obesity and Hormone Therapy on Surgically-Confirmed Fibroids in Postmenopausal Women," *European Journal of Epidemiology* 30 (2015): 493–99, doi.org/10.1007/s10654-015-0016-7.

CHAPTER 15: THE FOUNDATION FOR RESILIENCE: THE LIFESTYLE FACTORS THAT MATTER MOST

Jeannette M. Beasley et al., "Protein Intake and Incident Frailty in the Women's Health Initiative Observational Study," *Journal of the American Geriatrics Society* 58, no. 6 (2010): 1063–71, doi.org/10.1111/j.1532-5415.2010.02866.x.

Charlotte Elizabeth Louise Evans, "Dietary Fibre and Cardiovascular Health: A Review of Current Evidence and Policy," *Proceedings of the Nutrition Society* 79 (2019): 61–67, doi.org/10.1017/S0029665119000673.

Ghada A. Soliman, "Dietary Fiber, Atherosclerosis, and Cardiovascular Disease," *Nutrients* 11, no. 5 (2019), doi.org/10.3390/nu11051155.

Andrew N. Reynolds, Ashley P. Akerman, and Jim Mann, "Dietary Fibre and Whole Grains in Diabetes Management: Systematic Review and Meta-Analyses," *PLoS Medicine* 17, no. 3 (2020), doi.org/10.1371/journal.pmed.1003053.

Wendy J. Dahl and Maria L. Stewart, "Position of the Academy of Nutrition and Dietetics: Health Implications of Dietary Fiber," *Journal of the Academy of Nutrition and Dietetics* 115, no. 11 (2015): 1861–70, doi.org/10.1016/j.jand.2015.09.003.

Francine Z. Marques et al., "High-Fiber Diet and Acetate Supplementation Change the Gut Microbiota and Prevent the Development of Hypertension and Heart Failure in Hypertensive Mice," *Circulation* 135, no. 10 (2016), doi.org/10.1161/CIRCULATIONAHA.116.024545.

Weiwei Dong and Zhiyong Yang, "Association of Dietary Fiber Intake with Myocardial Infarction and Stroke Events in US Adults: A Cross-Sectional Study of NHANES 2011–2018," *Frontiers in Nutrition* 9 (2022), doi.org/10.3389/fnut.2022.936926.

Feifei Yao et al., "Dietary Intake of Total Vegetable, Fruit, Cereal, Soluble and Insoluble Fiber and Risk of All-Cause, Cardiovascular, and Cancer Mortality: Systematic Review and Dose–Response Meta-Analysis of Prospective Cohort Studies," *Frontiers in Nutrition* 10 (2023), doi.org/10.3389/fnut.2023.1153165.

Hamdi A. Jama et al., "Recommendations for the Use of Dietary Fiber to Improve Blood Pressure Control," *Hypertension* 81, no. 7 (2024), doi.org/10.1161/HYPERTENSIONAHA.123.22575.

CHAPTER 16: TALKING POINTS AND LAB TESTS: EVERYTHING YOU NEED FOR YOUR NEXT APPOINTMENT

Jennifer Wolff, "What Doctors Don't Know About Menopause," AARP, July 20, 2018, aarp.org/health/conditions-treatments/menopause-symptoms-doctors-relief-treatment.

M. S. Christianson et al., "Menopause Education: Needs Assessment of American Obstetrics and Gynecology Residents," *Menopause* 20, no. 11 (2013): 1120–25, doi.org/10.1097/GME.0b013e31828ced7f.

M. L. Brigden, "Clinical Utility of the Erythrocyte Sedimentation Rate," *American Family Physician* 60, no. 5 (1999): 1443–50.

J. B. Dwyer et al., "Hormonal Treatments for Major Depressive Disorder: State of the Art" [published correction appears in *Am J Psychiatry.* 2020 Jul 1;177(7):642], [published correction appears in *Am J Psychiatry.* 2020 Oct 1;177(10):1009], *Am J Psychiatry.* 2020;177(8):686–705, doi.org/10.1176/appi.ajp.2020.19080848.

J. M. Evron, W. H. Herman, and L. N. McEwen, "Changes in Screening Practices for Prediabetes and Diabetes Since the Recommendation for Hemoglobin A1c Testing" [published correction appears in *Diabetes Care.* 2020;43(9):2323], *Diabetes Care.* 2019;42(4):576–84, doi.org/10.2337/dc17-1726.

A. M. Freeman, M. Rai, and D. W. Morando, *Anemia Screening* (StatPearls, 2023), ncbi.nlm.nih.gov/books/NBK499905.

R. P. Heaney, "Vitamin D in Health and Disease," *Clinical Journal of the American Society of Nephrology* 3, no. 5 (2008): 1535–41, doi.org/10.2215/CJN.01160308.

L. Maxfield, S. Shukla, and J. S. Crane, *Zinc Deficiency* (StatPearls, 2023), ncbi.nlm.nih.gov/books/NBK493231.

N. R. Parva et al., "Prevalence of Vitamin D Deficiency and Associated Risk Factors in the US Population (2011–2012)," *Cureus* 10, no. 6 (2018) : e2741, doi.org/10.7759/cureus.2741.

M. Prasad et al., "Triglyceride and Triglyceride/ HDL (High Density Lipoprotein) Ratio Predict Major Adverse Cardiovascular Outcomes in Women with Non-Obstructive Coronary Artery Disease," *Journal of the American Heart Association* 8, no. 9 (2019), doi.org/10.1161/JAHA.118.009442.

P. M. Ridker, "High-Sensitivity C-Reactive Protein and Cardiovascular Risk: Rationale for Screening and Primary Prevention," *American Journal of Cardiology* 92, no. 4, S2 (2003): 17–22, doi.org/10.1016/s0002-9149(03)00774-4.

G. K. Schwalfenbergand and S. J. Genuis, "The Importance of Magnesium in Clinical Healthcare," *Scientifica* (2017), doi.org/10.1155/2017/4179326.

J. Watson, A. Round, and W. Hamilton, "Raised Inflammatory Markers," *BMJ*, 2012;344:e454, doi.org/10.1136/bmj.e454.

Index

abnormal uterine bleeding (AUB), 210–212
acetylcholine, 58, 59
Addison's disease, 50
adenomyosis, 212
adenosine triphosphate (ATP), 144
adrenal fatigue, 49–51
advocacy, 15, 73, 207–208
aerobic activities, 264
aging
    egg quality and, 202
    endocrine vs. chronological, 80
    understandings of, 19–21
alcohol use, 141, 202
Alloy Health, 18
Alzheimer's disease, 38, 82–83
American College of Obstetricians and Gynecologists (ACOG), 10–11
American Urological Association (AUA), 47, 181–183, 238–239
anabolic agents, 138
androcentric research models, 20
androgens, 59, 228–229, 240–242
androstenedione, 228
anovulatory cycle, 36
antidepressants, 17, 68, 70–71, 72
antifibrinolytics, 216–217
anti-inflammatory diet and nutrition, 252–256
anti-Mullerian hormone (AMH), 18–19, 111–112, 128
antioxidants, 254–255
anxiety, 16, 17, 67–69, 70–71, 168
apolipoprotein B test, 275
appointment preparation, 271–272
atomoxetine, 88
atresia, 27

attention deficit hyperactivity disorder (ADHD), 77, 86–90
Attia, Peter, 175

B vitamins, 263
back pain, 131–132
balance exercises, 264
barbiturates, 65
basal body temperature (BBT), 203
beta-endorphin, 58
bioidentical hormones, 235–236, 237
biomarkers, 19
bisphosphonates, 137
bladder pain syndrome (BPS), 46–47
bladder trigone, 46
blood sugar, 104–106
blood work, 273–277
Bluming, Avrum, 13
bone density
    bone mineral density (BMD), 129
    DEXA scans for, 101, 123, 127, 134
    fractures and, 123–124, 125–127
    FRAX (fracture risk assessment), 135
    hormone therapy and, 136–137
    loss, 19, 129–131
    pharmacological interventions, 137–138
    revised screening protocols, 132–134
    scanning recommendations, 21
    strategies for, 136–141
    use of weighted vests and, 138–139
    See also osteoporosis
bone health, 127–128. *See also* osteoporosis
brain
    cognitive function, 32, 77–78
    cognitive training, 91
    diet and, 74

brain (cont'd)
   endocrine system and, 57
   estradiol and, 72
   estrogen and, 58, 62, 79–80
   hormonal changes and, 16, 31–34, 55–56
   menopause brain, 87–88
   neurological symptoms, 32–34, 55
   progesterone and, 59, 62
   sex hormones and, 56–57, 62–63
brain fog, 32, 69, 76–79
burnout, 186–187

calcitonin, 137
calcium, 140–141, 260
cancer, 183, 213, 232
cardiorespiratory fitness, 251
cardiovascular disease, 99, 160
caregiving, 186
Casperson, Kelly, 13, 175, 185
CBC with differential and platelets, 274
CBT-i Coach, 166
cholesterol, 18–19, 21, 96, 98, 109–113
chromosomal abnormalities, 202
coagulopathy, 213
cognitive behavioral therapy for insomnia (CBT-I), 165–166
cognitive function
   ADHD, 77, 86–90
   brain fog, 32, 69, 76–79
   executive function, 78, 80
   hormonal changes and, 32, 77–80
   hormone therapy and, 84–85
   integrated approach to restoring, 88–89
   memory, 78, 80, 83–84
   obstructive sleep apnea (OSA) and, 160
   strategies for, 90–91
   trajectory of changes to, 82–84
cognitive training, 91
collagen, 263
compounded bioidentical hormone therapy, 237
comprehensive metabolic panel (CMP-14), 274
concentration, 32
contraceptive hormone therapy (CHT), 234–235
corpus luteum, 29
cortisol, 50–51, 69, 162–164, 168
cortisol awakening response (CAR), 50
COVID, 47–49, 78

Crawford, Natalie, 199, 202, 204, 205, 206, 207
creatine, 151–152, 263
cytokines, 99–100, 104

dementia, 82–83
denosumab, 137
depression, 16, 17, 32, 66, 67–69, 70–71, 160
desire, 185–187
DEXA scans, 101, 123, 127, 134
DHEA, 194, 228, 242–243
diabetes, 21, 99, 104–106, 112
diagnosis of dismissal, 40–41
diagnostic criteria
   ADHD, 87–88
   GSM, 182
   lack of standard, 15–19
   mental health concerns, 74–75
   PALM-COEIN system, 212–214
   sexual function, 188–193
diagnostic testing, 18–19, 273–277
diet and nutrition
   anti-inflammatory, 252–256
   bone health and, 140–141, 251, 258–259
   cognitive function and, 90
   fiber, 255, 256–258
   healthy eating tips, 260–261
   importance of, 252
   meal plan, 289–305
   metabolic management and, 118–119
   metal health and, 74
   muscle mass and, 151–152
   protein, 141, 151, 258–259
   sexual function and, 196
   sleep and, 166
   supplements, 164, 243–244, 261–263
   whole foods, 259–290
dilation and curettage (D&C), 217
doctors
   appointment preparation, 271–272
   knowledge-translation gap, 10–12
   lab tests, 273–277
   limited education on perimenopause, 7–10
   Menoposse, 12–13
   sexual dysfunction support, 191–193
   speaking up to, 272–273
dopamine, 33, 58, 69
doxepin, 167

INDEX 341

early-prevention measures, 20–21
eggs, 26–27, 34–35, 199–202
emotional intimacy, 183–185
emotional regulation, 61
endocrine system, 57
endometrial ablation, 217
endometrial problems, 213
endometriosis, 42, 244–246
estradiol, 29, 30, 50, 60, 71–72, 112, 144, 228
estradiol, extraction method test, 276–277
estriol, 228
estrogen
    bone health and, 127–128
    brain and, 58, 62, 79–80
    cardiovascular health and, 106–107
    cholesterol and, 109–110
    cortisol awakening response and, 50
    declining levels of, 33
    dominance, 35–36
    fat distribution and, 99–100
    genital and urinary organ impacts, 46–47
    insulin resistance and, 104
    liver health and, 113–114
    location of receptors in the body, 37
    in menstrual cycle, 27–29
    metabolism and, 97–98, 256, 257
    mood regulation and, 71–73
    multi-organ effects of changes in, 9, 37–38
    muscle mass and, 143–145, 152–153
    as a neurosteroid, 57
    pain modulation and, 44–46
    role of, 227–228
    sexual function and, 177
    sleep and, 156, 158, 160–161, 266
    unstable levels of, 229–230
estrogen therapy (ET), 84, 89
estrone, 228
Everyday Memory Questionnaire–Revised (EMQ-R), 83–84
executive function, 78, 80
exercise
    bone health and, 140
    cognitive function and, 90
    importance of, 263–264
    mental health and, 74
    metabolic management and, 118
    muscle mass and, 149–151

    routines, 265
    sexual function and, 196

familial hypercholesterolemia (FH), 112
fasting insulin test, 276
fatigue, 69, 158, 186
fats, healthy, 255
FDA-approved bioidentical hormone therapy, 237, 239
Female Sexual Function Index (FSFI), 189–191
ferritin test, 275
fertility
    after age thirty-five, 199–202
    egg quality and, 202
    evaluation, 205–206
    hormone therapy and reproductive planning, 206–207
    postpartum hormone monitoring, 205
    self-advocacy, 207–208
    tracking difficulties, 203
    unpredictability, 203–205
fiber, 255, 256–258, 262, 263
fibrinolysis, 216–217
fibroids, 212–213, 246–247
fibromyalgia (FM), 43–46
flexibility, 264
follicle-stimulating hormone (FSH), 27–29, 30, 32, 33, 128, 200, 203
follicular phase, 28–29, 34–36, 202
fractures, 123–124, 125–127
frailty, 143
FRAX (fracture risk assessment), 135
free T3 test, 277
FSH. *See* follicle-stimulating hormone
FSH test, 277

GABA, 59, 69, 161
gabapentin, 167
Galveston Diet, 254
gamma-glutamyl transferase (GGT) test, 275
gender health gap, 22, 249–250
generalized anxiety disorder (GAD), 67, 69
genitourinary syndrome of menopause (GSM), 46–47, 177, 180–183, 238–239
Georgiades, Kelley Sullivan, 260
Gilberg, Suzanne, 13
GLP-1s, 102–104, 119, 196

342 INDEX

glucose metabolism, 104–106, 146
glutamate, 59
GSM. *See* genitourinary syndrome of menopause
gut health, 114, 253, 255–256

health span, 22
healthcare system, sick-care model of, 19
heart disease, 38
hemoglobin A1C (HbA1c), 106, 275
high blood pressure, 106–109
high-sensitivity CRP test, 275
HOMA-IR score, 21, 106, 276
homocysteine test, 275
hormonal changes
   aging and, 19–20
   brain and, 16, 31–34, 55–56
   cognitive function and, 32, 79–80
   mental health and, 19–20, 65–67
   multi-organ effects, 9, 37–38
   sleep and, 32, 33, 162
   zone of chaos, 16, 30–31
   See also specific hormones
hormonal withdrawal bleeding, 204
hormone therapy. *See* menopause hormone therapy (MHT)
hormones, 226–227. *See also specific hormones*
hot flashes, 32, 38, 69, 158, 164–165
HPA. *See* hypothalamic-pituitary-adrenal axis
HSDD. *See* hypoactive sexual desire disorder
hyperplasia, 213
hypertension, 106–109
hypoactive sexual desire disorder (HSDD), 61, 179, 195, 229
hypothalamic-pituitary-adrenal (HPA) axis, 50, 69, 162
hypothalamus, 229
hysterectomy, 217–218

infertility, 207
inflammasome, 100
inflammation, 99–100, 102, 104, 253
insomnia, 165–166
Insomnia Coach, 166
insulin resistance, 98, 99, 104–106, 160
interstitial cystitis (IC), 46–47
intimacy. *See* sexual function

intrauterine insemination (IUI), 205
INVEST trial, 138–139
iron, 168, 260
iron, total and TIBC test, 276
irritability, 69–70
IUDs, 216, 231

lab tests, 273–277
lactate dehydrogenase (LD) test, 276
leaky gut, 253
legislation, pro-menopause, 9–10
leiomyoma, 212–213
leucine, 151
LH. *See* luteinizing hormone
libido, 61, 178, 179, 185–187
lifestyle interventions
   for bone health, 140–141
   for cognitive function, 90–91
   diet and nutrition, 252–263
   exercise, 263–265
   holistic approach to, 268–269
   for mental health, 74
   for metabolic management, 118–119
   for muscle mass preservation, 149–152
   for sexual function, 195–196
   for sleep, 166, 265–266
   stress management, 267–268
lipid panel, 275
lipoprotein(a) test, 275
lisdexamfetamine, 88–89
liver health, 113–117
long COVID, 47–49, 78
longevity, 21–22
L-theanine, 167
luteal phase, 29, 161
luteinizing hormone (LH), 27–29, 30, 32, 33, 203
Lyon, Gabrielle, 147, 149, 258

magnesium, 152, 167, 243, 263, 276
major depressive disorder (MDD), 66, 69
Malone, Sharon, 13
MASLD. *See* metabolic dysfunction-associated steatotic liver disease
Matsumura, Andrea, 157, 167, 168
McKinsey Health Institute, 22
meal plan, 289–305

medical gaslighting, 41–42
melatonin, 156, 167, 243
memory, 78, 80, 83–84
Menn, Corinne, 13
menopause
   average age of, 210
   defined, 10
   research funding, 14–15
   surgical, 107, 115, 236
menopause brain, 87–88
menopause hormone therapy (MHT)
   ADHD medications and, 88–90
   androgens, 240–242
   bioidentical hormones, 235–236, 237
   bone loss and, 129–130, 136–137
   cancer considerations, 183, 213, 232
   cholesterol and, 112
   cognitive decline and, 34, 84–85
   contraceptive hormone therapy vs., 234–235
   contraindications, 232–233
   delivery systems, 238–244
   DHEA, 242–243
   endometriosis and, 244–246
   fat distribution and, 102
   FDA-approved vs. compounded, 237, 239
   fibroids and, 246–247
   GSM and, 182
   guidelines, 85
   high blood pressure and, 108–109
   insulin resistance and, 106
   local therapy, 238–239
   MASLD management and, 116–117
   menstrual irregularities and, 215–216
   mental health effects, 17, 70–74
   metabolic dysfunction and, 119
   misconceptions about, 233
   muscle mass and, 145, 152–153
   progestogens, 240
   reproductive planning and, 206–207
   SERMs (selective estrogen receptor modulators), 240
   sexual function and, 194–195
   sleep and, 164–165
   supportive, 231
   for suppressing and replacing, 231
   surgical menopause and, 236
   synthetic hormones, 235–236
   systemic therapy, 238
   types of, 235–236
   unstable estrogen levels and, 229–230
   use of term, 227
menopause penalty, 80–82
The Menopause Society, 12, 209, 272
Menoposse, 12–13
menses phase, 28
menstrual cycle, 27–29, 199–201
menstrual irregularities
   diagnosing, 212–214
   expectant management, 215
   hormone therapy and, 215–216
   irregular bleeding, 210–212
   non-structural causes (COEIN), 213
   strategies for, 214–219
   structural causes (PALM), 212–213
   unpredictability of, 209–210
menstruation, stigma and shame surrounding, 25
mental health
   hormonal changes and, 17, 19–20, 65–67
   hormone therapy and, 17, 70–73
   strategies for, 73–75
   symptoms, 67–70
metabolic dysfunction
   amino acid homeostasis disruption and, 45
   cholesterol and, 109–113
   fiber and, 257
   gender disparities in research on, 94–95
   high blood pressure and, 106–109
   hormone therapy and, 119
   insulin resistance and, 104–106
   liver health and, 113–117
   markers to monitor, 117–118
   risk factors, 93–94, 98–117
   sarcopenia and, 145–147
   strategies for, 118–119
   symptoms, 93
   visceral fat and, 98–102
metabolic dysfunction-associated steatotic liver disease (MASLD), 96, 113–117
metabolic syndrome of menopause, 95–97, 120–121
metabolism, estrogen and, 97–98
MHT. *See* menopause hormone therapy
micronutrients, 152

344 INDEX

Midi, 18
mitochondrial dysfunction, 19
mood swings, 38, 66–67, 68
Mosconi, Lisa, 56n, 80, 83
muscle mass
   estrogen and, 143–145, 152–153
   hormone therapy and, 145, 152–153
   loss of, 145–147
   strategies for, 149–153
   testosterone and, 153–154
   See also sarcopenia
musculoskeletal syndrome of menopause (MSM), 43–46, 147, 148–149
myelination, 57, 60

Nagoski, Emily, 13, 175, 185
National Institutes of Health (NIH), 13–15, 116
natural remedies, 243–244
neuroendocrinology, 57
neurogenesis, 60
neurological symptoms, 32–34
neuromodulators, 195
neurosteroids, 57
neurotransmitters, 58, 59, 69
night sweats, 32, 69, 158, 164–165
988 Lifeline, 20
nocturia, 46, 47, 158, 159
nonsteroidal anti-inflammatory drugs (NSAIDs), 216
noradrenaline, 59
norepinephrine, 33
North American Menopause Society, 12
NSUN4, 19
nutrition. *See* diet and nutrition

OB-GYNs
   appointment preparation, 271–272
   knowledge-translation gap, 10–12
   lab tests, 273–277
   limited education on perimenopause, 7–10
   Menoposse, 12–13
   sexual dysfunction support, 191–193
   speaking up to, 272–273
obstructive sleep apnea (OSA), 158, 159–160, 168
omega-3 fatty acids, 243, 254, 260
oocytes, 26–27, 34–35, 199–202

oophorectomy, 107, 115
oral contraceptives, 215
osteopenia, 130
osteoporosis
   chronic back pain and, 131–132
   early onset of, 122–125
   estrogen and, 38
   fractures and, 123–124, 125–127
   screening guidelines, 126
ovaries, 27–29, 34–36, 203
ovulation, 29, 35–36, 161, 200, 203
ovulatory dysfunction, 213

pain
   back, 131–132
   bladder pain syndrome (BPS), 46–47
   estrogen and modulation of, 44–46
   during sex, 180–183
PALM-COEIN system, 212–213
pelvic floor physical therapy, 195
perimenopause
   changes in hormone level patterns, 31
   defined, 10
   diagnostic criteria, 15–19
   research funding, 14–15
   research on, 224
   symptoms, 5–6
   as a transition, 34–35
   treating, 224–226
PET hormones, 227
phosphate test, 276
phytonutrients, 255
pituitary gland, 27–29
polycystic ovary syndrome (PCOS), 114, 213
polypharmacy, 44
polyphenols, 255
polyps, 212
postmenopause, 10, 31
postpartum depression, 66
premenopause, 31
premenstrual dysphoric disorder (PMDD), 66
premenstrual syndrome (PMS), 29
progesterone
   bone health and, 128
   brain and, 59, 62
   declining levels of, 33
   in menstrual cycle, 27–29, 35

as a neurosteroid, 57
  role of, 228
  sleep and, 156, 158, 161–162, 265–266
progestogens, 216, 240
protein, 141, 151, 258–259

recipes
  Berry and Nut Bowl, 297
  Celery and Nut Butter Boat, 294
  Chicken Avocado Wrap, 293
  Chicken Crust Pizza with Side Salad, 301–302
  Chicken Hummus Bowl, 295
  Cottage Cheese Cup, 297
  Cottage Cheese Scrambled Eggs with Ezekiel Toast, 300
  Egg Roll in a Bowl, 298–299
  Guacamole with Carrot Sticks, 291
  Hot Honey Turkey Bowl, 291
  Hummus and Flackers, 294
  Kelley Salad, 260
  The Menopause Power Shake, 289
  Mozzarella Cheese, 292
  Overnight Oats, 292–293
  Pecan-Crusted Salmon, 293–294
  Sheet Pan Steak Fajitas, 296
  TPN Dense Bean Salad with Rotisserie Chicken, 290
  TPN Dense Bean Salad with Tuna, 298
reproduction, 26–27
reproductive system, 36–37
research
  androcentric models, 20
  funding for, 13–15
  gender disparities in, 94–95
  on perimenopause, 224
  sexual function, 192
resistance training, 140, 149–151, 196, 251, 264
responsive desire, 185–186
resting energy expenditure (REE), 100
restless legs syndrome, 158, 168
romosozumab, 138
Rubin, Rachel, 13, 175–176, 185

Salas-Whalen, Rocio, 13, 103
Santoro, Nanette, 30
sarcopenia, 125, 142–143, 145–147
satiety, 257

sedimentation rate test, 277
selective estrogen receptor modulators (SERMs), 137, 240
selective serotonin reuptake inhibitors (SSRIs), 17, 68, 70–71, 167
self-advocacy, 73
SERMs. *See* selective estrogen receptor modulators
serotonin, 33, 58, 69
sex hormones
  brain and, 56–57
  estrogen, 58, 62, 227–228
  progesterone, 59, 62, 228
  sleep and, 160–162
  testosterone, 59–62, 228–229
  use of term, 56n
sexual function
  communication and, 188
  desire and, 185–187
  diagnosing problems with, 188–193
  emotional intimacy and, 183–185
  estrogen and, 177
  Female Sexual Function Index (FSFI), 189–191
  genitourinary syndrome of menopause (GSM), 46–47, 177, 180–183
  GLP-1s and, 196
  hormone therapy and, 194–195
  hypoactive sexual desire disorder (HSDD), 61, 179, 229
  identity and, 183–185
  learning about, 174–176
  libido, 61, 178, 179
  nonhormonal therapies and, 195
  strategies for, 194–196
  testosterone and, 177–178
sexual motivation, 61
Sims, Stacy, 20
sleep
  architecture, 161
  cognitive function and, 90–91
  disruptions, 157–159
  estrogen and, 156, 158, 160–161, 266
  hormonal changes and, 32, 33, 162
  hormone therapy and, 164–165
  latency, 158
  memory and, 84

sleep (cont'd)
  mental health and, 74
  obstructive sleep apnea (OSA), 158, 159–160
  optimization, 265–266
  progesterone and, 156, 158, 161–162, 265–266
  sexual function and, 196
  strategies for, 164–169, 266
  stress-sleep spiral, 162–164
  supplements for, 167
  vasomotor symptoms and, 158, 164–165
Sleepio, 165
small dense low-density lipoprotein cholesterol (sdLDL-C), 18, 110
Smith-Ryan, Abbie, 149
smoking, 141, 202
social connections, 74
somatization, xv–xvi, 65
Somryst, 166
spices, 255
spontaneous desire, 185–186
SSRI. *See* selective serotonin reuptake inhibitors
Streicher, Lauren, 13, 175, 185
stress management
  cognitive function and, 91
  importance of, 267
  mental health and, 74
  sleep and, 168
  strategies for, 267
stress-sleep spiral, 162–164
suicide, 19–20
supplements, 164, 243–244, 261–263
support networks, 277–278
surgical menopause, 107, 115, 236
SWAN (Study of Women's Health Across the Nation), 110, 111, 145, 161
symptoms, 5–6
  dismissal of, 39–43
  mental health, 67–70, 73–75
  metabolic syndrome, 93
  misdiagnosis of, 39–40, 43–51
  most common, 5–6
  neurological, 32–34, 55
  obstructive sleep apnea (OSA), 159–160
  tracking, 271
  vasomotor, 32, 69, 158
synthetic hormones, 235–236

T3 uptake test, 276
Tavris, Carol, 13
telemedicine, 18
testosterone
  brain and, 59–62
  hormone therapy, 240–242
  muscle health and, 153–154
  as a neurosteroid, 57
  pellets, 241–242
  role of, 228–229
  sexual function and, 61, 177–178
testosterone, free and total test, 277
tibolone, 245
TPO and TG antibodies test, 277
transdermal estradiol, 71–72, 84, 153
trauma, 73, 168
triglycerides, 96
TSH test, 275
turmeric, 263
type 2 diabetes, 21, 99, 104–106, 112

uric acid test, 276

vaginal dryness, 38, 180–183, 195
vasomotor symptoms, 32, 69, 158, 164–165
visceral fat, 96, 97, 98–102, 146, 154
Vitamin B12 and folate test, 277
vitamin D, 140–141, 152, 168, 243, 260, 262, 263
vitamin D, 25-hydroxy test, 275
in vitro fertilization (IVF), 205–206

waist-to-hip ratio, 101–102
weight gain, 96, 98
weighted vests, 138–139, 265
Weiss-Wolf, Jennifer, 9
women's health
  deprioritization of in research, 41–42
  gender health gap, 22, 249–250
  research funding, 13–15
Women's Health Initiative (WHI), xvi, 126, 258
workplace menopause penalty, 80–82
World Economic Forum, 22
Wright, Vonda, 45–46, 147, 148–149

ZOE initiative, 255–256
zone of chaos, 16, 30–38, 201, 204

ABOUT THE AUTHOR

DR MARY CLAIRE HAVER is board certified in obstetrics and gynecology and is a certified menopause specialist through The Menopause Society. She is also a culinary medicine specialist through the American College of Culinary Medicine. She is a Louisiana State University Medical Center graduate and completed her obstetrics and gynecology residency at the University of Texas Medical Branch (UTMB). In her professional career, Dr. Haver has served as a clinical professor at UTMB and the University of Texas Health Science Center at Houston. In 2021 she opened Mary Claire Wellness —now The 'Pause Wellness—, a clinic dedicated to caring for the menopausal patient. Dr. Haver has amassed more than six million followers across social media platforms by posting evidence-based guidance for women going through perimenopause and menopause. She lives with her husband in Galveston, Texas, and is the mother of two grown daughters.